DESIGN FOR CARE
INNOVATING HEALTHCARE EXPERIENCE

Peter H. Jones

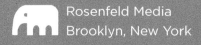

Rosenfeld Media
Brooklyn, New York

Design for Care: Innovating Healthcare Experience

By Peter H. Jones

Rosenfeld Media, LLC

457 Third Street, #4R

Brooklyn, New York

11215 USA

On the Web: www.rosenfeldmedia.com

Please send errors to: errata@rosenfeldmedia.com

Publisher: Louis Rosenfeld

Developmental Editor: JoAnn Simony

Interior Layout Tech: Danielle Foster

Cover Design: The Heads of State

Indexer: Nancy Guenther

Proofreader: Kathy Brock

Artwork Designer: James Caldwell, 418QE

ISBN: 1-933820-23-3

ISBN-13: 978-1-933820-23-1

LCCN: 2012950698

Printed and bound in the United States of America

DEDICATION

To Patricia, my own favorite writer, who kept me healthy while writing for three years

To my mother, Betsy, whose courage and insight in her recent passing from a rare cancer gives me empathy for the personhood of every patient

And to my father, Hayward, whose perpetual resilience shines through after surviving two cancers and living life well

HOW TO USE THIS BOOK

Design for Care fuses design practice, systems thinking, and practical healthcare research to help designers create innovative and effective responses to emerging and unforeseen problems. It covers design practices and methods for innovation in patient-centered healthcare services.

Design for Care offers best and next practices, and industrial-strength methods from practicing designers and design researchers in the field. Case studies illustrate current health design projects from leading firms, services, and institutions. Design methods and their applications illustrate how design makes a difference in healthcare today. My hope is that you will adapt the lessons, methods, and insights in this book to a product, organization, or service system in your own work.

Who Should Read This Book?

Design for Care was written for three audiences: designers and design researchers in healthcare fields; healthcare professionals and clinical practice leaders; and service, product, and innovation managers in companies serving healthcare.

Healthcare is complex, and learning even one vertical slice of a vast field is a significant undertaking. Learning and working across a second sector is a career challenge. Working effectively across sectors is unheard of. Designers, researchers, and practitioners across all three audiences typically work within a single sector—for a hospital, an information technology (IT) company, a medical products company, or a service provider. This book aims to inform design professionals across sectors (and design disciplines) and to contribute to their ability to design for the continuous life cycle of patient-centered service experiences. To ensure quality and manage costs across the whole system, a holistic view of healthcare and design is necessary.

For service designers, product, and innovation managers, I cover the most compelling information and service opportunities in healthcare with case studies and informed research. There are few guides for product managers in healthcare. Although this book does not specifically focus on product and project management, it weaves together many missing pieces overlooked in product and service innovation.

Most care providers work in one sector as well, deeply focused in a practice and an organization. This book helps inform clinical leaders of innovation methods, and encourages their understanding of the value of design thinking in health services, informatics, and organizational practice. Effective and ethical system design is not just making things work better for end users. Design leadership requires a collaboration at the practice level to contribute organizationally and systemically. I introduce health leaders to design and systems thinking approaches to help them innovate patient-centered service.

With the increased focus on improving the user experience in health websites and services, many designers new to the healthcare field will be learning about these users while on the job. *Design for Care* explores cases and methods for bettering human experience on both sides of the care experience, for both the patient and the care providers. It speaks to both new and experienced practitioners, and should be especially useful for those in transition between fields. For healthcare providers and those already managing projects "inside the system," adaptation of successful methods and patterns is encouraged between different cases and uses.

What's in This Book?

Part I: Rethinking Care and Its Consumers

The three chapters in Part I focus on the healthcare consumer. **Chapter 1: Design as Caregiving** presents a perspective on design as a way to provide care and addresses the problem of the fragmentation of design practice and engagement across the different healthcare sectors. **Chapter 2: Co-creating Care** focuses on design for health information seeking as a way of co-creating value in immediate care situations. **Chapter 3: Seeking Health** examines personal health decision making.

Part II: Rethinking Patients

The two chapters in Part II make the transition from health seeker in a consumer context to a patient-oriented perspective. **Chapter 4: Design for Patient Agency** presents agency and connectivity as alternative design factors to balance the traditional healthcare default perspective of *patiency*, which often treats patients as passive participants in their own care process. **Chapter 5: Patient-Centered Service Design** presents a systems approach to service design, and attempts to resolve differing concepts found across health service approaches. Human-centered approaches to service design focus on the primacy of patient experience, improving the touchpoints of care along the continuum of service responsibility.

Part III: Rethinking Care Systems

The four chapters in Part III look at care-centered service design in the complex systems of clinical healthcare and information-based work practices. **Chapter 6: Design at the Point of Care** is a service design approach to clinical decision making, medical education, and the four stages of clinical service design. The focus on medical education connects physician training, clinical work, and the care organization as designable services in a whole system. **Chapter 7: Designing Healthy Information Technology** looks at health IT as both innovation and system infrastructure at both the enterprise and practice levels. Lessons learned from electronic medical records and meaningful use provide a context for designing improved IT in clinical practice. **Chapter 8: Systemic Design for Healthcare Innovation** develops a systems thinking approach to designing service and organizational innovation in healthcare. **Chapter 9: Designing Healthcare Futures** presents methods and models for reimagining healthcare service from near- and long-term future perspectives, to enable strategic and socially responsive innovation.

What Comes with This Book?

You'll find additional content in this book's companion websites (http://designforcare.com and www.rosenfeldmedia.com/books/design-for-care/). Its diagrams and other illustrations are available under a Creative Commons license (when possible) for you to download and include in your own presentations. You can find these on Flickr at www.flickr.com/photos/rosenfeldmedia/sets/.

FREQUENTLY
ASKED QUESTIONS

Who are the stakeholders for this book?

The book is written to ultimately help health seekers—the patients and people who seek information, health services, and care from today's fragmented healthcare systems. We all rely on healthcare at some point, for ourselves and those we care for; therefore, everyone can be a stakeholder.

"We" are the user experience and service designers in healthcare, care providers improving healthcare service, and product and project managers in health industries. We are the ones who will ultimately employ design in healthcare transformation. Other stakeholders include design and medical educators, management of hospitals and companies providing healthcare applications, and policy makers.

How do you resolve the different terminology used in different design disciplines?

Throughout the book, references are made to concepts and terms that have distinct meanings in their own fields. Because the book presents a convergence of design methods and human research across the sectors of healthcare, a collision of perspectives is to be expected. The design disciplines have variations in design practice, research methods, and artifacts that cannot be resolved in one book. Research and medicine are divided by discipline, method, and legacy.

The intention of this book is to raise crucial issues of which designers should be aware. The common bond among all these disciplines is the compelling requirement to solve complex problems in effective and sustainable ways. See page 12.

What is health seeking?

The health seeker is any person aware of his or her motivation to improve his or her health, whether sick or not. Health seeking is the natural pursuit of one's appropriate balance of well-being, the continuous moving toward what we call "normal" health. For some, normal is just not feeling any symptoms; for others, it may be achieving the physical performance of an Olympian. See page 15.

What is Health 2.0 and Medicine 2.0, and is there a difference?

These designations are applied to coherent trends in Internet-enabled IT in healthcare and medical innovation. The implication of the release number

"2.0" signals consensus among IT vendors and innovators that a technology regime shift is being organized, similar to Web 2.0. Health 2.0 ranges from the conceptual shift in the management of patient care using online technology, to healthcare IT start-ups and Web services for health management. Medicine 2.0 was inspired by the shift in IT and data resources from academic medicine and biomedical sciences. See page 100.

How are design and medicine alike?

These two fields are similar in many ways. Both are performed as an expert-informed skilled practice that is learned by doing. And both are informed by observation and feedback, by evidence of their beneficial effects. Both disciplines are motivated by a deep desire to help people manage and improve their lives, individually and culturally. Modern medicine is guided by scientific inquiry much more than design, but then designers and engineers in healthcare often have scientific backgrounds. In medicine, evidence of outcome is gathered by measures of health and mortality, controlled experiments, and validated in peer-reviewed research. For clinical practice and organizational change, however, validation is often based on the social proof of adoption in practice. Design interventions in healthcare are often assessed by the analysis of empirical evidence, but in few cases would experimental validation be appropriate for service or interaction design. Different evaluation methods are valid in their contexts, a proposition that may not yet be acceptable across healthcare fields. See Chapter 6.

Why do you say "There is no user in healthcare"?

The designation of "user" privileges the use of a particular system and its functions, which promotes a language of efficiency based on "user tasks." It biases design toward optimizing for a specific set of use cases based on a strong representation of a primary user of IT. Healthcare is a huge social system with many participants and roles dedicated toward the recovery of individual and social health. Few of these roles actually require IT for their performance. A user-centered perspective risks isolating a single aspect of use and interaction, when nearly everything involves more than one of the primary participants: consumers, patients, and clinicians. If we take an empathic view, it becomes clear that *users* and even *patients* are names of impersonal convenience. The term *health seeker* is proposed as an unbiased way of understanding the person seeking care as a motivated actor making sense of a complicated system to achieve health goals. See page 13.

CONTENTS

PART I: RETHINKING CARE AND ITS CONSUMERS

CHAPTER 1

CHAPTER 2

CHAPTER 3

FOREWORD

In 2012, my wife and I were partners on a cancer journey. She was diagnosed with stage IIIA breast cancer in December 2011, and the cycles of chemotherapy, surgery, and radiation therapy filled the first seven months of 2012. As a clinician, I reviewed every order, every note, and every plan in her Beth Israel Deaconess online medical record. As a patient, she viewed everything written about her in her Beth Israel Deaconess PatientSite personal health record. I cannot imagine how care coordination, shared decision making, and communication would have been possible without ubiquitous patient–provider access to all the data, knowledge, and wisdom related to her care.

In *Design for Care*, Peter Jones outlines the critical role of design in the wellness care of the future, ensuring that every provider and patient is empowered with the services and tools they need for healthcare quality, safety, and efficiency. His thoughtful analysis includes all the core concepts that are driving the US healthcare IT stimulus—policies and technologies that engage the patient, eliminate disparities, protect privacy, and prevent avoidable harm.

When I mentioned that my wife's care required universal access to data, knowledge, and wisdom, what did I mean? *Data* includes the simple facts about her care—an appointment is made, a medication is given, a lab test has a result. *Information* is the interpretation of her data in a manner that is relevant to her care—her hematocrit at baseline is 39, and after chemotherapy it is 30. Her medications have caused side effects that may outweigh the benefits of the drug. *Wisdom* is applying decision support rules to her information that optimizes her care. Because her tumor is estrogen positive, progesterone positive, and HER2 negative, the best therapy is Cytoxan/Adriamycin/Taxol. Her accumulated radiation dose from all the mammograms, CT scans, and other studies is concerning, and thus ultrasound should be used when possible.

We clearly need better ways to move between data and information to knowledge and wisdom in today's complex healthcare world. This book illustrates these points and emphasizes the need for patients and providers to embrace a wise integration of technology into healthcare service.

Meaningful use and care improvements through universal adoption of electronic tools is just one of the major trends in the era of healthcare reform. "Patient-centered medical homes," "accountable care organizations," and "population health" are the new buzzwords. We need to rethink and actually design the new models of service, institutional practice, and patient engagement that ensure these new institutions become innovative alternatives to the care model, and don't simply replicate business as usual. The new concept is that care is no longer episodic, but continuous. Patients are engaged in their daily lives, and the emphasis is no longer on the treatment of illness but the preservation of wellness, maximizing functional status and care according to the preferences of the patient.

Peter Jones examines the kinds of innovations that are moving care away from academic health centers and into the community and homes. This trend is essential—healthcare in the United States consumes 17% of the gross domestic product. It is a poor value, with significant cost and less than stellar outcomes. To bend the cost curve and create high-value care, it is wise to follow the recommendations outlined in this book. Embrace technology, but design it well and consider its future trajectory and how it affects safety and interaction with patients. Engage the patient and innovate in ways that focus on longitudinal wellness rather than episodic encounters for illness.

I am confident you will find this book a helpful road map to guide your own journey to improve health and healthcare.

—John Halamka, MD
Chief Information Officer,
Beth Israel Deaconess Medical Center, Boston

INTRODUCTION

Care, and healthcare, is about taking care of humanity. Health is personal and universal—it may be the one value everyone cares about. Healthcare is the most hands-on of professions and services, and yet is extremely technical. As the industry intensifies the adoption of digital and electronic technologies, deeply informed design of services and systems becomes a pressing and critical need. At the same time, healthcare design does not yet fit into the conventional clinical organization, and institutional practices have not established meaningful positions for design. However, considering the increasing role of technology, the risk of errors induced by poor design, and the complexity of healthcare itself, designers from specialized disciplines should play critical roles in all technology decisions.

Healthcare in the United States is a mess. Technically, a "mess" is a complex set of problems with inextricable interdependencies. The overall system of healthcare—from services to payment to policy—has grown so complicated that a redesign of its components would not change the system substantially. New design thinking is called for, yet where do we start? Designers have no access to the system levers, and most of our work today is aimed at making the components run better and safer.

Healthcare has always organized itself around the patient encounter. Each human being with a healthcare need must be engaged in person and with respect to his or her unique biological and environmental circumstances. Healthcare services are designed to manage the flow of people from need to outcome, generally one at a time, according to the encounter formula. Services are aggregated into "big box" clinical solutions—hospitals and clinics—that serve as our "care malls" for full-service healthcare. Big box care is aggregated at the system level to regional and payer networks.

Healthcare is changing rapidly, attended by the increasing complexity related to its information glut. Consumer access to highly credible health websites has irreversibly altered the traditional equation, changing once-passive patients into stakeholders in the healthcare business. Their awareness of and access to health information challenges the hegemony of institutional practice. But innovations in healthcare and open information are also balanced by the inherent risks of institutional care, its systemic risk aversion, and its regulatory environment. As healthcare services undergo constant change, do we know how the numerous information systems are cooperating, and how different views of patient data are shared? How will new information infrastructures, systems, and configurations affect practice? How will changes in practice affect patients?

One intention of this book is to enable better communication, understanding, and knowledge transfer between healthcare fields and work experiences. The chapters are organized to reflect the human health experience and to discuss issues at the points of interaction where people seek and receive healthcare.

Designers (in general) perform systematic problem solving to formulate better ways for humans to interact with technology and services. Many designers work on systemic "big box" problems such as process workflow, information displays, and wayfinding; or behind the scenes on medical devices, health IT, or Web interfaces. As in the field itself, few designers are able to contribute in more than one healthcare sector. Therefore, better understanding between sectors will enable us to design better end-to-end processes and whole systems. This book aims to create awareness across these segments and sectors by indexing representative issues and powerful methods from successful applications.

Design, in all its disciplines and methods, is finally emerging in new and influential roles in all types of healthcare services. Medicine is not, in practice, an online and digital field, but the rapid development of digital technologies in care delivery and education is drawing new designers into all healthcare sectors, from consumer websites to clinic design. *Design for Care* speaks to these designers and health professionals about how, where, and why their fields connect at the many points of care and service.

Designing for Care Experiences

Care is a powerful value, one we all take seriously. When a friend announces that he or she is taking time off from work to "take care of" a spouse or other family member, we understand the empathic response to a life-changing situation that takes priority over other values. Care is not just a response in the present. We project concern and hope into a shared future, and hold both memory and expectation for the cared for. Caring extends over time, unlike the immediate empathy needed to understand user experience, for example.

Yet caring is not just temporal, based on need, it is considered an enduring and authentic characteristic of a person. People take care of the others in their lives. Direct design implications are revealed in this observation. There may not always be a single "user" for health information and services. The single-user persona may need to be updated to a family scenario and the "best-friend search" use case. As some informatics researchers are now pointing out, the health-seeking experience is a multiparticipant, multiuser circle of care. It is often familial, and inherently and intimately social.

The verb *care* has acquired different meanings in different health and caring professions, and each profession related to health and human development may subscribe to a different definition and view of care. When settling these differences in meaning and not just discourse, the problem becomes onto-logical, a question of the reality of caring. This is not simply a conversion of meanings from one field to another. The very meaning of care and caring differs between providers (health practitioners) and between providers and recipients (patients). Design has not yet taken a clear stand in the matter of care. Perhaps we recognize that we cannot own the core when we ourselves still live and work at the periphery.

Philosopher Milton Mayeroff defined caring as acting on empathy, as being able to understand another's world as if you were that person. Caring requires knowing, trust, patience, humility, honesty, and the primacy of life's rhythms. According to Mayeroff, for caring to take place, "there must also be developmental change of the other as a result of what I do; I must actually help the other grow."[1]

How the Design Industry Must Change

Design has never been a serious contender for service as a caring profes-sion. Across the full range of design fields, from communications and visual design to fashion and product design, designers are recruited to enhance campaigns that oppose values of caring. The recent vogue of design think-ing does nothing to alter the technological affinity of the design professions. Design, more than the sciences even, has been steered toward a values-neutral practice of creative product and service development. There are no core ethics of design thinking, no inherent barriers of duty or conscience that keep designers from switching from healthcare "content" to beverage industry clients. Design thinking's crucial test is not merely surviving the merger of design and business with its soul intact, but in transforming orga-nizational practices by continually repositioning real human beings in the center of design and service management decisions.

Learning from empathy is a first step toward caring, by allowing us to understand how other people experience the situations we are commit-ted to improving. Given the interest in emotional design and empathic research methods in recent years, this step may not be in doubt. Responding as professionals to the call of caring marks the current bright line between the caring professions and supporting disciplines, such as design, IT, and human research, that are not called to patient care.

The call to care suggests a possible primary design position. Caring confronts us directly with a question of human valuing that we—designers and health professionals—may believe we are already fulfilling in some way. As with all values, the way it is understood can and will differ significantly between people.

We might start from the assumption that, as designers, we do not know (yet) how the values of care are lived and acted upon. We must interpret without (yet) being expert. *Design for Care* presents scenarios for designers to consider the human and social value of caring, the various ways care shows up in health seeking and health making, and the systemic role of care.

Finding Your Place in the Story

Healthcare is a massively complex system that deals with at least two irreducible sources of complexity: the institutional (distributed provider systems and hospitals) and the personal (the biological and social setting of the human body). Furthermore, these realms cannot be isolated, because the purpose of the institution is to serve individuals. An infinite variety of possible problems arise in the relationships between these two spheres of purposeful behavior. The opportunities for design to have an impact are everywhere, from effective comprehension of materials and wayfinding to improving education and information resources. Healthcare systems provide designers a constant, endless challenge in helping clinicians and patients navigate complex situations. Where is your place in the larger story?

Design (of all disciplines) is not yet showing its impact in health services. For the most part, designers remain on the sidelines in institutions and practice, unsure of where and how to step in to make a difference. Compounding this position is the difficulty that designers are often not given the latitude to practice creatively and meaningfully in healthcare institutions. The medical and institutional care traditions do not offer a ready berth for design, and our traditional positions have little systemic impact if employed without strategic intent. Until we prove to be valuable contributing members of the care team, we risk being seen as specialists and even marginal players in the story of care.

User experience won over every other application field, after a decade or more of commitment to business and IT. But change and innovation happen differently in healthcare than in other sectors—the risks are higher, the funding is regulated, and the "users" are not paying (or complaining) directly. IT is not the front line of patient care. If we are not working together with a systemic strategy, we may be contributing to the fragmentation of the field by optimizing narrow bands of practice that sustain old habits. We have no way of knowing without reaching agreement on a common design language that aligns the levels of care, the organization, and its system.

"Designing for care" has several meanings. Each chapter in this book focuses on a different aspect of human-centered design for care practice, identifying design approaches for the activity. A critical opportunity for designers is to transform the value available at the front lines of healthcare practice. Healthcare is changing rapidly, dramatically, and somewhat chaotically, as any change pushes ripple effects through the complex system. Healthcare reform, creating better care services around the patient experience, and humanizing IT are opportunities for design to contribute as a field.

Rethinking Care and Its Consumers

The rapid diffusion of hundreds of Web resources for health purposes has created a gap between information quality and user expectations. Consumers can now pursue their own research into health issues by searching the vast collections of consumer-oriented health information on the Web. They cannot be expected to understand the complexity of health issues, but do expect health information to be truthful. Yet more information does not yield better information. In fact, quite the opposite may be true. Part I focuses on the health-seeking activities of the healthcare consumer.

Health-Seeking Experiences

A person's health seeking is a continuous process of taking steps toward better health—before, during, and after any type of encounter with traditional healthcare service. Health seeking, as with other human motivations such as pleasure seeking or status seeking, represents an individual journey, in this case toward relatively better health. For a very healthy person, the ideal of perfect fitness may be an authentic health-seeking journey. For a cancer sufferer, relative health may be a matter of surviving treatment and fighting for gains in remission. These are health-seeking behaviors with quite different personal struggles, achievements, care needs, and support requirements. Seeking health covers a set of fundamental human needs. Every person is a health seeker in their own way, even if not a "patient" or a fitness buff.

A person's progress in health seeking is measured by points of feedback sensed from their everyday lives and received from professionals. People with chronic health concerns such as diabetes need continuous feedback. Those in "normal" health may find health feedback only marginally helpful. (For example, I may measure my workout progress, but I weigh myself on a scale maybe only twice a year.)

People also have different timeframes of health feedback. Think of the health-seeking journey as occurring over a lifetime, a continuity that proceeds through youth, adulthood, and older age. The individual and his or her immediate circle of care (spouse or partner, family, friends) are co–health seekers in many ways (though never "co-patients"). Everyone travels this journey together with parents, children, friends. The health journey includes a lifetime of other encounters and experiences that can enhance responsible healthy behaviors.

Yet healthcare providers have little insight into the continuous health-seeking journey. Although doctors may see dozens of individual "cases" on any given day, they have little time and usually no formal payment mechanism to follow an individual's health journey after a professional medical encounter. Their brief touchpoint is but one opportunity for improving an individual's health among dozens in a given day. There are certainly different types of practices, and some do track and manage longitudinal health outcomes. Yet an individual's health seeking is his or her own journey.

For more than a century, Western healthcare has treated people as patients, as passengers in a complicated and mysterious train on rails governed by seemingly unknowable biological forces. Any degree of pathology is relative to a normal ("healthy") standard and to a person's own experience, which may be unknowably limited and limiting. The normal condition is one of relatively balanced health in a constant motion toward homeostasis. When facing conditions that require medical intervention, people are motivated to seek health as an end in itself, as well as supporting all other goals in life.

Clinicians might find the current mandate to improve the patient experience as the perfect entry point to engage design practices as full partners in providing better care. Designers have the advantage of not being doctors— they are not professionally bound to the same legal responsibility to treat people *only* as patients, subject to clinical intervention. By repositioning the individual health seeker as a deciding and knowing agent of his or her own experience, health services can be designed to facilitate a whole-person approach to health. Improving patient experiences is the just the first step in a cultural and historical shift. A person is a patient for a limited period, but the experience of seeking health is a continuous process throughout life. Care providers and resources can help restore natural and supported functions of life.

Health seeking is not just a "journey to normal" because there is no final state of health. People live with multiple conditions of relative health in a balancing system. Measures and indicators of "healthy" are not optimized; they are better or worse compared to an individual's own baselines. People may lose weight by dieting but not improve cholesterol levels; they may recover from a viral infection but have a cough for weeks. No health measures are static, and the numbers of good measures are not as "objectively healthy" as people might think.

Health journeys are *self-educating*—people evolve as they learn in stages of struggle, understanding, acceptance, and self-management. Health seeking is an evolutionary act of self-discovery, of sustainable improvements of behavior and experience that claim a personal stake in one's present satisfaction and future thriving.

The Health Seeker in Context

Beginning in Chapter 2, each chapter advances the scenario of a persona character, Elena, as she navigates complex health issues and pursues health outcomes over a series of setbacks and healthcare encounters. Her story serves as a baseline narrative to observe human responses to events, touchpoints, and likely decisions for care services. This health-seeking journey is loosely aligned with each chapter's content.

Health Seeking | Elena's Journey

	Caregiving	Health Incident	Diagnosis	Treatment	Living With
Situation	2 Years	2 Months	2 Weeks	2 Days	Future
Information Resources	Consumer websites (Everyday Health, WebMD, Mayo Clinic)	Consumer websites, physician references	Consumer/professional resources (Medscape, HealthKnowledge)	Physician references	Health communities and personal social media
Touchpoints	Web, e-mail, workplace, home	Doctor's office, Web, home	Specialist center, Web, home	Hospital, Web, home	Web, home, e-mail
		Mutual circles of empathy	Intimate circle of care	Personal circle of care	Social circle of empathy
	Relatives / Daughter / Father / Friends / Elena	Elena			
Journey	Seeking family health	Focus on personal health	Significant health concern	Seeking treatment	Helping others
Motive	Harmonious home and family	Sustain personal productivity	Recover health to at least former level	Best survival outcome	Share lessons learned
Chapter	2	3 4	6	7 8	9

Elena's scenario is not unlike a service journey map, except from the perspective of the health seeker, whose shifts in role and identity are based on health condition and goals. The journey map is based on a typical method for portraying the navigation of health seeking and clinical encounters (Figure I.1). Notice that over the entire span of roughly two years, significant health events happen in brief intervals of two months or less, with significant impact on future health and life outcomes.

Physiological measures indicating relative health are not shown on this timeline, but are suggested in other contexts to indicate correspondences between measures, acute incidents, and recovery. Design goals for the health seeker in this journey view might include:

- Connecting Elena to her immediate family to support her caregiver role (through electronic media, printed artifacts such as notes and reminders, and multisensory media).

- Giving her direct support to inform and manage her family's health needs, and connecting her with any services for which she has regular touchpoints.

- Providing her with emotional support as a caregiver to help sustain her motivation and keep track of health progress.

- Enabling her to easily update and track her interactions with clinical services and healthcare systems.

Part I, with its focus on consumer contexts, describes Elena's personal sphere as she seeks information, support, and resources from her immediate circle of family and community to meet her health goals. Part II describes her choices and outcomes experienced as a healthcare patient, and Part III shows her as a participant in the healthcare system.

FIGURE I.1
A health seeker's journey.

CHAPTER 1

Design as Caregiving

Can Healthcare Innovate Itself?

Whether you choose a story from your own life experience or from that of a friend or family member, or just Google "healthcare horror stories," the problems in healthcare today are clear and all too common. Urban emergency rooms are overflowing, medical devices have misleading interfaces that lead to errors, doctors order too many expensive and unnecessary tests, and medical records are confusing and unreadable. Private health insurance is complex, expensive, and fragmented, sometimes resulting in crippling financial difficulties. Pharmaceutical wonder drugs are pulled off the market after a few years as emerging harmful side effects show up. Healthcare has optimized every function in the system, but the system grows more complex as these functions overlap and compete. As Harvard management professor Rosabeth Moss Kanter recently wrote,

> Supposedly, everyone working in health care wants the same thing: to help people get and stay healthy. . . . The problem is that everyone can have a different view of the meaning of getting and staying healthy. Lack of consensus among players in a complex system is one of the biggest barriers to innovation. One subgroup's innovation is another subgroup's loss of control.[1]

Because healthcare problems are so complicated and messy, they cannot easily be untangled once they appear. Mike McCallister, CEO of insurance provider Humana, described the US healthcare sector as a gigantic mix of varied players that is "broken, but can be fixed. We don't actually have a healthcare system. We have a lot of different systems that are glued together."[2] Alex Jadad, founder of Toronto's Centre for Global eHealth Innovation, calls for immediate innovation in person-centered healthcare and collaborative development of IT to help Canada's high-functioning but stressed healthcare system: "This technology can help us transcend our cognitive, physical, institutional, geographical, cultural, linguistic, and historical boundaries. Or it can contribute to our extinction."[3]

Designing for care brings a holistic and systemic design perspective to the complex problems of healthcare. We are already improving services by designing better artifacts, communications, and environments. What remains missing is the mindset of professional care in designing for people, practitioners, and societies. Like clinicians, designers in the health field can take responsibility for helping people and societies become healthier in all aspects of living.

Technology Will Not Save Healthcare

Technologists advocate for disruptive innovation in healthcare, a call that envisions radical change for consumers as well as the largest institutions. The two targets of disruption are typically hospital-based institutional healthcare and the medical care model itself. The cure is envisioned to be a future of low-cost networked computer technology owned by consumers, not clinicians. A kit can be imagined consisting of embedded sensors connected to a handset, cloud-based data collection with instant analytics, and continuous-learning algorithms that diagnose individual conditions based on rapid sensor tests and genetic analysis. Possible new treatments are not described clearly, but still an accountable person will be needed to administer injections and judge the appropriate therapy and medications. A problem with such scenarios is that they project a future driven by technological determinism—because it can be done, it will be done.

The decentralized "future of medicine" scenarios articulate radical changes in technology but fail to address changes in cultural meaning. As pictured by Silicon Valley, healthcare could be decentralized and fragmented into defined care streams that the "user" (the patient) would navigate as self-service interfaces. In effect, these scenarios shift care decisions to "consumers" who might be existentially vulnerable to their own poor decisions (as well as to new types of usability risks). If patients are forced by economic changes to trust a technology instead of a physician, the ethics of "brave new healthcare" scenarios become socially problematic.

The technologically determined scenarios suggest a sociological change more radical than any other system designed in human society. Healthcare is the world's largest employment base, with national health systems among the largest employers in their respective countries. Such a disruption would ignore the sociotechnical foundation of healthcare that underlies practice, education, policy, employment, and the very meaning of care. It risks replacing medicine with a new corporate system devoid of human socioculture or caring, treating diseases as functional states mediated by robots. Although the enabling technologies can and will be developed, their implementation will look very little like the visions of computational "personalized" medicine imagined by technological utopians (and investors standing to benefit).

Another focus of disruptive change is the US private insurance model, which turns on policy innovation and not technology. Innovation in insurance-managed payments to guarantee equitable care services might make the single largest difference in people's everyday lives. If patients did not have to worry about going bankrupt to pay for the noncovered costs for healthcare services, they would view their health and self-care differently. Although not a perfect policy for either citizens or providers, the Affordable Care Act (Obamacare) established a new framework for policy innovation to occur, to meet the goals of covering uninsured Americans and managing aggregate costs. If the system were not based on profit-seeking business models, innovative new care practices would be designed and implemented. In the United States today, however, with multiple layers of cost accounting and payment review, stakeholders distrust one another, and patients lose out. Unfortunately, the ultimate fix is not technological but political, the results of policy innovation to ensure universal coverage and appropriate technology support.

Major policy changes will be necessary to encourage the risk-averse health industry to accept system-wide innovation. Today, healthcare systems and their management are the biggest barriers to meaningful innovation, as they have so much to lose in a paradigmatic shift.

Even the most radical breakthrough technologies often demonstrate only incremental improvements to the service and experience of care. As new clinical services are developed around emerging medical technologies, the form and function of current practice will change only modestly, perhaps not even perceptibly to patients. Due to culture, risk, payment, generally accepted practices, and other systemic factors, technological change is often not leveraged as an opportunity to change policy and practice.

Both of these envisioned "disruptions" shift profits and costs, winners and losers. Only the disruption of the insurance industry guarantees a beneficial cost shift to consumers in the near term. There are no guarantees that technological disruption will pass end savings to consumers. Though low-cost systems can be developed, there are no social provisions for regulating the resulting business models and new corporate entities that could manage health technologies. If the pharmaceutical industry (which is rarely mentioned as a target for disruption) cannot innovate new business models, it seems misguided to believe that emerging technologies slated to replace physicians will be priced any differently than pharmaceutical products.

In a market-based system, disruptive innovations create real competitive value by making long-established services obsolete. But even if many healthcare services are profit-based, should innovation best be envisioned as enabling a competitive economic outcome? How does disruption help healthcare? Human lives are at stake, not merely profits.

Innovation of Human-Centered Care Systems

All-out radical technological change is not the only way to create value for health seekers and reduce exponential costs. A better way to innovate might be found in designing human-centered care systems.

The human-centered design of healthcare has never been more necessary. Leading innovation provocateur Don Norman, with designer and author Roberto Verganti, proposed a concept and solution to the paradox of "merely" incremental innovation from human-centered design.[4] They position radical and incremental *technology innovation* against radical and incremental *innovation of meaning*. The position emerged from Norman's observation that only new technologies were found to trigger radical change. And yes, he found that human-centered design research (studying users in their native habitat) rarely, if ever, led to disruptive innovation. Though essential to incremental improvements in technological systems from airplanes to software, design research fails to find breakthroughs, due in part to the fact that radical changes cannot be extrapolated from observing practice. Further, user evidence tends to reinforce the very practices being studied, as user behavior is defined by its goals and productivity, not the experimentation that might lead to completely new practices.

The shift to cultural and practice innovation is found in the other half of the Norman-Verganti equation: the radical innovation of meaning. What Verganti calls design-led innovation involves redefining the socially recognized meaning of technology or a practice. Sociotechnical practices in healthcare may be reframed (without radically changing technologies) to shift the social purpose. The accountable care organization (ACO) model promoted by new US legislation carries the seeds of new value propositions that have yet to be tested. The essential meaning change is that of localized care centers with more attention to patient life needs to reduce readmittances. Although ACOs might become radically patient-centered, perhaps the most significant value will emerge in the social meaning change, with new types of care practices being envisioned that reinvent the relationship of providers and health seekers. These practices and their business models offer fertile ground for the new types of designers being trained in socially aware innovation.

Disruptive innovations that we see in other industries may have less of a role in healthcare, even though the opportunities for new technology are clearly present. Healthcare facilities are not early adopters. New software, devices, and systems take time to learn and socialize, and the investment of professional time and budget in training and ramp-up is quite expensive. The expense of these social costs can outweigh the benefit of adoption. For example, desktop computers took years to infiltrate hospitals, and by the time they were ubiquitous in the clinic, they had become common in homes. Minimal training was necessary because the technology was already pervasive. The use of mobile devices is following the same late adopter cycle, allowing for a more natural (less forced) introduction of new devices into high-performance, high-risk clinical environments.

Even information systems require mammoth projects for system-wide implementation. The *adoption* of new services and systems is by no means a given. Breakthrough medical technologies are also not adopted immediately by institutions. New technologies, devices, and therapies require extensive review and evaluation through animal and human trials, developmental testing, and regulatory approvals. Changes in practice may take months or even years to filter through an institution or system diffused across regions and affiliation. For example, the truly disruptive da Vinci robotic surgery system did not change medical practice as we know it. It allows skilled surgeons to operate on remote and special-case patients who were previously underserved. Da Vinci signals the start of a new trend that might increase capital costs (as hospitals must all acquire it to compete) as well as lower surgery costs, potentially having a democratizing effect of equalizing the quality of routine surgeries across regions.

Da Vinci is a disruptive technology that shows significant yet incremental effects. Organizations absorb the new system into the current business model. For now at least, hospitals remain big box clinical institutions. Technology and product design have only incremental effects on the patient experience. Patients must still be prepped and undergo an invasive procedure, yet now with the much greater convenience of being able to show up at a community-based clinic in the healthcare network. Change is difficult for doctors, and adaptation to changes can be discomforting for patients.

This perspective of redesigning existing practices explodes one of the most treasured myths of innovation. Many authors suggest that disruptive interventions have the highest impact and are therefore the aim of innovation. Innovation theories celebrate the value of "disruptive" innovation as the most competitive form of innovation. Yet what are the purposes of disruptive healthcare innovation? To improve efficiencies, costs, practices, or patient experiences?

We might reframe the purposes of disruptive innovation in institutional healthcare based on the experience with platforms and devices. The da Vinci system performs operative functions that surgical teams can understand and integrate within well-defined routines. It doesn't disrupt the function of surgery, but rather the way routine operations are physically performed. Information technologies tend to disrupt clinical work in ways that may *reduce* efficiency of performance. New systems require training and ramp-up time (away from patients). Additional time must be allocated for electronic entries for the purported benefit of administration, not patients.

Consider the societal value of an innovation from the perspective of those most affected by the results. Does a simple value analysis show benefit to all direct stakeholders? Will health seekers benefit from the change?

Are There Users of Care?

Healthcare is a complicated business, and can be a complicated context for design. Multiple *stakeholders* (from consumers and patients to clinical staff, administrators, and insurers) interact with multiple *services* (from primary care to academic institutional networks) in multiple *sectors* (from clinical practice to insurance and government). Traditional user-centered design practices are insufficiently powerful to solve problems at this level of complexity. We can easily and mistakenly design a perfect product or service for "our users," yet remain disconnected from the other systems and stakeholders the service may affect.

In health contexts, the risks to health and the effects on practice are always considered. Healthcare environments require the use of far more rigorous design and development methods than the contemporary trend in user experience (UX) and service design. Involving both significant financial and human life impacts, investment decisions are based on evidence, with a strong organizational bias toward statistical evidence.

Designers face a recurring challenge in every healthcare project—to envision the scope for service sufficient to meet future needs and growing complexity. We design for situations that have multiple interacting workflows, poor integration, layers of legacy infrastructure, and highly dispersed applications. These legacies constrain the ability to design services across departments, institutions, or at any level we consider as "the system."

Healthcare is a large-scale distributed system dedicated to serving individuals with health needs but who are not the paying customer. This is a classic dilemma of service and experience design: the patient (the end user) has little decision-making power but a life-critical need; the institutional customer (who pays) has significant power but little understanding of need.

Patients and practitioners are changing the balance of power through improved transparency and access to information. But these social, human, and information interactions magnify the technical complexities because they introduce new uncertainties to decisions and transactions.

UX design advocates understanding and designing for the optimal user interaction. It often supposes an interactive product with specified uses in a work (or point of care) context. User-centered design has served as a sufficiently powerful methodology for a generation, and health informatics and technologies have improved significantly, if incrementally. A generation of experience designers has been trained to represent the interests and needs of users, and we have institutionalized "the user" as shorthand for design (user-centered) and usability (user-friendly). However, there is no single user in healthcare, and the convention of referring to users may be misleading in the context of care.

In healthcare practice and design, the vocabulary and perception of the human subject is dominated by three primary frames: user, patient, and consumer. All three designations are passive, objectified representations that constrain a person's significance as a "health actor" to a transactional role. These roles designate people as users of products (user), clients of institutions (patient), or recipients of services (consumer). If we examine critically the ways in which designers participate in projects, advise on the design of IT and systems, and select research methods, the attendant design values of these roles show up in dialogue and decision making.

A user-centered service design perspective leads us to focus on the *patient*, the recipient of care and the human actor most vulnerable to "disruptive" technology impacts. By focusing on patient outcomes and processes, design decisions are unassailable and credible. Presenting a case based on real patient needs and experience can move a room of mixed opinions to consensus agreement.

The patient-centered perspective has become a significant movement in medical practice, and is central to healthcare service design. Yet people do not see themselves as patients; it is not a persistent role or identity that people choose. The patient identity is not persistent across the continuous experience of health seeking. Also, as readily observed in healthcare institutions, not all service problems involve patient behavior. The patient is not central to every function in healthcare systems and organizations.

We have also been conditioned through years of professionalization to accept a medical view of wellness and sickness, a view in which people show up as patients within a largely corporate healthcare system. As designers, we unwittingly follow this model when we adopt a conventional approach to workflow and personas. We even risk this perspective when making claims for "improving the patient experience." That is, we are still framing a clinical encounter as a "patient experience," making the inevitable more comfortable or efficient. We risk representing a supply-side (vendor-oriented) perspective, which only simulates empathy or care, regardless of the humanizing intent of the methods. If not working within a clinical organization, we may not be able to speak with real patients in actual care situations. Designers and health professionals need better methods for understanding experience and making design claims with often limited access and data.

A market-based viewpoint defines people as customers and receivers of health or information services that others produce and supply. The *consumer* designation fixes our attention to a transactional service relationship inimical to the values of care. Critiquing the consumer persona or mindset frees up the capacity to innovate with fresh perspectives. Human health is not the result of a service transaction; rather, it flourishes in the context of care, drawing on personal, familial, professional, and community resources.

In a complex system such as healthcare, naming any persona as a *user* privileges just one role in the system. It also assumes something to use, and traditional modes of use are often not the case in healthcare. In care situations, everyone participates at some point in a human system of health seeking from which we produce care and support. By enlarging the scope of health seeking to view it as a social context of health seekers and caregivers, we expand beyond our narrow (and professional) point of view that wants to designate people as "users."

Each of these three frames (user, patient, consumer) has relevance in certain circumstances, and they are useful to indicate to designers the differences in identity and activity across the spectrum of health services. Yet real people do not experience themselves as these roles, especially in health situations.

We might actively replace the old mental models with a fresh perspective based on the *lived experience of health*. What should designing for care establish as the perspective for care-centered practices? To answer this, let's ask higher order questions: Why are people in the healthcare system? What motivates people who seek care and health?

The health seeker may not be a patient or even a consumer, but any person aware of her motivation to improve her health. A health seeker may be any person desiring better health for his own life circumstance, for a family member, or a friend. A family or community might seek health. It is not necessarily an individual experience. People do not always follow medical advice, take their prescriptions, or take the most rational steps when dealing with a disease condition. People make sense of their life concerns together with their specific questions when seeking health and health information. As such, health seeking is not just looking things up on Dr. Google. It is a process of organizing one's experience and trusted resources, including materials from the Web and advice from health professionals and family and friends, to address partially formed questions. If health seeking can be understood as a continuous lifelong process, a care-centered design orientation can span the different needs of patient, professional, and service, and help us define priorities for intervention and redesign.

A Caring Design Ethic

Caring design requires a change in meaning, as the design professions have no tradition of care practices. True care goes beyond the appreciative and participates with the personal feelings and social concerns shared by both patients and practitioners. Beyond the instrumental empathy "in order to" understand the user, care seeks to understand the senses and feelings of a person, as they really matter.

An honest, empathic interest expressed in care will be challenged by the typical organizational commitments of a designer's IT company or agency. When we use project management language to structure our product requirements and define our shared goals, we may fail to even acknowledge the other values calling for attention in a care situation. In healthcare, care design may then part ways with both the individualistic approach to creativity and the brutal efficiencies of project management in design execution.

The values and ideals promoted in a caring design ethic are drawn from the humane arts and sciences of health and medicine. These include empathic care, doing no harm, health for the whole person, and helping people live sustainable lives. Devoting a new focus of care in design practice requires an innovation of meaning for designers, and it may change our methods, tools, and engagements. The narrative for this next generation of humane design practice has yet to be formed. How will the meaning of value to clients, communities, and health seekers change?

Shifting Focus from Product to Person

New systems are not always the answer. Consider the cumulative impact of the thousands of cognitive interactions required of users for every new service, system, interface, device, or billing statement. Doctors are too busy to adopt more than a few essential services, and they often maintain older systems that are safely committed to memory, rather than invest time in learning a new system that may introduce transition risks and fail to improve care or costs. Patients may be confused by the sprawling range of Web services and competing arrays of redundant online health information.

Consider the many new products, interfaces, and tools for individual healthcare that may be innovative but have no accepted mandate. For example, personal health records (PHR), such as Microsoft HealthVault, have been available since 2007, but adoption has been hampered by the lack of basic usability, limited utility, and "understandability." Most people do not yet understand the PHR and its possible value. Google ended the Google Health PHR in 2011 due to a lack of general acceptance and process (not just interface) usability. An application only used by individuals who *must* use it is not a basis for mass adoption.

Issues such as information privacy, caregiver accessibility, and care team collaboration are also significant design factors. Technical and usability concerns are also daunting impediments to acceptance and adoption. The early adopters of personal health technologies are people motivated to use these tools for daily needs, but patients living with significant health concerns may—due to age and multiple conditions—find it more difficult to learn and use these tools than people with less need for them.

The Case for Caring Design

Although each design discipline differs in its methods and targets, most designers work at understanding problems of human use of a thing or a system, and innovate to make effective changes that people desire. Since the dawn of medicine and physical care, people have designed artifacts to enhance practice, comfort, and communications. Nurses "designed" the Kardex documentation system, and medical librarians contributed to the formal design of medical charts. But until very recently, people trained as designers have largely been absent from the health professions, and very few programs educate designers in healthcare practices.

In the 1980s, first in architecture and then (much later) in device design human factors, specially trained designers began focusing on health applications. Human interface design for medical devices only improved after problems were reported with control interfaces in devices (such as drug infusion pumps) that had been designed by engineers with no user interface design training. With the recent explosion of informatics and health websites in the last decade, it would seem the entry point for service and experience design has finally arrived.

Design is not taught or (in practice) led from a caring perspective. Design is a creative practice that employs empathy as a method for designing better, more usable products and services. Empathy is a *temporary* caring, and becomes instrumental when invoked as a means to improving the design of things or services for sale. Although we may care about the impact of our design work, we do not usually follow and care for the lives of our users, or the patients affected by our systems. We may care about users and patients, but we are not called on to care about any particular person. How we might "care more" is a question that requires rethinking the role of design and human-centered research. The difference may entail moving from performing as contributing designers to coordinating patient-centered service projects. In these scenarios, the health outcomes of future patients are now at stake. Yet the imperative for innovation and service change means organizations will accept a higher level of creative and participatory design.

The Design Thinking Divide

Healthcare practice and institutions have no common voice, and few "whole system" advocates are followed. Ranking just after the prime directive of "help all and do no harm," institutions care about cost and risk. Because change incurs both costs and risk, healthcare has significant incentives not to change the system. These values and incentives powerfully determine the scope of design impact. Traditional UX and service design methodologies may be necessary, but are not sufficient.

Design proposals require sponsors to weigh care, cost, and risk. Institutional sponsors deal in quantitative evidence where possible, and designers make qualitative arguments based on human experience. Making matters worse in practice, design and implementation decisions are fraught with competing interests, often imposing near-term decision making on the IT team and changes in practice, and design and research professionals are often isolated in narrow bands of problem scope.

The complexity of healthcare IT applications requires that designers make a personal and usually long-term commitment to the domain, involving years of learning, practice, and patience with slow progress. In institutional or commercial healthcare IT development, designers have much less control over the delivered experience than in other fields. The opportunities for creative influence or enhancement may not be apparent (and may need to be courageously co-created in the organization). Healthcare as a domain is strongly influenced by empirical scientific tradition and evidence-based practices. Designers will be expected to understand and adapt to the language of the domain rather than the language of design and user experience.

Large-scale healthcare applications are based on enterprise IT architectures, which may take many years of development cycles to significantly change. And ethnographic or field research is hampered by limited access to the different "users," especially patients, due to privacy and immediate care considerations. Most research studies take months, not weeks, because they are carefully designed and then reviewed by ethics boards. Due to these factors and the hierarchical and highly managed healthcare culture, a design team must be committed to making a difference over the long term.

Healthcare applications—at least institutional applications—are not designed by means of creative ideation, participatory design, or even iterative prototyping. There are few national-level design advisors or advocates from the design or even the industrial engineering fields. Publications are dominated by physicians and informatics specialists, whose work is often based on tightly focused, feasible research agendas fitting institutional mandates. Conferences are highly specialized within medical or educational discipline (professional societies), technology (health IT and informatics), technology-oriented research (the Medicine 2.0 movement), and disease specialization (e.g., the American Diabetes Association). There are no regular design-oriented conferences in the healthcare field yet, and few tracks within conferences to encourage discourse between design professionals across different fields. Our current lack of standing is also evidenced by the subordination of design practice to every other field we support. Yet the situation is changing, and many new points of entry have opened.

Lost and Found in the System

How do designers build a more systemic approach? We are not typically engaged at the level of healthcare reform or practice, but serve in problem-solving teams for well-framed issues. Our points of entry to the system level are not clear. The advisors and policy advocates in healthcare are distinctly separated by problem area (disease management, medical education, health insurance reform) and separated by problem-solving approach (policy, practice innovation, patient-centered medicine, information systems).

Due to the complexity of healthcare practices and the compelling urgency of narrow-focus concerns, individual designers and design teams are often unable to design solutions to address root causes. It is rare to design any application that scales across institutions or practice areas. The Web does not count because most applications are piecemeal, insufficient, or one of many similar sites. Universal access is not a solution for scaling across domains or services.

Given the serious design risks of unforeseeable design error in health practice and the hazards of liability, designers, researchers, and engineers are obligated to understand the systemic problems in the field. Small oversights can lead to consequential errors. As a patient you may have noticed an irritating but inconspicuous oversight, such as the overly small text size on a prescription label or a long wait in an examination room. Or you may have experienced the frustration of poor information organization—or even intentional obfuscation—as you attempt to decipher your insurance coverage before phoning for an appointment. You may have been the hapless recipient of an everyday medical mistake, such as a slightly misplaced needle insertion that leaves a well-liked muscle tender for weeks. Chances are these irritants, on their own, would not be considered worthy of special design attention. Are they symptomatic of systematic problems?

From an outsider's perspective—and designers are still outsiders—the system that connects these particular incidents may not readily disclose itself. However, once inside the health-industrial complex, significant design concerns will show up that overwhelm these trivial annoyances. Do not lose sight of the seemingly minor inconveniences; frustration is one of the leading causes of innovation. Frustrations with wayfinding, communications, or documentation may reveal underlying systemic causes that have been completely overlooked.

If your intention is to apply design thinking and skills to make a difference in healthcare, start with your own history and perspectives. We are all health seekers. Uncover your personal interests and biases, your beliefs about life and health, and your positions on scientific evidence and the art of medicine. Unlike other fields of design and management, personal experiences and common sense may harness your motivation and inform a sense of genuine empathy.

Designers and researchers work with and deeply appreciate the abstract— our building blocks include information, artifacts, interaction, aesthetics, methods, templates, personas, and so on. The healthcare field, which has become automated and intellectual, is centered on embodied subjects— people with health concerns. Healthcare itself is a hands-on practice of continual and practical problem solving. In few other worlds of design do we find such a difference between our maps (our products) and the territory.

Design Thinking in Service and Policy Sectors

People working on the front lines of healthcare are overloaded with well-intentioned information services. Research has identified the prevalence of platform fatigue, when busy professionals become weary of maintaining an institution's multiple systems for patient records, billing, orders, and decision support, each of which requires access, password control, login sequences, and learning a new interface. Future healthcare problems are not solved by the introduction of a better user experience.

Scalable services—service systems—require rethinking IT, not just as an integrating resource in a whole system but as a team player that is as trusted as a human member of the clinical team. Clearly, IT has not achieved this level of reliability and resilience yet. The implementation of IT "solutions" should never become a default management decision. Multidisciplinary clinical service design teams are called for to determine the appropriate allocation of technological, organizational, and individual role functions in care service systems. At the very least, a regular practice of critical evaluations can assess that care provision is not impeded or complicated.

The societal waves of change happening now are driving the need for better design. We should expect a historically large shift from other fields into healthcare, due to the near-term political and institutional attention on implementing electronic patient records. Driven by the push of the 2009 Health Information Technology for Economic and Clinical Health (HITECH) Act in the United States, and the general mandate of ready funding for technology, health centers continue to rush to implement and integrate medical records, hospital management, billing, and insurance in massive institutional databases. These systems are complex, unwieldy, and at some point, necessary. Yet their interfaces are intended for practitioners working in hectic care settings who usually consider computers an administrative chore.

Outside of the United States, healthcare requires a complete rethinking of our experience with health services, providers, costs, and innovation. Whereas developed nations may be faced with an overabundance of choice, emerging economies require consideration of how design can help the very basic outcomes of healthcare services. In the United States, we expect an exchange of ideas and methods between the consumer and professional sectors. In global healthcare, we cannot expect to transfer knowledge and the easy fixes learned from North American successes. In developing nations, culturally appropriate innovation might require a integration of traditional practices with guidance from mainstream healthcare procedures and medications. Automation may be a helpful but secondary concern, with health centers enabled by off-the-shelf software and sufficiently reliable computers, while allowing for unreliable grid power and Internet access.

We might also acknowledge how the technological imperative is implied in innovation thinking. Not all "systems" in healthcare are computer-based; the technical work of care is performed as a hands-on human process. Diagnosis, treatment, procedures, aftercare, and care planning are not (yet) automated, and the human-to-human relationship of care never will be. Yet healthcare process and procedure generates a massive amount of data helpful in analysis and management of services. The allocation of human and automated tasks remains a moving target as IT and sensors expand the possibilities of public and individual care, and the designers of service and experience have rights to the negotiable intersection between human and information. Unfortunately for interaction and UX designers, the healthcare IT market has not matured to the point where UX factors significantly affect purchase and implementation decisions. We are only now getting a hearing, and with the rapid pace of newly installed databases, we may be appearing on the scene much too late. Yet these systems still need our help.

Wicked Problems in Healthcare Design

Healthcare is not only a "mess," it technically entails many *wicked problems*—complexities with no clear and immediate resolution. Wicked problems are generally large in scale, affecting unknown numbers of people with unknown levels of risk and effect. They include most persistent social and environmental issues that have emerged from multiple root causes over time. In truly wicked problems, original causes (such as bad regulatory decisions) evolve into new effects (corrupt agencies and regimes), interventions have no testable solution (How do you determine whether the situation has been resolved?), and the very acknowledgment of a "problem" results from the earlier effects of embedded, interconnected, complicated problems.

Systems scientist Horst Rittel reserved the term for systemic social problems that defy analytical problem solving, are not understandable by any single individual, and have no single best solution.[5] In healthcare, wicked problems are the most critical (and costly) issues, such as aging populations, multiple chronic diseases, interacting conditions in persons living longer, and rapid changes required of practice based on constant updates to (and conflicts in) research. They occur at a scale that can have devastating financial and societal impacts that increase over time. Reaching agreement on how to solve these problems remains difficult, but they also require action in the face of incomplete knowledge and limited foresight, meaning that we often do our best and then live with the consequences.

Problems that do not meet the definition of wicked are commonly framed as simple, complicated, or complex. *Simple* problems are those situations with a clear cause and a reliable response in most cases. In healthcare, these include well-understood routine conditions such as broken bones and lacerations. Many more health concerns are *complicated*, requiring iterative tests and observations. Surgical operations are complicated, with many moving parts and many ways to fail. *Complex* problems are interconnected and entangled issues with uncertain outcomes. Chronic, interacting diseases are complex, such as asthma, allergies, and many cancers or autoimmune diseases. *Wicked* problems are complex problems with uncertain interventions as well as uncertain outcomes. These can range from healthcare system reform to facial pain management.

Design Strategies

Design strategy is necessary to align any radical innovation with organizational purposes. A design strategy, spanning every role from communications to services, reframes the meaning of change to stakeholders, and creatively aligns a new concept with implementation. A design strategy determines whether managers will risk changing the meaning of healthcare services or merely adapt technology to current practices. Because the tradition of professional care has become so culturally embedded, few institutions risk taking the road to radical meaning change.

Over the last two decades, a small number of progressive frameworks for design thinking have been found applicable for the selection of strategic design options. Design theorist Richard Buchanan's orders of design is an influential schema for problem framing, as well a definitive reference to the contemporary view of design thinking.[6] He proposed four placements that designers employ to compose integrated design strategies across four classes of design targets:

- Symbolic and visual communications
- Artifacts and material objects
- Activities and organized services
- Complex systems and environments

Buchanan observed that designers draw upon placements as ways to creatively reconfigure a design concept in a new situation. All designers build their own vocabularies, as well as a set of skills and styles applicable in their domains of work. Rather than following a fixed series of orders to reach an outcome, the placements are a strategy for creative invention. An information design problem for a website might lead to a discovery of a better wayfinding information scheme by adopting the new Web information categories and shifting across types from one placement to another.

We can find a range of problem types in every healthcare sector, but things become complex when defining problem boundaries. An individual health problem can be viewed as a matter of self-care or as interacting with multiple institutional systems. Where we draw the line matters. Designers and strategists Garry VanPatter and Elizabeth Pastor defined design geographies—four essentially different design domains, Design 1.0 through 4.0, that represent an evolution of design practice, research, and education to develop new knowledge bases necessary for increasing complexity (Figure 1.1).[7]

The stages are not replacements of former paradigms (as in *Health* 2.0). They are based on observations from practice settings, and their "proof" is not theoretical but comes from application. Managing complexity is not just a matter of increasing scope. Different skills and methods apply in each domain that are generally transferable up, but not down, from one level to the next.

The four stages embody design processes for the following contexts:

1. **Artifacts and communications:** *design as making,* or traditional design practice

2. **Products and services:** design for *value creation* (including service design, holistic product innovation, multichannel, and user experience), or design as *integrating*

3. **Organizational transformation** (complex, bounded by business or strategy): design for transforming work practices, strategies, and organizational structures

4. **Social transformation** (complex, unbounded): design for transforming social systems, policies, and communities

Because of the magnitude of complexity difference in each stage, they are not interchangeable. In any given design process, the skills and orientations from *all* levels might be employed. Each higher phase is inclusive of the lower levels as the problem complexity expands from Design 1.0 to 4.0. An organizational process (D3.0) can design communications in line with the quality of the best D1.0 work. The process itself follows the methods and practices of a D2.0 service.

The four domains differ in their strategy, intention, and outcomes. Each requires skill and coordination of distinct methods, design practices, types of collaboration, and stakeholder participation. These are not fixed requirements but merely entry criteria for performing in the capacity of that "geography" in practice. The domains are described as follows (Figure 1.2):

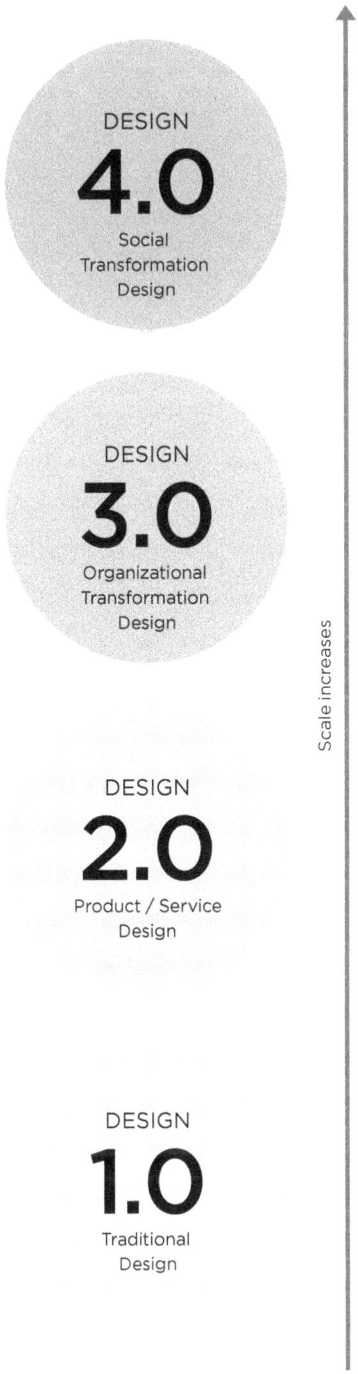

DESIGN

4.0

Social
Transformation
Design

DESIGN

3.0

Organizational
Transformation
Design

Scale increases

DESIGN

2.0

Product / Service
Design

DESIGN

1.0

Traditional
Design

FIGURE 1.1

Mapping design process to challenge complexity. (Courtesy of Humantific)

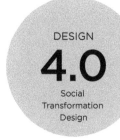

DESIGN 4.0
Social Transformation Design

- Focus on change-making
- Health policy
- Healthcare affiliations
- Social innovation
- Multistakeholder networks
- Participatory action research

DESIGN 3.0
Organizational Transformation Design

- Focus on change-making
- Organizational processes
- Business system design
- Participatory leadership
- Clinical practice and research
- Cross-function action teams
- Business, process, and practice innovation

DESIGN 2.0
Product / Service Design

- Focus on differencing
- User experience design
- Service design
- Product design
- Informatics and decision support
- Product team collaboration

DESIGN 1.0
Traditional Design

- Focus on differencing
- Consumer and institutional products
- Communications, websites
- Promotion and advertising
- Brands and identities
- Patient literature

FIGURE 1.2
Design 1.0–4.0 approaches in complexity scale.

Design 1.0: Traditional craft design processes. This is a typical creative practice approach in which the design of artifacts and products is led by a designer with ingenuity and experience. This stage relies on individual design skills in form-giving, illustration, and representation to define and finish desired products, such as publications, simple websites, or advertising. It is performed as an invisible process to stakeholders.

Design 2.0: Industrial and interactive product design. This stage includes the vast majority of all design-led projects in a clinical organization, including all types of IT, interactive services, and most services design. A design and research process is published for the specific purposes of the project (such as a process and style guide). Clinical stakeholders have representation in a multidisciplinary team. User behavioral research is necessary to ensure useful and usable products for effective interaction in the intended environment.

Design 3.0: Organizational level transformation design. This stage co-creates the organizational change necessary for the increased complexity of services that change clinical work practices or institutional policy. Organizational research and workflow analysis are compatible with sociotechnical systems approaches,[8] such as activity theory and cognitive work analysis. Design 3.0 integrates health IT and practice change as part of social systems. The project teams are extended with clinical stakeholders and patient representation. Processes are not only published, they are developed by the extended team with consensus and made universal across projects. Advanced internal skills (collaborative facilitation) and design/research skills are required to lead, conduct, and communicate the full cycle of design and research for complex problems.

Design 4.0: Social transformation. This stage is the highest order of complexity, in which multiple social systems intersect. The large healthcare institution can be seen as a nested social system, with many different social systems overlapping in the cause of health and care provision. Because this stage typically has no single fixed boundary, the scope and problem are defined through socializing agreement. Even the problem definition requires mixed, multidisciplinary stakeholders. As the design intent reaches beyond the organization, research approaches informed by social systems design[9] and participatory action research[10] are compatible with this scale of design.

Design across Healthcare Services and Sectors

Shifting the target of design from a print or material artifact (D1.0) to a product or service (D2.0) may not require a significant change in design practices, but represents a shift in artifact complexity and certainly in user or organizational involvement. More stakeholders are necessary to inform design, and product teams deal with multiple competing requirements and interpretations of value and quality. An increasing requirement for stakeholder collaboration and technology integration is shifted up to each subsequent level.

Many integrated services or complex Web products have made the shift from individual to social interaction, and D1.0 and D2.0 are often combined within the same product. But healthcare practices occur in distributed settings and require more than well-designed apps. In the institutional setting, IT applications require organizational integration (D3.0), and new clinical services may address community health concerns (D4.0).

One series of transformations moves from part (function) to whole (system) up the levels of ordering. In diabetes management, for example, a D1.0 solution might entail a public service advertisement for a D2.0 diabetes information website. Moving to D3.0, a hospital might offer a specialized clinic to serve the growing demographic of patients with diabetes and related issues. Moving to D4.0 might co-create an online community organized for diabetes aftercare staffed by live clinicians for asynchronous responses to questions and even review of personal health data to minimize the burden and expenses of in-clinic appointments.

Figure 1.3 shows a relative scale of problem solving, from simple design problems to wicked social concerns, and the design strategy consistent with the needs in each problem area. As complexity increases, the demand for sensemaking of the problem itself increases. Sensemaking, considered here the consensual understanding of the functions of a problem area, becomes a critical requirement in situations of high complexity (D3.0 and D4.0). In a social design process, multiple stakeholders, managers, and experts come to agreement or make sense of the situation together.

Strange-making is a process of differentiating form to capture attention. It consumes the larger proportion of D1.0 and D2.0, where novelty and provocation is expected for product design, commercial communications, or sophisticated Web services. In a competitive consumer marketplace, the need for design differencing is absolutely clear. Distinctive value propositions are embodied with differentiating design values. In D3.0 and D4.0 contexts, however, there is no need to differentiate. These contexts share a high degree of social and process complexity and interconnectedness among problems. For organizational and social systems, deep problem understanding (through processes of collective sensemaking) comprises the majority of the design engagements over the development life cycle.

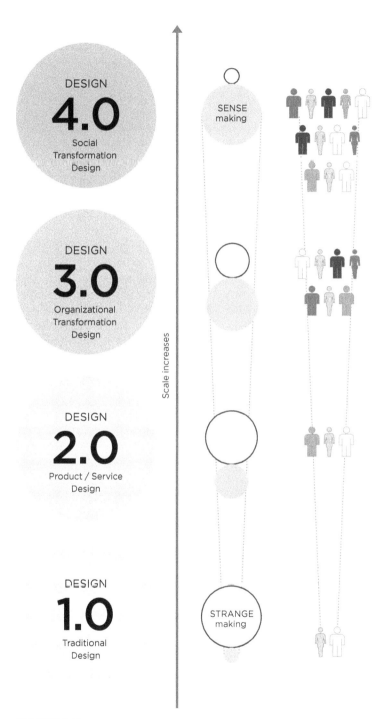

FIGURE 1.3

Design geographies and complexity scale. (Courtesy of Humantific)

The framework gives designers the ability to make a case for systemic design. Consider a consumer website such as WebMD. As a conventional Web content product, WebMD provides valuable information to searchers of health information. Yet it does not connect the individual socially to other users (D2.0); to institutions or business processes (D3.0), except through advertising or embedded content; or to larger-scale social transformations of healthcare (D4.0). Its advertising-based revenue model, although commercially lucrative, inhibits the site from growing into a broader service with institutional or societal impact.

D3.0 expands the target of design to the organization itself—one that is already structured to function as a repeatable production system. D3.0 facilitates practices within an organization that help multidisciplinary teams and functional groups reinvent their work and rethink innovation as a direct management concern. D4.0 facilitates design and innovation owned by multiple stakeholders in a complex situation, a transformative design perspective that engages people from across organizations in a much larger social system. Few design projects are defined at the level of D4.0, but some organizations face challenges that are better framed this way. The strategies of top clinics and diversified organizations such as Kaiser Permanente reach beyond the organizational boundaries to government, universities, patient groups, and clinical research, expanding the boundaries of design. They are not solely organizational programs, and can be facilitated as multistakeholder social systems problems.

Design thinking at the social and cultural scale is collaborative and cross-organizational. Designers become conveners, sharing the process and co-creating artifacts, research methods, and local decisions. The distinction between D3.0 and D4.0 is one of boundaries—when the institutional boundary of D3.0 is crossed to the societal realm of 4.0, design intent changes to policy and social action. Responsibility for the process is transferred to the stakeholders, not just for effective collaboration but as a normative practice, following the principle that social and policy design is owned by the stakeholders who live with and benefit from the outcomes.

Design thinking—and design strategy—are not development processes. Buchanan's paper was among the first to employ the term *design thinking*, and it avoided any suggestion of the popular stepwise frameworks that characterize current approaches to design thinking. His proposition was that designerly thinking afforded ways of flexibly addressing intractable (wicked) design problems through a creative process of shifting solutions through the levels he called placements. This reminds us that systemically complex problems are not "solved" as much as they are addressed through thoughtful and often disruptive interventions. The geographies model reveals that higher orders of complexity require different skills, practices, and languages.

Designing No Harm

Collaborative design attention is most needed where the probability of harm is increased by poor design decisions. Nobody dies from a bad website, but patients can and do die from information display errors and counterintuitive device interfaces. Thoughtless design is magnified greatly when it shows up in a healthcare process or medical device.

The healthcare system presents us with an ongoing and interconnected family of problems that no single person can understand and navigate. A fix for a local situation (such as online scheduling for long-term care) could destabilize the larger system in unforeseeable ways (such as increasing the demand for nursing homes when a mixed-residency alternative might be promoted instead). We are responsible for outcomes, whether or not we accounted for them in our local projects. We cannot always know in advance how systems will interact in practice, and yet we must act in any case.

Every activity in the healthcare setting is interconnected and tightly coupled to measured health outcomes and highly professionalized practices. Any artifact, document, and interaction in a care situation can introduce a systemic effect. However, we also cannot conduct institutional research or user research studies for every intervention and new product. We need new ways to learn, think, and work quickly to make sense of the human, system, and organizational problems that co-occur every day in the morass of healthcare.

The fastest growing markets are electronic health record systems, billing and management systems, and Health 2.0 start-ups (often just Web applications). This trend may draw a large proportion of talent from information architecture, interaction design, software design, and user research from other fields into the healthcare arena. These innovations give hundreds of new ideas a chance to be heard in the field.

Designers have a unique opportunity to advance local and systemic change by empowering caregivers to enhance their ability to deliver caring. Together, the possibility emerges to design and campaign new service systems that enable people to better express caring in the system.

The convergence of design research, service and UX design, and human factors has led to fusions of practice and methods. Designing for care helps improve the *experience of being human*, and not necessarily the user experience. Consider that the aim of healthcare is to free people from a disease condition and help them live with chronic situations, and at the same time to create independence from the medical system. Caring design looks for systematic opportunities to create this independence, which may then lead to new products. Aligning with the values of caring professions may lead designers to new careers that are only just now being envisioned.

CHAPTER 2

Co-creating Care

Elena's Story: The Family Caregiver

Elena Reiser is the primary caregiver in her household. She takes care of her ailing father, Ben, and is an active mother of a preteen girl, Andrea. She spends nearly an hour overall in an average day seeking health-related information for her father, her daughter, or herself.

Late last year, Ben experienced congestive heart failure, a severe attack that imposed the requirement to downshift his lifestyle, take several pills a day, and watch his diet. Ben was out of shape after two decades as an active executive who worked long days and ignored increasing signs and symptoms of physical difficulty. After a golf outing with friends, he experienced angina chest pains and extreme shortness of breath. Widowed and living alone, his first thought was to call his daughter, Elena, not an ambulance or other emergency assistance. She has been helping manage his care ever since.

Today Elena searches for authoritative materials to inform herself about her father's recent cancer diagnosis. She hopes to find trustworthy articles and posts from other people dealing with cancer in their families. Ben faces colectomy surgery to remove and resect a cancerous section of the lower bowel discovered after a fortuitous colonoscopy. Less than a week ago, a gastroenterologist removed and biopsied polyps discovered in the examination and determined their malignancy in on-site tests at the outpatient surgical center. The physician immediately scheduled a surgical intervention.

Ben is scheduled for additional imaging and tests prior to the surgery, and Elena's contact list of clinicians will soon grow to five different providers necessary for her father's care—a private family physician, a practicing oncologist, a gastrointestinal specialist (a senior resident), a general surgeon, and a nurse practitioner—not to mention the anesthesiologist, pharmacists, visiting residents, and shift nurses.

Ben's surgery is another major health situation in the family, coming 4 years after Elena's mother succumbed to lung cancer, and bearing the responsibility for her father's care is taking a toll. Caught between the emotional concern for her father and the complex medical system she navigates on his behalf, Elena has become a primary care manager. She spends time on the phone seeking advice, manages appointments and travel, helps Ben manage his complicated medication schedules, and scans materials online.

Busy taking care of others and keeping up with her full-time job, Elena is continually stressed, and she is neglecting to take care of herself. She has stopped exercising regularly, and fast food meals have become common as her daughter's schedule and her father's medical needs crowd her time. Elena has found it necessary to postpone nearly all other priorities while taking care of her father. Keenly feeling the possibility of losing both parents to cancer within a short time, she has taken great pains to learn about the situation and negotiate the healthcare process as her father's caregiver. ■

ELENA REISER

Demographics

Elena Reiser, 42, divorced, lives in a St. Louis suburb. Owns a three-bedroom ranch, lives with her 12-year-old daughter, Andrea. Ukrainian Jewish ancestry. Bachelor's degree in business accounting from University of Missouri.

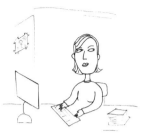

Culture and Psychographics

Midwestern Generation X professional. Has worked for 9 years at a large regional bank as corporate accountant; started her career as an accounting clerk.

A food hobbyist who explores recipes and likes to cook meals for Andrea. Vacations with her daughter at beaches and resorts in Florida, North Carolina, Hawaii.

Drives a Ford hybrid SUV, listens to iPhone podcasts more than the radio, and goes out for lunch 2 or 3 times a week with office friends. Goes to movies frequently with her daughter, and watches TV series and movies at home, up to 25 hours a week.

Elena at Work

Elena works at least 40 hours a week in a salaried job in the credit card division of a bank. She often works an additional 10 hours since a recent promotion. Overall, Elena likes the predictability of her work and the regularity of the tasks. She often leaves the office early to attend her daughter's activities or to bring her father to his doctor's appointments.

Elena at Home

Elena's job is not stressful, but being a single parent and taking care of her widowed father during his recent health episodes has put additional burdens on her time.

Health and Wellness

Elena experienced good health through her early thirties. She gave birth to Andrea at 30 and maintained a workout schedule during her daughter's early years. In her late thirties, she stopped exercising and eating regular meals, and she gained 20 pounds. Although her health is not bad, her physical energy and immune resistance have dropped.

Technology Habits

Elena has used computers at work for years. She is comfortable with Microsoft Windows, Word, and Excel, accounting applications, and common Web services. An avid Web user for most of the decade, Elena joined Facebook in the last year, but does not use other social applications. Elena uses e-mail daily, and uses Internet Explorer on a 2-year-old laptop for online magazines, news, shopping, banking, and recipes.

Goals and Aspirations

Elena hopes to provide a good family life for Andrea and has been in a serious relationship for nearly a year. Coworkers like Elena, and she likes working with the people in the office—affinity more than achievement is a motivator for her. She aspires to manage another department so that she might earn bonuses, but she's happy with the recent promotion.

Infocare

As the largest demographic cohort in history ages and calls for special care, Elena's situation will be increasingly common. Therefore we are all stakeholders in personal, institutional, and community healthcare. Will the next generation of health services be sufficient to handle this historical shift? How might we better design the way care is delivered and experienced?

People have always sought to learn more about a health condition they or a family member are experiencing. In the past, information and advice were sought from doctors and other people experiencing the condition. The Internet has enabled global access to a massive amount of basic health knowledge, creating a vast database of published work and an accessible ecology of information resources associated with disease conditions, therapies and treatment, personal experiences, and research.

In less than a decade, an extraordinary shift has occurred in the information behaviors taken by individuals seeking to learn about and improve their health. Instances of *health information seeking*, as with the health concerns they reflect, are associated with a person's experience of ill health. The *health seeker* is a person acting on the intention to pursue or sustain health, and *health seeking* is a purposeful activity that aims to restore or improve health. This new, neutral term gives context to the full range of experiences a person encounters in the pursuit of a homeostatic balance of relative good health.

Designers who build resources to help educate, inform, and enable individuals to make effective health decisions might start by understanding the situations of health seekers and their cognitive and affective participation in their own journeys to health.

People often do not consider their health until it is threatened by an incident or concern. Then their health-seeking journey begins by recognition of a knowledge gap, or need for further understanding, a *health information need*. A practical view of information needs comes from clinical practice researcher Paula Ormandy, who defined health information needs from a patient's perspective as "the recognition that their knowledge is inadequate to satisfy a goal, within the context/situation that they find themselves at a specific point in time."[2]

People in reasonably good health are not typically online every day seeking health information, and are generally unconcerned with the crush of resources available to inform decision making. People with chronic conditions (such as pain, diabetes, or cancer recovery) may seek a more or less continuous flow of information to help with their everyday concerns.

When any concern arises—whether it's sleeplessness, an unusual internal pain, or a chronic condition—our perspective changes, our information activity becomes focused and intentional, and in some cases our identity changes. A personal mood shifts from the indifference of everyday health to that of relieving a concern. Health seeking begins in earnest. People may undergo a significant change in identity—from a nonmedicalized self to that of a patient or even of a disease sufferer.

Consider the patient's entire *circle of care* when designing for a patient context. The circle of care includes not only immediate family and increasingly responsive providers but also extended family and friends as direct caregivers. Patient-centered philosophy recognizes that serious illness touches everyone in the health seeker's life. The notion of a disease "survivor" or "living with" a disease has expanded from patients to their entire circle. Everyone is caring, cared for, and a "survivor." According to Peter Pennefather, research director of the University of Toronto's Laboratory for Collaborative Diagnostics, "the term 'cancer survivor' has evolved from 'patients who survive treatment for more than 5 years' to 'persons diagnosed with cancer and their relatives, friends, and caregivers.' A similar shift in emphasis from curing a disease one person at a time to collaborative coping with general symptoms has occurred with other chronic diseases."[3]

How do we co-create care across these separate domains? We have few guidelines to help us design services for distributed care because most of us have lived our entire lives under a doctor-patient model of care. Care support and medical decisions are typically shared between patients and their immediate caregivers. In the "consumer" health context, where the design team has no contact with dedicated or frequent users, it is increasingly important to give caregivers centrality when making product design decisions. Although the goal of a consumer health site or product may be to inform or support the "patient," there may well be multiple health seekers involved in any given episode.

Health Information Design Is Personal

Healthcare design draws extensively on knowledge and methods from the human and social research fields, more so than other vertical design domains (such as finance, retail, or entertainment). A broader literature base is necessary when attempting to describe and design across the complex functions of body system, clinical service, and community health. When designing for other complex services in other fields, design research representations (personas, customer journeys, user models) can often be general and sanitized with little loss of fidelity. But in health scenarios, these narratives become personalized. If we generalize, we risk underestimating the complexity and emotional issues involved in the actual situations being addressed.

The risks are higher when lives are on the line. When we recognize that a persona could be a relative and a scenario might occur in our own family, our tools become less abstract.

Health Information Needs

Information needs are a presumed cognitive state wherein an individual's goal state triggers information seeking in a given context. The concept of information need helps understand user motivation and provides a lens with which to view behaviors that focus on motive, goals, and activities.

Information scientist Robert Taylor originated the concept in a 1962 article, "The Process of Asking Questions," which describes four types of needs:

- The actual but unexpressed need for information (*visceral* need)

- The conscious, within-brain description of the need (*conscious* need)

- The formal statement of the question (*formalized* need)

- The question as presented to an information system (*compromised* need)[4]

Taylor's four information needs have been cited continuously for 50 years and have acquired validity due to influence perhaps more than science. They were defined long before cognitive psychologists researched human information interaction. For our purposes in the consumer health sector, we can say individuals seek information to inform the many issues that arise in the context of a health situation.

Care professionals are increasingly interested in the health-information-seeking behavior of patients because these patterns reveal the patients' interests, of which healthcare practitioners should be aware. What information is involved in health seeking? Oxford researcher Angela Coulter's research[5] identifies 12 recurring needs and aims that hold true whether people obtain information from professionals or libraries or the hundreds of health sites that have emerged on the Web. These 12 motivators for health information seeking define a sequential series of information needs relevant to the patient experience life cycle:

1. Understand what is wrong.

2. Gain a realistic idea of prognosis.

3. Make the most of consultations.

4. Understand the processes and likely outcomes of possible tests and treatments.

5. Assist in self-care.

6. Learn about available services and sources of help.

7. Provide reassurance and help to cope.

8. Help others understand.

9. Legitimize seeking help and their concerns.

10. Learn how to prevent further illness.

11. Identify further information and self-help groups.

12. Identify the best healthcare providers.

Information seeking is often expressed in terms of a need and is defined in relation to need satisfaction. Health seekers are attempting to achieve personal health goals; they make sense of emerging situations and have critical decisions to make. Elena's scenario introduces new information needs in every chapter. Her father is facing multiple, interconnected medical, health, and life choice situations with his impending cancer surgery. Elena, as his caregiver, is motivated to understand her father's disease condition, medical treatment details and options, and post-treatment care.

Making Sense of Health Information

Information seeking can be a messy process in reality. Searches and sources lead a seeker to unexpected resources, information "places," and objects that draw attention and bias or bend the journey to different perspectives. How is a searcher to vet the validity of a government site (such as CDC.gov) versus an advertising-sponsored site (WebMD) or an independent activist information site (ThinkTwice.com)? Information seeking is value-laden. Objective representations of a site's credibility are not sufficient—health seekers are emotionally guided and may not embrace a scientifically informed view of evidence or facts.

Designers must learn to recognize the power of *confirmation biases* in information seeking and health issues. Confirmation biases, hundreds of which have been identified, are cognitive frames—essentially beliefs about a situation—that orient seekers toward locating and confirming opinions from sources that agree with their expectations. Often, these biases are rooted in a context of hope or the expectation of a positive outcome. Others seek clues and support for a negative concern. Hypochondriacs, for example, seek confirmation for negative health outcomes, such as every facial mole having the likelihood of being a melanoma.

Outcomes of information seeking can be thought of as information objects. In search activity, these are often discrete texts or pictorial representations that may be separated from their original context. The separation of objects from context renders them the equivalent of discrete factoids that present actionable information to some readers. We might recognize that consumers may not stray far into the details of the digital health domain, and they may attempt to supply meaningful contexts (domain URL, authority citations, brand) to health information at the page, article, and paragraph level.

Encounters with information are informing and multidirectional. That is, a health seeker engages in *sensemaking*—actively pursuing resources that contribute to learning and building knowledge—to help in reaching certain goals in response to the disruptive and consequential situations of a health issue. Sensemaking describes the cognitive and affective processes by which people navigate and repair breakdowns and ambiguous situations, relying on recognizable cues and acting on patterns that fit into current or changing mental models. People encounter information not as a goal, but as an aid to making sense of their situations by adapting behaviors to new learning.

Designers structure information as *content*, as factual data that can be optimally presented for effective visual appeal and readability. Consider treating information not as static data (as a *stock*) but rather as a series of encounters in a *flow* toward health goals. Information has a fluid quality, as it conforms to the biases of perception. People construct information in constant interaction with their needs, contexts, experience, and background. Information can be treated as *informing*, a verb and activity rather than an object. While Elena is seeking answers for her father's condition, she may find stories that appeal to her various contexts in life. Her personal (and unexamined) motives for informing will also emerge in the context of resolving an issue about her father's cancer treatment. These encounters help people make sense of their world as they choose materials that support a perspective and help them repair the many gaps between their worldview (or mental model) and the world as presented in the informing process.

From a practical perspective, the convention of information need is assumed with a consumer scenario. For a consumer, health-related information needs are not substantially different from shopping or news information needs. People optimize their available time by conducting a limited number of searches using minimal effort (using the fewest search terms) to locate sufficient responses. In the trade-off between time and information value or quality, observations show that people maximize the utility of efficiency, or time value. Quality of information remains difficult to evaluate in any context, and the demands of time pressure create value relativity.

Regardless of whether the searcher is a consumer or a doctor, cues that indicate authority or trust are used as shorthand to navigate answer sets and articles. Consumers may evaluate quality based on a trusted institution (Mayo Clinic), whereas physicians may assess quality based on recognition of a top-ranked journal (*New England Journal of Medicine*) or a clinical brand (UptoDate) with which they have extensive experience. In these different contexts, the impact of brand as a recognized entity aids the assessment of expected value in information decisions. The market value of brand in health decisions is found in optimizing time during information seeking.

From a patient perspective, the value of information may relate to one's personal condition or self-diagnosis (or any of Coulter's information needs). Consumer and patient contexts differ because these are states of identification with a disease or concern. Information design can be sensitive to all stakeholders, not just those assumed to be users. In designing a consumer or public website, we cannot assume visitors are patients or, more superficially, information consumers or buyers. If we consider the designed outcomes as enabling health seeking, all types of activities and needs can be supported.

Health Search Behavior

How might we characterize the consumer's health-seeking needs for information and product design? Personas and scenarios can be misleading because they only present a synthesis of the design team's current knowledge and research (at best). How do we discover what we don't know or have access to knowing?

There are ways to exhaustively examine the information tasks and health activities that we might have missed in first-pass or limited-access research. Among them are literature reviews, which are recommended for producing well-grounded classifications of tasks and information uses such as Coulter's. Taking into account the information needs presumed for Elena in this scenario, we can include the following:

- To better understand her father's condition

- To identify risks in treatment and care

- To learn how to care for her father's condition at home

- To be prepared to converse with care professionals

And although these needs may be presumed important to disclose at a "persona" level of description, in reality each person's situation is different and a situated context will not be so readily described. Whereas a consumer's search for the best deal on a laptop computer might be easily defined, health situations are unique, changing, and can be complex.

Although the definition of *consumer* may be inappropriate in this context, it helps in describing Elena's scenario. Adopting a consumer frame helps map design practices from consumer online services to the other healthcare sectors. It illustrates the changes in role and identity that occur when a person moves from a "nonpatient" state to the institutional definition of *patient*.

Elena's information seeking starts with simple term searches and scanning the results. Based on an information use model I developed,[6] a sequence of information tasks includes the six shown in Table 2.1.

TABLE 2.1 INFORMATION-SEEKING TASKS

Information tasks	Activity outcome	Information object
Simple search terms entered in Google	Scanning to find	Search terms (1 or 2)
Skimming search results for candidate articles	Scanning to select	Search results page
Selecting salient titles	Scanning to inform	Online articles (less than one printed page each)
Printing key articles	Selecting and printing	Printed article set (for father or doctor)
Reading and annotating articles	Comprehending for learning	Printed article
Sharing printed or PDF articles	Exchanging meaning with others	Printed, linked, or e-mailed artifact

In simple searches, terms matching disease conditions return high-ranking results from Mayo Clinic, WebMD, MedicineNet, and dozens of disease-specific sites. People searching for critical health information often require the output of a simple printable factsheet. But websites are formatted for online browsing, and printable articles require time to find.

The best resources anticipate these needs and offer a range of media formats. The National Cancer Institute provides online pamphlets in both printable sections and as full PDF articles. Major institutions require registration to retrieve printable articles, which discourages rapid access or noncommittal use, because competing articles can be located within seconds from the same search results.

The majority of these resources have not been designed for the most effective use by consumers or patients. They are simply not designed as *services*. But many of their users may not especially care because health information needs are immediate and compelling responses to inform urgent concerns. With the vast majority of all health information seeking being initiated by a search, most of these resources display to their visitors as landing pages, indexed and linked to a search results page. Site-level navigation, site-promoted related content, and advertising become superfluous to users as ever more users reach pages directly through searches. These intrasite navigation and content features can actually interfere with information use and can be counterproductive to use if not designed with deep site page access in mind. This issue is described in more detail in the case study that follows.

From a design perspective, institutional healthcare may be one of the last frontiers (along with education and government) to accept the necessity of visual aesthetics and typographic layout. Reportedly, a recent increase in hiring UX designers has occurred across healthcare information services, as evidenced by job notices from healthcare information/IT providers. This trend promises to improve interaction, visual design integration, and information usability. Yet the industry has to overcome its blindness to good design. To encourage that trend, designers need the explicit support of physicians and administrators in healthcare services.

DESIGN BEST PRACTICES

- Better design for information seeking requires new ways to think about constituents. The health seeker is proposed as the individual actively seeking to recover his or her health or to help care for a loved one. This orientation motivates health information behavior.

- When identifying information needs, treat them as provisional (temporary and dynamic) and even speculative. We can never really know why a person is seeking information unless we understand their context through observation and feedback.

- By treating healthcare information as a dynamic flow rather than as static objects, designers can formulate more communicative and contextual resources that dynamically update information, build on social interaction, and build narratives from finer-grained information objects.

- Health-information-seeking needs should be treated as starting points, not end points. Designers should always ask "So what?" and "What's next?" to any defined information "need."

Case Study:
WebMD—Health Information Experience

Consumer websites typically have similar presentations of the most basic background information on their landing pages, requiring diligent internal site navigation to locate advice or topics of specific value to a user. In this case study, WebMD—the most popular consumer-oriented health site—is critiqued to examine contextual usability issues as well as perspectives, biases, and design concerns from a health-seeking perspective. WebMD was selected because of its high profile with the public and its professionally developed content. This critical review is transferable to other health sites.

WebMD presents a full spectrum of health portals covering a range of interests and levels of depth. The different segments its products serve represent the most critical stakeholders in the health marketplace. Each portal presents a slightly different design and brand, but a strong family resemblance is apparent in brand prominence, color, navigation, and information architecture. Bringing together a range of consumer and professional resources, WebMD leverages a single organization's knowledge, reach, design and development, medical advisory team, and content management. The WebMD family has consolidated five major portals (and includes at least three others not listed):

- WebMD: a general-purpose, consumer-facing Web portal

- MedicineNet: clinical information translated for consumer use

- Medscape: the most popular general medical professional website in use by US physicians in 2011

- eMedicine: a higher-end professional website cited by more specialists (now part of Medscape)

- TheHeart.org: specialist portal for cardiovascular health and cardiologists

WebMD is a platform-level innovator, a first-mover service that captured a consumer niche early and extended its position by building out a spectrum of services on an extensible content platform. Its second leading innovation among healthcare information portals was to define and structure an information marketplace using a graduated presentation of health activity. No other service provider has developed and maintains a unique resource for each of the following:

- Consumer health information seeker (WebMD)

- Health seeker with specific health information needs (MedicineNet, eMedicineHealth)

- Immediate consumer or family health queries (MedicineNet, eMedicineHealth)

- Drug information for consumers (RxList)

- General medicine website (Medscape)

- Specialty portals for specialized, evidence-based information (eMedicine)

- Specialty portals for professional topical currency (TheHeart.org)

- Personal health record (WebMD Health Manager)

A typical Web search results in a top-ranked link landing a health seeker on a view such as the one shown in Figure 2.1. Within this page of heart disease–related information, multiple levels of navigation are presented, and the user may not know which link, button, or tab to execute to advance to the next logical step. Although the decision-aid tabs may seem logical to younger, Web-literate readers, older and infrequent users may feel lost when too many options are presented.

The navigation column presents three blocks of content links related to heart disease in general. Nearly all of these are of the "See More" type and are not hierarchical subtopics or facets of the immediate subject searched (Arrhythmia). The next steps are not clear. The first navigation block presents different content types by "type label" but with no semantic information relevant to types of arrhythmia or medical actions. The second block presents a "Heart Disease Guide," which would apparently remove the user from the current context and present an entirely different set of features. The third block, "Related to Heart Disease," presents several links relevant to arrhythmia, but mixed in a flat list, not in an ordered information hierarchy.

Accessibility would be a problem with such a page. A screen reader for a visually impaired user might be forced to scan and read each line before reaching the main content, including any duplicated navigation.

Although arrhythmia may be a common symptom of heart disease, the presentation of the topic as part of the Heart Disease Guide joins these two together. The reader may not be able to separate the two descriptions at a later time, and may form a mental model that arrhythmia is "heart disease," a catchall term that may frighten the person with mild arrhythmias.

The information of most value to a patient, or health seeker, is a clear description. On WebMD, competition for content placement has created a dense panoply of text and links. The excess of design sophistication will lose many users due to its complexity, and the actual user's experience may be precisely the opposite of what was intended by the design. Health seekers oriented to one or more of the 12 information needs discussed earlier will find their experience fragmented.

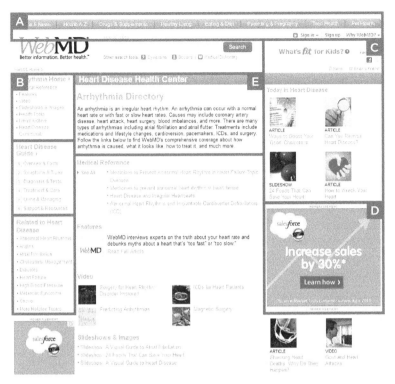

FIGURE 2.1
WebMD topic page.

If a user is in a hurry to learn about a heart condition from the industry's leading resource, what information behaviors might we expect from his or her health-seeking activity? Consider the following five sections of the page highlighted in Figure 2.1 as a wireframe model:

A.   The global navigation shows eight functional groups (most of which are compound, making this a lengthy scan). But where are we located in the site? The current context is not indicated by highlighting the label.

B.   The navigation trail at left enables contextual site navigation. The topic searched (Arrhythmia) shows the top set of content links, none of which are highlighted to current context. The list requires the user to observe and negotiate between types of content (video, slideshows) and features (health tools, news archive). The Heart Disease Guide might be helpful, but is placed between the topic navigation and a list "Related to Heart Disease." There are too many choices.

C.   Content that may be related to the topic is highlighted in the right column, but until the reader understands the implications of the destination topic (Arrhythmia), these may only be distractions.

D. An advertisement totally unrelated to the topic is the most visually dramatic object on the page. The ad is echoed by a small mirrored segment below the left navigation, eliminating any white space from the crowded layout.

E. Finally, the content of supposed interest, the Arrhythmia Directory, is squeezed into the remaining area constrained by these features and links. The only relevant content is a single definitional paragraph, with sections titled Medical Reference and Features below it. In summary, the health seeker is compelled to read many of the text links before being able to make a decision about the next step to take in following the search.

This example illustrates an integrated analysis and critique for a single page of a given resource. Nearly the entire service can be evaluated based on a single page—the navigation, brand, coherence, page layout, information architecture, messaging, aesthetics, and nearly every other heuristic. In a thorough experience critique, a sample of pages and interactions within the service would be selected by consensus for review (see "Experience Critique" on page 48). The heuristic process tends to cover most of the evaluation indicators and elements in the first page selected, with other pages chosen and described to ensure completeness, consistency, and additional details not discoverable on the homepage and an example content page. The deliverable for this process is typically a consolidated report presenting the findings of all reviewers, merging duplicative findings, ranking findings by priority and impact score, and concluding with recommendations and discussion.

Consumer Use Models

Web information design for consumers may be ignoring the lessons learned from research in human interaction with print content. As sponsored or ad-supported health websites become more popular (due to their ability to buy placement and to purchase superior content), the total experience will suffer as users require more time, attention, and recovery from false starts in the dense, attention-demanding online experience. This may be the trade-off necessary to provide credible information to the health seeker, yet the possibility for ineffective communication is heightened by this complexity.

In contrast to the WebMD experience, professional medical information resources usually lack advertisements and present technical details in compact and concise encoded formats. Information providers of subscriber resources understand that physicians have no time or patience for distraction in their search for information to aid clinical decision making. The easy revenue generation of commercial advertisement has been shifted to an institutional sponsorship or personal subscription model.

Is it worth paying for the preservation of a physician's time and attention? Should there be an equivalent public resource with simple, clear presentation of health information for health seekers as an alternative to ad-revenue-driven commercial sites? Although numerous specialist sites exist for different disease conditions and health concerns, one site in the public sector clearly meets these criteria and yet does not display in the top results of most health term searches.

Health.gov is the US Department of Health and Human Services' public resource for information seeking about most supported health contexts (Figure 2.2). Because the site is a portal, indexed to link to partner organizational sites, and most of its content is referenced to other domains, it fails to display in open Web searches. Yet the undeniable simplicity and quiet authority of the resource shows a meaningful contrast in brand identity, communicative style, and intent compared with WebMD.

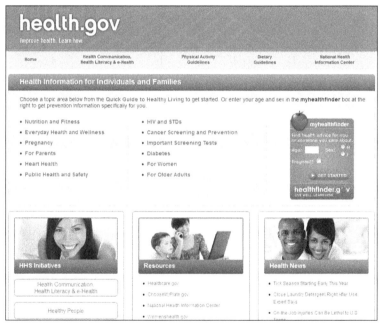

FIGURE 2.2
The Health.gov information portal.

- Start by empathizing with health seekers. Imagine whether they would ever encounter such information density and complexity in any other situation in their everyday experience (other than on the Web).

- As a reality check, assume the health seeker is a person concerned with an immediate, perhaps painful experience at the time of information seeking.

- Consider the disruptions and confusions a person may experience and whether the site's values and priorities differ noticeably from those of a health seeker.

- Ask whether the information architecture presents an optimal model given the total competition for limited attention.

- Recognize that every large-scale information service presents design dilemmas as it grows. With more customers, sponsors, and content, every feature and link creates a claim on limited real estate.

Methods:
Consumer Service Design Research

Three models help in selecting research methods for understanding people, their behavior, and their thinking:

- Systems: healthcare applications and processes, from websites to the institutional system

- People: the range of personal and social identities that change in health situations

- Methods: the types and functions of design and research in these domains

The "consumer" context in healthcare is not that of a retail consumer. Design research for consumer healthcare requires a closer engagement with people's *everyday* activities than for health practice or education. Choose methods that help develop an understanding of the complexity and problems of the everyday lives in which people make health choices.

In consumer research, the most typical research methods are not design or innovation methods, but are market and business oriented. In consumer healthcare design, both families of methods are needed, along with scientific social research (e.g., well-designed hypothesis-testing surveys or ethnography). Typically, exotic innovation methods are not called for in low-risk and broad-market consumer services, which serve a wide range of popular content needs. Method selection and use should be a judgment based on the product offering, its context with consumer health seekers, and the possible access to real users to deploy the research technique.

Table 2.2 lists common consumer-level innovation research methods and their relative applicability across four canonical phases of deployment. The remarks in bold indicate the most prevalent or recommended use of the method in consumer-oriented research.

The selection of a design research method in a consumer health context is contingent on project goals and product outcomes. In a consumer world, the primary goals are to reach the right health-seeking consumers and to satisfy their information and action goals. The consumer context always raises the problem of representative users—in a large unknown user base, research participants are always proxies and not committed users. The lack of a meaningful sample and the need for validity can confound the outcomes of using a single method. Multiple methods are nearly always recommended. Of these methods, the technique discussed here is the experience critique, a variation of heuristic evaluation.

Experience Critique

The experience critique is a hybrid technique developed from methods of heuristic review and interpretive assessment. The method provides a validated tool for rapidly evaluating an interactive service. It extends the classical heuristic review with an empathic framework for relating an interactive experience to a persona's information-seeking behavior and activities. Informed by systems thinking, experience critiques evaluate the systemic relationships of an interface to the user's practice and needs. Yet experience critiques are simple enough for practitioners to modify as a practical technique for service or information design applications. The method is based on:

- The *methodology* of heuristics (especially Werner Ulrich's critical system heuristics[7]).

- The *method* of adapted heuristic evaluation (developed by Jakob Nielsen[8]).

- The *technique* (way of doing the method) of experience critique, an expert review with evaluative questions.

(For more on Ulrich and Nielsen, see the sidebar on page 53.)

Experience critiques help a product team evaluate usability and experience issues from multiple perspectives to support interface and feature decision making. The process is intended as an early-stage research exercise for engaging multiple stakeholders meeting the selection requirements of the innovation of interest (e.g., your personas).

The experience critique delivers a collaborative review of a service or system with prioritized assessments and both expert and user value judgments. Typical applications of the technique include evaluation of product portfolios, websites, or Web services; multiperspective review of an existing service for a planned redesign; and user experience audits.

TABLE 2.2 CONSUMER DESIGN AND MARKET RESEARCH METHODS

Consumer design research methods	Stage 1: Ideation and market analysis	Stage 2: Research and concept design	Stage 3: Product development	Stage 4: Beta and launch
Market surveys	**Important**	Critical	A little too late	Good for assessing market response
Focus groups	A little early	**OK, but not sole method**	Too late, except for pricing	
Direct customer feedback		**Initial product idea from users**	Useful for validation	Are we on track?
Sales and service feedback	Address emerging market issues	Useful to know desired features		Help with early feedback from beta
Customer demonstrations	**Is product acceptable?**	**Interactive prototype demo**	Useful for validation	
Concept testing	Generate concepts	**Build and test concepts**	Compare concepts to product	
Heuristic evaluation/ experience critique	**Very helpful**; analyze existing sites and products	**Helpful**: analyze and compare concept with current product		
Usability evaluation		Usability testing of current product to set baseline	**Early product tests**	**The earlier the better**
Web surveys		Gather and evaluate ideas		Helpful for early release feedback
Participatory/ generative methods	Gather range of ideas and latent needs	**Create and elaborate on concepts**		
Contextual inquiry user interviews	Very helpful; fit concept to user need	**Combine with concept walkthrough**		

A group of appropriate experts are identified and invited to participate in a critical review process. This reviewers' circle performs individual reviews and audits, and the coordinator collects and integrates the reviews and convenes a live dialogue about the findings. The critique asks each reviewer to consider two perspectives—their own domain of expertise and that of a selected user persona. By explicitly representing goal states and values, a critical evaluation is carried out on behalf of that desired experience.

The experience critique identifies four dimensions, some questions that probe each dimension, and indicators for an empathic design inquiry (Table 2.3). Indicators are measures by which each evaluator scores the dimensions and questions (variables) for each factor being assessed.

TABLE 2.3 EXPERIENCE CRITIQUE PROCESS FRAMEWORK

Dimension	Empathic inquiry	Indicators
1. Current system (as is)	Describe your current goals and practices.	Evaluate current system
		Resource lists
	What resources and services do you use most often?	User-specified values for activity and operations
	Describe activity: What do you do to accomplish goals?	
	Describe operations: How many/How often/How long?	
2. Relevant system values	What do you consider a good experience?	Open-ended or comparative feature evaluations
	Evaluate/score different features of the system.	Score or rank preferences
	Specify preferences for the system's behavior.	
3. Ideal system	Describe the ideal system from a user's perspective.	Provide guidelines
		Lists of value points
	List significant points of value.	Rate competing services
	Evaluate other references that provide similar value.	
4. Ideal values	Identify ideal values applicable to the system of concern.	Values scale assessment
		Values comparison
	Compare current values with the ideal.	Values card sort
	Rate the strength of value or concern.	

A critique examines user values and needs, as well as system functions and interactions, from an external and detached perspective. As an analytical process, the critique allows the design team to deconstruct elements of a service and evaluate them from both an expert and a consumer/human-centered perspective.

Conducting the Experience Critique

An experience critique is a coordinated process guided by a research leader and managed in five main steps:

1. The conceptual framework is used by the coordinator as a reference for ensuring the critical variables are identified and selected as questions in a review template.

2. A template is designed as an electronic file and provided to reviewers as a survey form, along with instructions for conducting an individual review of a system or service.

3. After individual reviewers conduct their personal critique of a service or system, the individual surveys are aggregated into a common review, and findings are presented and discussed in a roundtable review.

4. The coordinator annotates the compiled report with findings from the roundtable, including strategic recommendations and solutions for identified interaction or usability problems.

5. The coordinator provides the comprehensive experience critique as a formal, actionable review of the service.

In step 1, the framework maps the priorities and objectives of the review or audit in a template such as the example shown in Figure 2.3. Heuristics are selected based on their value in the review, and weights are assigned to heuristics based on user, system, or market goals.

The results of a combined experience critique, based on heuristic evaluation, supports stakeholders and designers to jointly make grounded assessments of not just usability, but the artifacts and services.

DIMENSION 1. EVALUATE CURRENT SYSTEM

What do users predominantly do or seek with WebMD?	To locate consumer-level health information quickly to better understand a condition or symptom and its impact.
What are the *primary* goals and tasks of WebMD?	To get information from a rapid search and to assess whether action is needed.
How else might these tasks be accomplished? (competitors)	List of five competitor sites/services: Mayo Clinic, Everyday Health, disease-specific sites, Wikipedia
What is the main value proposition?	WebMD: Single comprehensive resource for personal health information.
How well is it met?	Current site confuses this value with distracting related resources.

INDICATORS	TYPICAL HEURISTICS WEIGHTS	
A. Establish heuristics for current system review.	Match to users' world and language	5
	Navigation and action visibility	5
B. Evaluate current system using heuristics.	Readability (prose) and legibility (type)	4
C. Assess the impact, frequency, and persistence of issues discovered:	Page layout and information structure	4
	Branding, aesthetics, and design	4
	Process guidance (helps users in process)	3
0 = Not an issue	Consistency and standards	3
1 = Cosmetic problem only		
2 = Minor	Flexibility and efficiency of use	3
3 = Major issue		
4 = Usability catastrophe	Access and usability of advanced features	2
D. Score competing systems.	Error recovery	2
E. Assign weightings to user priorities (multipliers).	(Weights are indicated based on the criteria of importance to the specific project.)

FIGURE 2.3

An experience critique review template. This example shows how an expert reviewer might evaluate WebMD.

Heuristic Evaluation and Critical System Heuristics as Design Critique

Although heuristic approaches may appear to be loosely constructed on opinions rather than empirical observation, they have a solid footing in human factors psychology, systems thinking, and human sciences. The experience critique is based on several references in well-established procedures:

- Jakob Nielsen's *heuristic evaluation* is a staple of rapid usability assessment. The method is based on a series of heuristics, or interpretive questions, that elicit informed opinions from individuals selected to evaluate a product during a stage of design.

- Nielsen's heuristic evaluation is part of a complete usability engineering methodology, yet is also one of the most *interpretive* of usability methods. Experts and multiple reviewers make interpretive judgments in a cooperative setting, allowing expert opinion to be presented and minds to be changed in the review.

- A practitioner gap exists between human factors (the "usability school") and design research methods, with little crossover. Even though significant development has occurred in participatory and critical methods such as these, such techniques are rarely used in design research, even though their value has extraordinary impact on client understanding and decisions.

- Werner Ulrich's *critical system heuristics* is a systems thinking evaluative process based on critiques of a system and its impact on human and social systems. It presents more of a framework than a process methodology, and it has no published applications in product design. Critical system heuristics offers guidelines for reflective evaluation of systems in their pragmatic and humanistic contexts. Ulrich suggests, unlike Nielsen, for example, that nonexperts are not only helpful but necessary in the critical decision processes by which systems and design decisions are made:

> Our judgment of the merits of a proposition . . . depend heavily on this context, for the context determines what "facts" (e.g., consequences) and "values" (e.g., purposes) we will identify and how we assess them. With respect to this crucial issue of boundary judgments, experts are no less lay people than ordinary citizens. Surfacing and questioning boundary judgments thus provides ordinary people with a means to counter unqualified rationality claims on the part of experts or decision makers.[9]

- Designers in other fields may not need to specify methods appropriate to the domain, but in the high-risk world of healthcare, it helps to have grounding in human factors and empirical methods. Methods such as the experience critique incorporate the best of both worlds.

- If the scientific worldview does not represent your stance toward knowledge, refresh your understanding of both evidence-based research and design methods, as these are essential to bringing real innovation to healthcare problems.

- Become conversant with a sufficient variety of methods in order to become method agnostic, allowing you to choose the right research technique for the problems and opportunities you face. Selecting the best methods for the problem is a design process in itself.

- There are many appropriate methods for conducting evaluations of processes and systems in healthcare, representing an extensive body of methods on their own. The methods identified in this book are used in practice, but are not recommended as sufficient to all situations.

CHAPTER 3

Seeking Health

Elena's Story: It Can Happen to Anyone

Less than 6 months after her father's cancer diagnosis, Elena suddenly feels faint and passes out on the couch after the brief exertion of vacuuming the carpet in her living room. She comes to after a couple of minutes, still feeling faintness and lethargy, rapid heartbeat, and heaviness in her legs. She calls Ben and tells him about the occurrence. Her first impulse is to attribute to overwork, being out of shape, the stress of dealing with his condition, and worry about giving enough attention to her daughter.

Elena is reluctant to see a physician after just a single incident. Because nobody was at home to witness the episode, Ben encourages her to see her doctor. Elena realizes her fainting and rapid heart rate may be of concern, but because it hasn't recurred and there was little pain, she feels she can safely "wait and see." However, at Ben's insistence, she calls her primary care physician, Dr. Fran Martin, a general practitioner in a family practice.

A nurse handles the call and asks Elena to describe the incident. The nurse then asks a series of specific questions: Do you have any relevant medical history? What medications are you on? Are you wheezing? Do you have an elevated heart rate? Because the family practice follows a consistent routine for patients calling in with potentially critical issues, the nurse has been trained to use an interactive checklist system following current clinical checklist practices. The checklist serves as an information model for patient intake, so that clinicians in the office are prepared for the possible conditions Elena may present. If it had been an emergency, Elena's responses to the checklist would have triggered immediate treatment. Because it is not an emergency, the nurse asks Elena to take an appointment for 8:15 the next morning.

Concerned by the urgency of the nurse's questions, Elena reflects on her episode. She had not thought it significant at first, but she now sees a pattern. She had stopped exercising about a year earlier, hasn't been watching her diet, and smokes about a pack of cigarettes a week.

After spending hours reviewing information about her father's condition, Elena is quite familiar with consumer health websites. She runs searches on her symptoms and is quickly overwhelmed by the volume and variety of health sites. Although some top hits seem reliable by virtue of being prominent "brands," such as Mayo Clinic, WebMD, and Family Doctor, others are offbeat and amateur in appearance.

She finds dozens of links to brief articles on syncope, heart disease, and stress. There are more than 10 different diagnoses she could follow. Although her symptoms seem simple, teasing out a clear condition is impossible. Ironically, the more informed she becomes, the more complex her situation appears to be. The many aspects of her condition (if she even has a condition) are daunting. Elena grows worried and frustrated. ▪

Information First Aid

Although consumers can and will use whatever information they can find online or find easily, mere use does not mean that their problems are being solved. Health information seeking is much more complex than goal-based information seeking. Information seeking presupposes the goal of an *answer*, which facilitates a real-world action. Health seeking can be a long, continuous journey with an elusive goal. How do health seekers know when their goal of health has been achieved?

Consider Elena's scenario, which appears to be a simple information-seeking case. As an individual with an emerging health need, she queries the Web in an attempt to understand her situation and determine some possible causes. At this point, the activity revolves around a consumer choice situation, as Elena has not yet been diagnosed by a doctor. Interactions with information (searches leading to websites) are incomplete and inconclusive.

Designers accounting for this "consumer" activity might consider a normal person's limited knowledge of their situation. Recognize that participants will "not know what they don't know" by the end of their search. A design scenario can never fully address an end-to-end situation in health, as the individual's end state is not a predictable outcome—it is unknown and unknowable. Health is also a biological and cultural function; it is not an end result guaranteed by the service provider.

Information seeking is the first intervention most people take when considering their health options and undertaking a course of action. It defines the point at which a person acts on a motive and locates an online (or other) resource. From a user-centered design perspective, information seeking is an activity that breaks down information tasks into specific actions and guides tangible design options in interactive product design.

Do not assume that information seeking represents the core user behavior your interactive design or product is concerned with. Taking action on that information must be assumed, in most cases, to be the outcome. It is easy to overemphasize the significance of information seeking as a central activity. It seems to represent the most salient point of a consumer's engagement with an information resource or service. If health-seeking behavior is studied *only within the scope of a product or service*, the risk of confirmation bias increases greatly. That is, we are likely to discover what we are looking for because we have offered users no other choice! How do we evaluate beyond the boundaries of our product scope when information seeking explains the behaviors we observe?

There is no single best UX methodology, but some approaches may fall short. For example, a strong task-oriented design approach may fail to capture and represent the activity system of which information seeking is just a part. A focus on interaction usability may optimize the website interaction and fail to discover missing or ineffective content.

The design and testing of consumer sites and services encounters risks that professional and in-house systems do not have. The primary risk may be called the "home court disadvantage." An existing system is considered to have a public user base that can be sampled by drawing on local self-selecting participants. A confirmation bias is promoted when interaction design is evaluated with positive outcomes from small samples of nondedicated users. The generic use case may ignore the vital and urgent necessities real people have for information. Yet all the user actions hidden from observation—prior and forgotten searches, family interactions and conversations, encounters with professionals—are inaccessible to a *product*-focused design orientation. The real life of the health seeker comprises much that cannot be easily reduced to personas and scenarios.

This chapter identifies the stages of activity in a goal-directed journey, scenarios wherein people learn, decide, and take action. Is there a "user" in the conventional sense, as the subscriber to a service or active user of a product? When people are motivated to recover health to restore normal life, their health activities are oriented to health seeking, which describes the persona's intent and suggests the primary context designers might consider in making product or service design decisions.

Information Is Insufficient

Elena's scenario points out how real-world problems can show up in one's lived experience as a jumbled mix of personal concerns—disease symptoms, emotional feelings, the wearing signs of stress, and the cognitive shifts experienced as different information sources are considered. Although information seeking may seem like a rationally guided task to a designer or professional, the *felt experience* of the person living with a health concern is not experienced rationally. Information-seeking tasks demand a rational mindset, at least to compose effective queries and evaluate results. Yet for health seeking, information seeking is only an aid, and one that is subjugated to the necessity of identifying health options, considering actions, and recovering health.

Health seeking invokes numerous trade-offs, options that may constantly shift depending on how sense is made of their fit to circumstance. A person with employer health benefits might explore all options available to her economic situation. An unemployed individual with no health insurance might attempt to mitigate the near-term effects of the disease process until he has coverage or can afford treatment. Someone else in the early stages of a disease might not be motivated enough to "seek" a healthcare response.

Health is always a relative condition, and there is a wide range of "normal" across the population spectrum. A health concern may be experienced as a bundled emotional mess, as a mix of worry, anger, or confusion; frustration over the lack of knowledge or choice; and the physical pain compounding this emotionality. Or it may be experienced as nothing more than a physical performance problem interfering with one's plans. Although the emotional response of individuals may vary widely, significant cognitive and emotional overload may be experienced by anyone merely by accomplishing the first of many health-seeking actions. Any one of dozens of personal concerns and habits could tip the balance of action toward a different outcome.

Most human decisions are not as rational as we like to believe. As cognitive scientist Gary Klein has shown, decision making even under optimal conditions is nonrational and emotionally biased.[1] Under the stress of health concerns, decision making may be colored significantly by known cognitive biases implicated in information seeking, especially:

- Confirmation bias (seeking and filtering information to support one's preconceptions).

- Loss aversion (attempting to mitigate perceived losses, inferred from seeking information to learn about or confirm/eliminate severe risks).

- Anchoring (focusing attention on salient points of information rather than considering all relevant views).

- Pessimism or optimism (believing in biased outcomes that may not be probable based on prior attitude).

Individual health decisions are often made as the result of uncertainties, emotional contexts, hopes and fears, and serendipitous conversations. People are not predictable users of systems. They "muddle through," recruiting information and other helps in ways that uniquely fit their life situations. Human beings are motivated to negotiate and bridge gaps or perceived discontinuities in their access to reality. They have many and shifting priorities, which are redefined in their making sense of a situation as it appears to them, in the context of the other issues in their lives.

Information Seeking as Self-Diagnosis

Health breakdowns are clearly experienced as "gaps" in the continuity of life and represent a motivated occasion for sensemaking. People attempt to understand the impact and options for a health condition on their own (unaided by health providers) by information seeking.

Yet diagnosis is a complex cognitive task learned through experience by consolidating memories over hundreds of cases. Except in trivial instances, health seekers are not likely to reach a correct diagnosis on their own. Even if health seekers do identify their condition correctly, they would be unable to determine the best response given the range of tests and examinations, traditional and emerging treatment options, or possible comorbidities related to other health concerns. Yet people seek information to evaluate their situation and to deal with (not minimize) uncertainty.

Searches on individual symptoms are highly unreliable, because symptoms (awareness of feelings from internal states) and signs (externally presented indications of disease) are just the outward manifestations of an internal process. People act on symptoms, but mistake them for the disease. Guesses are likely to be unproductive at best, dangerous at worst. A general design axiom might be formulated with this precautionary principle* in mind: Expect that people seeking health information will have insufficient knowledge to conclude the information is valid in their case; design accordingly.

Searches aimed at guessing a diagnostic outcome are even more unreliable because individuals cannot run simple tests and take consistent measures without training or calibration of the measures against a standard. People also have insufficient understanding to compare and trade off "differentials" to narrow down and identify the most likely condition from several alternatives that might match symptoms.

If designers know the rationale for health information seeking and recognize that traditional websites can be misleading, what are the best alternatives to consider? This chapter's case study describes a diagnostic tool using a decision tree mode, which shows that for some conditions and situations, a thoughtful experience design can meet the demands of health seeker's inquiry with information first aid.

Making Sense of Health Decision Making

Taking care of one's own health is ultimately a series of decisions to take healthful actions, decisions assisted by medical guidance, trusted information resources, and personal social networks. Decision researchers still debate how people actually make decisions. Some decision theories assume individuals choose the best action according to unchanging and stable preferences and constraints. The classical, *rational choice* model assumes that humans are rational actors, and that they choose options consistent with anticipated economic interests. *Behavioral* models are grounded in empirical observations of human decision behavior, and their theories start from observations of decision behavior, revealing decision making as significantly biased and experience-based. *Naturalistic* models of decision behavior are developed from consistent in situ observations and analysis of the cognitive tasks being performed by the decision process. All three offer value and need to be understood to relate to the different contexts referred to as "decisions" in healthcare. But only the naturalistic model requires that we recalibrate our notion of how decisions are actually made in real life.

---

* The precautionary principle states that if an action or policy has a suspected risk of causing harm to the public or to the environment, in the absence of scientific consensus that the action or policy is harmful, the burden of proof that it is not harmful falls on those taking the action.

The classical model has been debunked at least since Herbert Simon's explication of bounded rationality.[2] Rational choice provides a formulated schema for making the "right" decision when faced with several alternatives. But the model is untenable in reality, failing to account for the cognitive and emotional biases that have a significant influence on choices and actions.

Yet the classical model has been widely implemented in corporate and organizational practices. Kepner-Tregoe and the Analytic Hierarchy Process are two well-structured decision tools that enable people to perform a factor analysis of decision components to facilitate more effective final choices.

What people actually do in practice differs significantly from these best-practice models. Humans consistently make decisions based on an emotional response, a felt understanding of a given option path. In group decisions, emotional persuasion rather than true consensus is the norm. In short, what we call "going with our gut" rules in all types of decisions—personal, business, financial, and health.

The Branching Metaphor of Decision Trees

A venerable decision analysis method—the decision tree—has been taught to healthcare workers for years and is gaining support for individual decisions. Nurses, physicians, and specialists learn to read and memorize "algorithms" or decision structures that visually portray decision options as a series of steps (Figure 3.1). The decision tree approach to structured decision making discussed by science writer Thomas Goetz suggests that decision trees are effective for making better everyday health decisions.[3]

Decision trees have two problems, however, that reduce their efficacy in health reasoning. First, they are formulated on the assumption that health decisions can be made by assigning inputs and outputs to determine a preferred course of action. Better inputs—food, exercise, lifestyle decisions—lead to better outputs, which are improved health measures and a healthier experience of life. In practice, however, these inputs are a matter of degree, not either/or binary decisions. The extent to which a given action improves health does not show directly as an output.

Second, decision trees by their design are retrospective constructions, not prospective. They are a proposed path of choice based on someone else's past experience with a similar choice scenario. For a decision about a personal unknown situation, such as choosing between surgery and drug therapy to treat a heart condition, decision makers are faced with a quandary. They are required to enter options for each pathway on the tree's branches of decision logic based on past data from other people's situations.

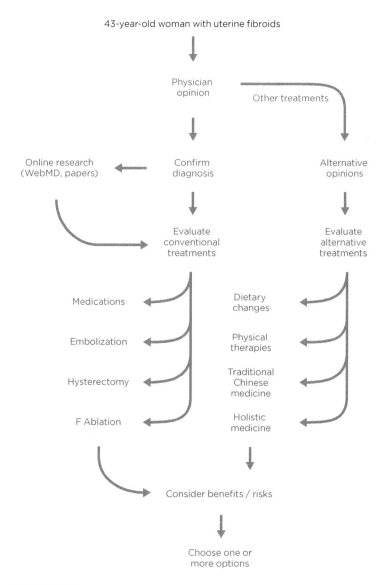

FIGURE 3.1
Decision tree for a health problem.

The goal of decision trees is to empower health seekers to make up their own minds and to be less reliant on their physicians in personal health matters. Yet the physician will have seen and intervened in perhaps hundreds of similar cases, compared to the health seeker's single (and highly biased) case. The emotional freight attached to each micro-decision in a tree can also bias the application of the tree. A significant role for any physician is to help guide patients to health decisions that are in their best interests. Analytical methods such as the decision tree do not enable the inexperienced health seeker to formulate a decision based on context. As the science of decision making suggests, such a practice is too rational for most individuals.

A key difference in Goetz's application is using the tree for *personalized* decisions, so that the option paths are constructed for an individual's situation. But the form of the tree in most applications is as a clinical guideline that presents a set of rules that can be universally applied. These are similar to clinical algorithms for selecting drugs and dosages, or specifying the correct diagnostic procedure. Devising decision trees as tools for guiding complex health decisions is based on the classical model, and they may fall short as a self-diagnostic tool. Instead, these structured decision support tools might be used as ways to visualize and categorize options so that eventual decisions are based on effective personal research and trade-offs.

The approach is simple, but can be misleading if health seekers attempt to self-diagnose following its steps. The tree tools may not be helpful outside of the context of a diagnosis for which the guidance applies. By the time health seekers receive a clinical diagnosis, they usually have guidance from their physician on the decisions and steps necessary for their individualized situation. A generic decision tree for a disease may present a range of options the physician has already considered and dismissed.

In addition, by the time one gathers and analyzes the information necessary to construct a decision model (or an accurate decision tree), the best path among those options would become obvious because of what was learned in the process, not because the variables were organized in tree form. Important life and health decisions are more complex than input-output relationships. Over time, people change their valuation of different options, which are not balanced evenly on a simple flow diagram. In life, valuation of personal options is tested through a dialogic process (e.g., sensemaking). People speak with others who had similar experiences and judge the same variables in personal terms. Attempts to simplify the process by reducing it to a pathway may help, but may not actually aid in a significant decision. Also, a personal decision is not a simple act performed at a given time; it takes place over a series of smaller decisions. It is a mix of actions and new options that are opened up due to actions taken.

Human beings are notoriously poor at envisioning the future and making good prospective decisions. They are driven by prevailing emotions and fail to consider trends, countervailing evidence, and exceptions. When people face a life decision, they may wish for a certain outcome (e.g., to lose weight or regain a youthful physique), but what they choose on a moment-by-moment basis may contradict the desired outcome. Health choices beneficial in the long term compete with short-term choices that have significant emotional resonance and psychological benefit (e.g., smoking or eating dessert).

Although the decision tree represents a road map of best options, it is a rational model that assumes a rational decision maker. People need more than the motivation of future prospects to maintain a commitment to a personal plan for health recovery. So although decision trees could be used to describe prospective, anticipatory decisions, they are not the best tool for the way people actually reason about the future.

Expert Decisions Are Intuitive

A physician's experience with numerous cases leads to a decision-making style that appears intuitive. Intuition is not a magical synthesis of ideas or a leap of creative thinking. Intuition is largely based on responses to new configurations that trigger recognition of similar situations from the past. Intuition emerges as personal (tacit) knowledge and can lead to effective pattern matching in a problem-solving situation.

Professional clinical decisions often draw on intuition and demonstrate the problem-solving style of sensemaking. Sensemaking is both retrospective and prospective; it allows for trial, testing, and learning by considering possible narratives in the face of a situation.

Sensemaking (as Gary Klein defines it[4]) attempts to understand the causes of recent events and anticipates the outcomes that may occur at that time or in the near future. Klein presents the example of a group of anesthesia residents attempting to assess and repair the hidden source of a ventilation tube blockage in a patient simulator. Of 39 trainees, only 9 were able to solve the simulation. In all cases, these "adaptive problem solvers" jumped to an intuitive conclusion about the situation, quickly tested the hypothesis, and kept an open mind.

Sensemaking describes the style of expert problem solving in medical disciplines characterized by evidence-based decision making, although this is only now beginning to be recognized.[5] Research in clinical informatics shows that residents and trainees use decision tree approaches for diagnostics and treatment decisions. Trainees do not have sufficient experience to make expert judgments, and they are required by agreement and liability to "go by the book." Senior physicians, on the other hand, have a huge repertoire of experience to draw on, and do not need to look up decision algorithms for common diagnostics. Because the resident can manage the majority of cases using the standard algorithm, a senior doctor can help with unforeseen and complicated situations that trainees cannot and would not address. If a complex patient situation challenges an expert, would he or she even try to resolve it by using a decision tree? If the problem is not common, it is solved by an unfolding process of discovery, trial, and iteration—sensemaking and not decision making.

We cannot always design for sensemaking because the resources recruited in a problematic occasion are things like memory cues, images, and references that connect to personal gaps. Professionals will not stop and read a student-level guideline in every tough case to catch a rare exception. The exceptions are caught by *decision triage*. Decision triage simply enlists another knowledge resource (person or system) to mediate in the decision, especially for a complex situation, such as one in which multiple drugs could interact or diseases co-occur. It is also a designable process whereby a second health professional (nurse or physician) relies on a trusted information resource as a check on the decision practice.

Design for Consumer Health Decisions

How well can product or interaction designers understand a consumer's health-seeking options? Designing for websites or services may be based on very limited research, small samples, and usability studies. Without experience in the healthcare domain, service and information design approaches may "underconceptualize" the problem. Designers often treat online services as equivalent in function and as though an information product that is successful in another domain (such as Mint.com for personal finances) will translate to healthcare applications. Sometimes this works if a concept is presented with good navigation and information architecture principles. But the complexity of health problems and information context suggest otherwise. People do not manage their health like they track investments, and they could not if they wanted to.

Designers creating healthcare scenarios for a service design may be tempted to envision objective, "clinical" perspectives to describe expected health-seeking behaviors. For example, a linear series of events, decisions, and actions may be traced from a person's information seeking to a service touchpoint (Figure 3.2).

From a health seeker's perspective, concern for a disease condition drives the journey and leads to contact at the physician's office. The actual touchpoint is a coordinator or receptionist, triggering an exchange of information. The clinical service process may involve extensive independent preparation for a day's appointments, allowing the physician to manage a high-volume practice and to maximize patient interaction while satisfying the necessary patient scheduling for emergent situations.

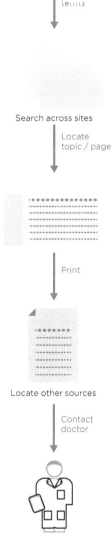

Health Question

Formulate terms

Search across sites

Locate topic / page

Print

Locate other sources

Contact doctor

FIGURE 3.2
Health-information-seeking pathway.

Social Construction of Healthcare Services

What is the requisite "standard of care" for designers in a consumer health-care context?* How do we know we have helped health seekers? In specifying content and interaction, the respected design values of simplicity, clear communication, and visual and content hierarchies are necessary but insufficient. Healthcare services at every point are designed and guided with respect to health outcomes.

Health content intersects social practices, scientific validity, and current medical knowledge. Accepted practices and both core and referenced knowledge can be changed or overturned abruptly, requiring revision of related health issues in online and archived sources. A good example of currency is the US Centers for Disease Control's website, a public resource but not (strictly speaking) a consumer context. Consider the precise language and comprehensive categories found on a given page structure (Figure 3.3).

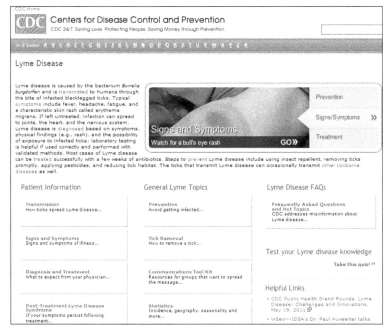

FIGURE 3.3

A public context health information site under the highly usable URL www.cdc.gov/Lyme.

---

* The standard of care must reflect the art (consensus of opinion of clinical judgment) and science (published peer-reviewed literature) of medicine and must be uniform for all healthcare personnel, whether they are providing direct clinical care or reviewing the medical necessity of past, present, or future medical care. (American College of Medical Quality. [2010]. "Standard of Care." Ethics and Professional Policy 3.)

Retail healthcare is no different than retail sales. As an online service grows its user base and market value, new features are launched and evaluated for customer engagement. The content page sprouts multiple lists and navigation areas as the various features (articles, tags and indexes, related content, external resources) compete for attention. UX and design decisions get squeezed between these competing interests in the internal decision-making process for commercial or sponsored websites. For designers, creating realistic end-user scenarios and defending appropriate diversity and user-sensitive information can become political, almost adversarial actions. Although the application of user scenarios is a design process, their construction requires *content* knowledge, which verges into the claims of core content disciplines (e.g., medical, biological, publishing, product). Arguments to resolve the narrative, validity, and veracity of scenarios are typical among disciplines, often resulting in compromised or mediocre narratives.

Building Up the User Experience Catalog

Intense project schedules (as typical in Agile development) sometimes require the compromise of some design values on behalf of product delivery. Trade-offs between schedule and quality are frequent in consumer-facing healthcare products; in most cases the designer loses the trade. Of course, user data is needed to win the argument, not merely Web analytics.

UX practitioners have learned to adapt user research and discount usability to support the rapid turnaround required in today's product development cycles. The primary UX research methodologies—ethnography, interactive interview, usability testing, remote observation—now have official rapid versions documented in the literature.

Within healthcare disciplines, however, the rapid mindset is not highly valued. Rapid research can be perceived as unreliable and not evidence-based. The health sciences research tradition recognizes rigor, and requires the ability to publish findings in the public research literature. The original UX field of human factors psychology established scientific norms and experimental methods for hypothesis testing and evaluation that remain the standard in healthcare. Healthcare processes, medical devices, control and dispensing devices, and internal information systems are validated by human factors research. Designers in the human factors tradition rely on strong empirical methods, validated measures, and statistical analysis to support high-reliability and safety values in design decisions. Human factors methods are consistent with producing the types of evidence deemed valid for healthcare decisions in current institutional and scientific practice.

These are appropriate methods in the contexts of clinical research, and due to their general acceptance in medical contexts, these hard empirical methods and the presentation of statistical data have become mandated in most clinical situations, including informatics. If lives or significant investments are at stake, industrial-strength human factors experiments and validations are necessary. However, these methods are typically summative, applied *after* innovation and in an evaluation context, and are better for validation and hypothesis testing than for generative or conceptual design of new informatics concepts or clinical services.

In UX and service design for healthcare applications, we readily adapt standard methods from the UX toolkit. These include observational and interpretive methods, which may be untested or even untrusted in health institutions. Yet these methods may be necessary for a robust innovation strategy and can be defended in terms of their near universal applicability in information product design.

DESIGN BEST PRACTICES

- A newly acquired illness or injury is a novel experience (in most cases). Expect all health seekers to be uncertain in their knowledge, options, and decisions.

- Health seekers may only rarely interact with your product, so rapid comprehension is vital.

- Do not presume people know what they are looking for in a healthcare situation. There are design trade-offs between providing a clear pathway to an answer or multiple options (which can be confusing).

- Design information to help health seekers meet well-defined information needs. Describe these need states with task-oriented labels that relate to the needs and possible decision outcomes.

- Clearly indicate the end result of your service or process so that people know when value satisfaction has been acquired.

- In activity design, help people make health decisions by indicating steps or status in a series or timeline, provide references to related information, and when possible, link to a variety of cases illustrating a range of options a health seeker may want to know about.

Case Study: Healthwise Decision Aids— Personal Health Decision Support

Healthwise is a US-based nonprofit organization specializing in complete information solutions for healthcare, which the company refers to as "information therapy." Healthwise provides decision aids and custom content to hospitals, health management companies, and health websites. It also serves clinicians—nurses, doctors, and health coaches in a variety of settings—who can adapt content provided by Healthwise to "prescribe" this information to a patient or health plan member. Healthwise specializes in providing current, scientific, evidence-based information to the point of user need, using innovative channels and interactive formats.

Healthwise has been in business for more than 30 years, but their focus on improving the user experience of information products is much more recent. In just 5 years, a 15-person UX team has grown to include interaction, visual, and production designers with a range of specialized skills (usability, information architecture, medical illustration, and multimedia art and production). Healthwise interaction designers recently partnered with Indi Young, author of *Mental Models* [6] and co-founder of Adaptive Path, to establish a mental model methodology in the organization. Healthwise works closely with leading decision support researchers from both the International Patient Decision Aid Standards (IPDAS) group and Ottawa Hospital Research Institute to help ensure IPDAS decision aid standards are met. The Healthwise UX team reports that their methods for understanding users include continual user testing, user interviews, observational field studies, and focus groups. They have developed analysis methods based on card sorting and mental models for representing and mapping decision patterns for interactive aids. Unlike many other information providers, Healthwise maintains an in-house clinical advisory team, and staff work closely with behavioral health psychologists and doctors to review and advise on clinical content and prototypes.

Healthwise Decision Point

The Decision Point resource is an embedded decision aid created for a wide range of conditions. The example in Figure 3.4 shows an individual's decision steps to proceed with surgery when faced with a herniated disc and its attendant daily pain.

Becky Reed, UX interaction design manager at Healthwise, described the evolution of the Decision Point tool:

> The previous version of this [tool] was a hypertext system that was very much in a physician's mental model. It looks very much like you would see in a nursing protocol book that over the years would be filled with lots of supporting information. We redesigned

these with the goal of being able to assess symptoms, and there are two different users conducting this: one user on a health portal trying to figure out what they should do about their symptoms and the other a nurse in a call center talking to a patient.[7]

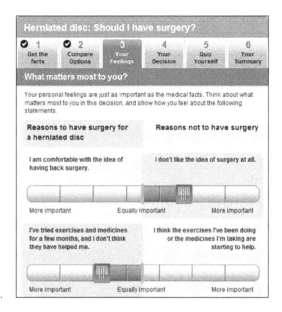

FIGURE 3.4
The Healthwise Decision Point decision aid.

Healthwise designed the consumer and clinician tools in parallel because, according to the designers, they have the same clinical logic behind them. The consumer information model was adjusted slightly to emphasize the simpler language and steps. Reed discovered early in usability testing that consumers often misperceive symptoms. For example, people often assume that a tightening in the arm requires an emergency visit. Reed wanted to make sure sufficient education went along with the tool to help consumers interpret the severity of their symptoms correctly: "The intent was to make this tool action-oriented so that the person knows the next step [he or she] should take to better control . . . or resolve the situation."[8]

Although the underlying content is essentially the same, the clinical version employs rapid interaction design for nurses and triage coordinators, who can use the tool during a phone call to assess and guide patients. Clinicians use these decisions aids not for informative purposes, but rather as active guides, checklists, and language support, so that they have specific language at their disposal without having to translate for each patient in phone calls. "From a clinician's point of view, the symptom topic tool allows nurses to use it as a support tool so that they are able to give consistent recommendations. Nurses are highly trained users, so they would be using this tool to make sure they are delivering consistent care," Reed explained.[9]

For a related project, the Symptom Triage tool (Figure 3.5), the Healthwise UX team conducted contextual inquiry interviews with floor nurses at clinical sites, and also interviewed representative nurses who worked in call centers and were using competitive products or traditional paper-based nursing protocols for triaging clinical situations. A significant period of user research led to prototypes and revisions, then evaluations of the tool on client websites. Reed continued,

> We noticed that [nurses] had a good sense of the types of questions that should come up, but the order of which is often debated. It was important they proactively get a sense of what was coming up in the triage. And then, finally, we knew that nurses are working against the clock, with time being a huge issue. Call time, wait time in discovery, and system time, like scrolling and waiting for windows to start, were completely unacceptable because they contribute to call time and increased cognitive load for nurses. So we addressed these issues with this model. With progressive disclosure, they are able to see the questions that are coming, so they have reassurance that the question they were thinking of has already been afforded in the design.[10]

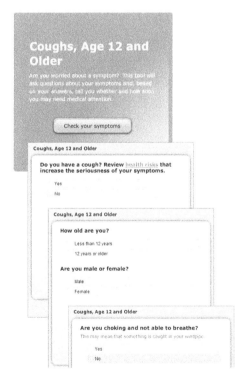

FIGURE 3.5
The Healthwise Symptom Triage decision flow.

To strengthen their method and approach, Healthwise staff are returning to the user sites to gather outcomes data and perform additional task analysis to inform design of related applications in overall symptom triage.

The latest direction of Healthwise UX design involves engaging users in interactive dialogue. The Ix Conversation multimedia product uses a virtual coaching methodology to help people understand health conditions. Through branching logic questions, Ix Conversation helps people find the best answers and next steps. In turn, health seekers/consumers are encouraged to seek better targeted or appropriate care from their physicians.

The development of a more personalized approach to health content with a focus on user experience and better design requires significant organizational investment. Julie Cabinaw, Healthwise's former director of user experience, described the critical role of organizational support and investment in design research in enhancing their competitive advantage through usable and engaging services:

> Good design is so critical to user engagement and usage. We can create the best content in the world, but if users can't or won't use it or read it, we have not fulfilled our mission to help people make better health decisions. We consider our investment in design extremely strategic for Healthwise.[11]

LESSONS LEARNED

- Healthcare information can be leveraged into multiple products, serve several constituencies, and increase the opportunities for revenue and brand recognition.
- Insightful product research requires a holistic outlook to identify possible opportunities that would be missed by following a project plan to the letter.
- Get out and play! Early stage field research, on-site and with truly representative people, leads to insights or iterations that guide design, messaging, product plans, or strategy.
- Small-sample interviews and observations can be conducted to acquire "early warning signals" to identify emerging or overlooked needs for public and consumer uses.
- Rapid research and task-oriented usability evaluation may not be sufficient for product teams to identify and develop the right response for needs discovered through cycles of research and iterative refinement.

Methods: Empathic and Values Design

Empathic design research methods are selected for understanding the everyday life contexts of people. Though based on user-centered design traditions, empathic design inquires further into lived experience, with the aim of understanding the authentic perspective of people.

Service and product designers research the experience of individual health and information seeking from a mediated distance, often at best through field research or recruited interviews. In the consumer context (typically Web and interactive digital design), *interpretive methods* from UX research have currency in gaining user understanding. Perhaps because lives are not at stake in website design, a commitment to business and design performance outweighs validity or scientific values. Partly because hybrid, mixed methods are now used frequently, design research has become more applied and informal.

Complexity Demands Interpretive Research

Several years ago, strongly interpretive, empathic, and even ethnographic methods were considered too "soft" for business decision making. In clinical and professional contexts, empirical methods (measured observations in controlled settings) are well respected. A commitment to *evidence-based practice* is often expected in institutional research, requiring adherence to a medical definition of evidence as verifiable objective observations in a controlled setting. Though we might argue the validity of human and social forms of evidence, the healthcare environment expects careful sampling, control for variation, structured data collection, and quantitative if not statistical analysis of data.

Medical, nursing, and administrative practices and procedures converge at the point of patient care, and these perspectives may conflict on many issues. When empirical, evidence-based approaches are fully adopted in institutional culture and reasoning, complementary perspectives are screened out, and the patient's perspective is filtered out as well. Empirical studies that measure the outputs (such as outcomes, length of stay, and satisfaction) ignore multiple and unknown input variables (such as prehistory, unique conditions, and cultural or individual differences). Although necessary for high-confidence decisions affecting populations, such as randomized clinical drug trials, empirical and experimental studies are not intended or useful for design and interaction decisions. Narrowly scoped, isolated variables in such studies cannot reveal the emerging patterns at the heart of the complex situations across the spectrum of personal and institutional care.

However, in the consumer context we have more freedom of research design. We can first recognize that people's experiences and meaning as consumers in healthcare, in personal health, and in caregiver relationships are forms of personal knowledge. Experience has direct meaning for individuals, and in empathic design research we can elicit and represent meaning veridically— as true to their experience.

Interpretive UX methods are tools for engaging design research participants in creative, subjective expression of their understanding. These methods are biased toward eliciting individual experience, the projection of creative ideas, or subjective narrative expression to better understand and empathize with the varieties of human experience or to formulate creative ideas in early innovation.

Focus groups and in-depth interviews are not typically interpretive. *Group* interpretive methods are often generative, not directly eliciting individual expression but deriving it from creative artifacts. Design-led workshops are conducted to co-create images and artifacts in a semistructured setting, allowing for individual expression while engaging participants in a novel group exercise. Co-creative techniques for consumer-oriented research include:

- Facilitated group processes for eliciting ideas and generating proposals.

- Storytelling and narrative techniques.

- Embodied methods for acting out scenarios with low-fidelity mockups or concepts.

- Individual projective techniques (such as collaging or sketch imagery) for subjective expression.

In the early stages of design, identifying the right problem context calls for patience and tolerance for ambiguity. It is called a "fuzzy situation" for a reason—the initial situation is perceived as complex, and problems may be described by stakeholders in terms of deficiency rather than opportunity.

When we are not immediately sure of the best solution or intervention, UX methods are more readily employed and more effective than experimental methods that require a hypothesis and statistical sampling. Dealing with complexity calls for us to carry out multiple observations and iterations, not experiments with premature hypotheses and unknowable constraints. Rather than avoiding human complexity, interpretive research helps identify the scope, boundaries, people, practices, barriers, and opportunities in the situation. They are meant to help *understanding*, not prediction and control.

Intuition and Insight

An *insight* is a penetrating observation about a situation. In design research, an insight is an actionable interpretation; it reveals understanding and relates an observation to a design decision. The right observation in context can make the difference between a great user experience and a poor showing in the marketplace.

Insights are claims drawn from the analysis of research data. They may appear intuitive, but are selections of salient observations associated and framed by other relationships in the study. Although intuition can help frame the construction of insights, intuition is not a magical synthesis of ideas or a leap of creative thinking.

Rather than a mysterious personal capability, intuition draws from a person's largely tacit repertoire of experience and patterns from which to match a current situation. It is the result of experience and reflection on experience in a given domain. In other words, people with healthcare, patient, and industry experience are likely to have better "intuitions" about health seekers than designers without experience in the domain. But designers might have better intuitions about the practical approaches that might be formulated to design and present the solution.

Powerful insights are also produced from iterative working theory. Simple theories, or working hypotheses for understanding, are categories with a guiding proposition that direct observations toward meaningful features. A working theory is not a hunch (although hunches may help). It is an explicit proposal that can be applied by others to test their own observations.

For example, a working theory for field testing a clinical information concept was that mobile applications would find limited adoption in hospital settings for in-depth clinical decision support. Even though most hospital-based clinicians have mobile devices or smartphones by now, their use in clinical settings has been limited by the legibility of text, images, and tabular information. With the prevalence of desktop computers in hospitals, doctors and nurses recognize that the shorter amount of time spent reviewing information on a larger screen outweighs the benefits of handheld convenience. The insight drawn from the data was not just that this claim was supported (in more than 90% of the observations), but that some types of content (images and figures, rather than long text passages) would be used on mobile devices if they were specifically designed for the point-of-care context. Although not a universal finding across applications, the realization allowed product managers to adjust their innovation strategy to focus on current adoption trends and not to overextend resources to accommodate a very small (and nonpaying) market position in mobile technology.

Empathic Design Research

Empathic design comprises a point of view and a methodology, a collection of interpretive methods applicable to human-centered design and research. Empathy is consistent with the innovation theory of designing products from knowledge gained by deeply understanding consumer behavior and aspirations. Harvard's Dorothy Leonard first gave shape to this innovation theory in an influential *Harvard Business Review* article, which promoted highly qualitative, open-ended empathic research for understanding real customers and their concerns.[12] Empathic design was proposed as first-person research to discover real behaviors in the field, as opposed to hypothesizing through questions in survey research. Empathic design helps designers create a common understanding of the *person* for which an innovation is planned. Empathic research ranges from first-person methods (e.g., simulating the user or donning impairments to experience aging or weight factors) to participatory design, inclusive design, and ethnography.

Empathic methods seek to understand an individual's authentic experience in a real-world context, so that design options for enhancing experience or resolving difficulties might be located and attempted. A study by Froukje Sleeswijk Visser of Holland's Delft University of Technology reviewed the psychology of empathy and described four phases of engagement with participants:

1. **Discovery:** establishing initial encounters with participants, usually targeting a specific user segment, and selecting situations to engage with curiosity

2. **Immersion:** expanding knowledge of and appreciation for a person's situation and life by participating, hanging around, and absorbing information without judgment

3. **Connection:** making an emotional connection by relating to one's own experiences, forming associations with situations in the participant's life, and understanding both feelings and meanings

4. **Detachment:** detaching, reflecting on insights, and applying them to ideation[13]

Of these four phases, the most crucial to learning and meaningful ideation is immersion, wherein the designer takes significant time to "wander around in and be surprised by various aspects of the user's world."[14] The immersion period enables the designer or researcher to identify with the everyday life and objects, the tempo and pressures, and the conversations and language of the person being shadowed. Sleeswijk Visser is correct in noting that the opportunity to "hang out" is usually given insufficient emphasis in design projects with tight schedules and budgets.

Personas present concise snapshots of representative users or constituents in a design project. Typically, personas are drawn up to match the characteristics sought in the primary participants in a research sampling frame. In consumer projects, user profiles are often generalized to different customer types and are frequently exemplars associated with market segments defined by a business team. In informatics research, personas might be defined for specific professional roles and contexts that determine different levels of expertise, information need, content, or usage patterns.

In a consumer context, an online product or service may be public and fully accessible to all. A full range of health seekers for which a service is being designed may be impossible to characterize, and attempts to project preferred "example user personas" may institutionalize certain expectations. De facto personas (and scenarios) might overemphasize the role of health seekers as users.

Personas are ubiquitous artifacts in the business applications of UX research, and are often presented in flattened, stereotypical ways when invented from representations that have no basis in field research. Ethnographer Steve Portigal advocates for the use of *stories* instead of stereotyped personas. He makes the case that reliance on personas can create a false intimacy and pretense of user knowledge, preventing the organization from really looking at its customers and considering the reality of their behavior:

> Any process based in falsehood takes you away from being genuine. If this is the best way we have to keep the organization focused on a "real" customer, then we have larger organizational problems that need to be addressed. With personas, we're going down the wrong path. Rather than create distancing caricatures, tell stories. Don't deny the need to do in-person research with real people. Look for ways to represent what you've learned in a way that maintains the messiness of actual human beings. And understand that no tool, no method, and no shortcut, can substitute for real, in-person interactions. People are too wonderfully complicated to be reduced to plastic toys.[15]

In the best cases, personas are prepared as an outcome of ethnographic research as a tool for presenting and describing salient characteristics of people and their behaviors and interests relevant to a product. However, especially in online consumer healthcare services, access to real patients can be difficult due to privacy issues and the expense of recruiting even small samples for field research. Design teams therefore often make up semi-realistic personas that are adopted as proxies for user research. When proxy personas are adopted by a product team, their limitations may be overlooked and the personas may travel beyond the original utility of standing in for real customer research.

Personas are given context and depth when supported by descriptive stories or narratives, which can be created to follow one of several formats:

- Narrative scenarios involving the personas (similar to Elena's scenario in this book).

- Rich picture scenarios that illustrate the persona's relationship to functions in use cases.

- Story narratives that bring the persona to life by presenting an authentic narrative based on real interview data, making the persona an indisputably real person.

Stories based on observed experiences present the most compelling warrants for design decisions because they portray vivid emotions and details that help people remember the salient issues in the research.

Storytelling Personas

Stories (all stories) embody a particular shortcoming that personas overcome—stories are nontransferable in their original richness as a performed narrative. Ethnographers are trained (and often talented) storytellers. They become steeped in interview and contextual data so that their stories are embodied artifacts and part of an overall compelling narrative. This unfair advantage of the ethnographic researcher is not conferred to the product team receiving the stories. When the team tells the same story to management, much may be lost in the translation because team members will not have been immersed in the collection of the field data and will not be trained in the expression of story narratives. Organizational recipients of the research products are better able to work with a set of succinct capsule profiles (i.e., personas) that reflect a composite of salient characteristics of customers (based on real people where possible).

A central problem in human factors psychology is that of identifying and representing a valid range of behavioral and physical (anthropometric) characteristics in the target population. Human factors shows us that designing for the "average person" actually designs for nobody. In healthcare situations, the range of consumers (and patients) is considered extremely diverse. Designing for the average user is not only futile, but impossible. Ranges of characteristics based on relevant distinctions can be used to articulate user profiles. If presenting a range of ages, they can be marked by life stage rather than chronological age or decade. If documenting a range of patients based on type of disease, their touchpoints with the clinical care system (initial presentation, diagnosis, admission, treatment) might be the defining order.

Values Design and Research

A values framework affords insight into essential needs and drivers that motivate emotional and felt responses from people. Psychologist Abraham Maslow's hierarchy of needs provides a guideline to mapping meanings to observations (Figure 3.6). Maslow's well-known framework offers a hierarchical formation of values, where underlying physiological concerns (e.g., health) must be resolved before basic safety and social needs can be fulfilled, all in the pursuit of betterment or self-actualization.[16]

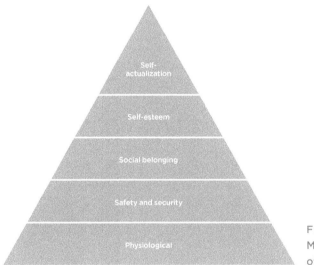

FIGURE 3.6
Maslow's hierarchy of needs.

Farther Reaches of Empathy

Critics have often missed the essential role of the Maslow hierarchy.[*] The model describes the normative development of healthy personality, a road map of values for the formation of a strong center to guide life decisions. Whether it is "true" or not is irrelevant. A working theory must first be useful. In an interpretive research context, if the framework is defined and supported by precedent, and if the content it elicits builds understanding and provides insight, it shows sufficient strength for the purpose.

Value-based empathic insights provide a scale to identify a point of intervention for a human concern, starting with the level of needs most important to a participant and the research purpose. Maslow's hierarchy allows us to identify a position and trajectory from fundamental personal care to self-transcendent values. Though the pyramid form suggests a structural perspective that ends

---

[*] For more on Maslow, see the *Design for Care* website (http://designforcare.com).

with self-development, a healthy person may be actively meeting needs at any or all levels, as well as seeking self-actualization, at any time throughout life.

Basic health needs are met at the base, but healthcare experience research should explore health seeking at all levels. The hierarchy levels are also "units of analysis," and clinical research typically focuses inquiry and analysis on solving a problem defined within a scope at one level. Table 3.1 lists empathic design methods that can be selected at each level to inquire into and understand the human needs of a situation. Mapping methods to needs to human values enables the design team to formulate a clear rationale and create a robust case for their research approach.

Any of these methods appropriate for the purpose might be chosen and used in concert with other techniques. The design context—service, website, interior/environment—determines the frame for inquiry and the staging of a series of engagements in the field or online. Any method will be integrated within a design process of iterations, prototypes, and critiques, usually contributing to another phase. An example of a process for redesigning a visiting home health service might include the following:

- **Customer profiles and segmentation:** Initial sampling frames and categories of clients are used to characterize the primary groups of clients in the service area. Initial (nongrounded) personas and scenarios are created.

- **Home audits:** Physical audits using checklists and observations are conducted to characterize the living situations and unique needs and requirements in the customer segments.

- **Customer understanding:** Interviews for physiological and safety needs are conducted using observation frames, checklists, and photographs to characterize the range of people and their needs by segment.

- **Service system mapping:** To determine the most appropriate new service functions and to maintain the best of existing service processes, initial specifications of service processes are generated as a series of interactions with clients, with differing stakeholders and services by class of service, location, or segment.

- **Health experience understanding:** To characterize the aspirations and health needs for a range of clients and the service interactions, in-depth interviews are conducted, and observational and empathic methods (such as ethnography and diary studies) are used to understand current and evolving behaviors, trends, and aspirations.

TABLE 3.1 RESEARCH METHODS BY NEED/VALUE

Human need	Values inquiry	Empathic design research methods
1. Physiological	How and where do participants live?	Interviews
	What is their physical health status and story?	Observations, checklists
		Personas, scenarios
	How are food, dress, and sleep needs cared for?	
2. Safety and security	What are the probable safety hazards?	Observations
		Physical audit
	How do people experience safety and comfort?	User diary studies
	How are environmental and material hazards mitigated?	Incident surveys
	How confident and secure do people feel?	
3. Social belonging	What groups and communities are people engaged in?	Scenarios, storyboarding
		Participatory workshops
	How do participants express their social identities?	Photo journals and diaries
	How do people relate and work together?	Context mapping
	What are their cultural events, practices, and social goals?	
4. Self-esteem	How do people experience their sense of total health?	Sensemaking interviews
		Hermeneutic inquiry
	What stories do participants express about their health?	Video diaries and storytelling
	What achievements, values, and life goals are valued?	Appreciative inquiry
5. Self-actualization	How do people frame and express their highest ideals?	Generative design research
		Appreciative inquiry
	How do participants seek transcendent experiences?	Video diaries and storytelling
	How do people want to be remembered for their lives?	

A selection of methods can be chosen to research empathically at each level. Questions (and related research methods, such as interview and observation) are chosen for the situation, not from a template. Needs and values are chosen for the insight they contribute in design.

Empathic research requires access to people matching the profiles in a population sample's range. In consumer health products, a team is often limited in its ability to reach authentic participants. We often have to make do with reasonable estimates of experience.

TIPS ON TECHNIQUES

- Access to real patients is rare. Academic researchers and clinicians require ethics board approvals to conduct even informal research with patients. Researchers rely on proxies for real patients as needed, who can be recruited for nonclinical design research and product evaluations.

- If collecting multiple forms of data in a research interview, establish safety and comfort with the participant. Ask permission (and use informed consent and releases when appropriate) if taking photographs or video. Some people may prefer that only manual notes are taken if discussing personally sensitive issues.

- Find additional time to observe and hang around the locations where interviews are scheduled. Additional and unexpected insights emerge from making connections between the interview content and observations in the field.

- Empathic research can be presented in formal or creative artifacts. Before conducting empathic research, identify the expected outcomes or artifacts to communicate the findings to the team. A client may have expectations for traditional personas in document form, whereas a design studio may prefer to co-create new presentations from photographs, interview snippets, sketches, and symbolic maps.

PART II

Rethinking Patients

Health Seeking | Patient Journey

Situation	Caregiving 2 Years	Health Incident 2 Months	Diagnosis 2 Weeks	Treatment 2 Days	Living With Future
Care Providers	Father's care team: surgeon, oncologist, pharmacist, chemotherapy nurse	Primary care physician, Nurse	Attending physician, Staff resident	Cardiologist, Electro-physiologist, Nurse practitioner	
Touchpoints	Family and friends, Web, clinicians	Social media friends, doctor, pharmacy	ER, lab, insurance, pharmacy	Hospital, family, clinical team	Social media, health communities
		Hypothyroid, metabolic syndrome, anxiety, multiple medications	Medications—cardiac condition	Medications—SVT ablation	Medications
Journey	Family caregiver	Primary care—initial diagnosis	Emergency care—cardiac diagnosis	Specialist care—cardiac treatment	Health community advocate
Patient Role	Caregiver/consumer	Ambulatory	Outpatient	Inpatient	Advocate

Part II transitions from design for consumer health seeking to a patient-centered perspective. The focus of design shifts to services designed for people with health problems who seek professional care to improve wellness. Health seekers are presented not as patients in the system, but as active agents in charge of recovering their health, relying on and partnering with the care resources of their providers, in their community, and in digital services. Five views of patient experience are explored in the context of health service innovation:

1. The patient as *health seeker*, a self-directed agent responsible for his or her own health and well-being

2. The patient as a *participant* in the healthcare system and subject to the rules and roles this entails

3. The patient as a *customer* of a service, who seeks and pays for treatment directly

4. The health seeker or patient as a *subject* of user research for innovation

5. The patient as a *person* under care, located in a community in a particular society and culture

With respect to service design, healthcare is different. Theories of service define value as co-created, in the delivery and active acceptance of expected service. In clinical care, however, the direct service of treatment is only the *potential* value. The *realized* value of care is in the full relief of symptoms or the outcome of treatment. If the health service provided is a simple intervention, such as a wart removal, value realization may be immediate. If the service is iterative for a complex diagnosis, value realization may be diffused and may arrive in stages. Although people may inherently understand this to be the case, the responsibility of the patient to co-create "realized value" of their health is not typically acknowledged.

The Patient Experience as Health Seeking

Elena's health-seeking journey is presented in the context of patient experience in Figure II.1, an overlay of the primary map shown in Figure I.1. Here Elena is concerned primarily with the experience of managing the consequences of medical diagnoses and treatments, and the personal experience of "being a patient." Figure II.1 shows a summary view of the changes in life situation over time; thus the most pressing common concerns that consume time and attention and promote worry and frustration are not displayed.

FIGURE II.1
The patient journey as health seeking.

Elena's *patient* scenarios in Chapters 4 and 5 evoke the stages of her journey through the clinical world as ambulatory patient, outpatient, and inpatient. Her experience as a health seeker contrasts with her role as a type of patient. Her patient touchpoints are related to navigating the healthcare system and making sense of her diagnosis, treatment, and resolution. These are touchpoints Elena might recognize:

- Managing clinical appointments and making sense of diagnoses, tests, prescriptions, and options

- Making sense of health conditions, symptoms, and emotions, and communicating about these

- Managing insurance, bill payments, doctors' orders, and other patient business

The patient journey is a complex individualized pathway to navigate resolution of health needs. This is not a service process path (as will be described in Part III) or a journey of workflow or standard disease protocols.

Elena is locating information to help make sense of specific health questions and personal support, so here information *use* is more important than the actual sites and services used. Information in use results from following the patient information motivators or needs described in Chapter 2.

There are many resources Elena could use to satisfy information needs. Information needs associated with each stage in the journey are suggested, not as exclusive information tasks but needs for facts, research, and reassurance that result from having to navigate each stage's new problem setting. (This series of encounters and resolutions is referred to as sensemaking, a process described in the Methods section of Chapter 4.)

Design goals for the health seeker as patient might include:

- Improving the continuity of service experience: finding common information touchpoints and aligning data types, date-driven events, providers, and communications across resources and sites.

- Enhancing the information architecture and visual presentation of patient records, tests, and instructions.

- Discovering ways to indicate personal and "patient" status meaningfully in online communications, to establish a personal buffer zone during care and recovery and to facilitate social and work transitions.

- Developing simple medication and schedule reminders that maintain currency and continuity with the clinic.

CHAPTER 4

Design for Patient Agency

Elena's Story:
A Personal Health Journey

Elena shows up at the family practice for her 8:15 appointment, but still has not reached any conclusions about her condition. She had spent over an hour browsing online the night before, jumping from articles on heart disease and healthy diet to blood pressure and stress management. Although Elena had hoped to be more informed for her visit, she was confused by the abundance of details about conditions for which she had little evidence or insight.

Her doctor's suburban medical office is a group practice that serves as both a primary care and outpatient surgical center. Elena is welcomed by an office receptionist and is asked to fill out several pages of forms and interview questions. She is told that updated information is needed because the office is switching to electronic medical records. Elena would not have noticed the change in routine otherwise because the existing paper records are still taking up an entire wall of the open office area. Prompted by one of the questions, Elena retrieves her smartphone to look up the date of her last visit to the office. She has no personal health information stored on the phone or accessible through an app. Nearly all the information requested—from her medical history to the facts of her current condition—is duplicated on old paper and new electronic records. Yet Elena has no personal copy of her own records.

The primary care practice retains five physicians, four nurse practitioners, and six registered nurses, who either work in teams or are assigned to patients based on the procedures and clinical tasks required. Specialists and anesthesiologists are scheduled and on call for procedures as needed. The backstage management of clinical task assignments is handled by a medical director and coordinated by an office manager.

After an initial weigh-in, a nurse briefly interviews Elena in the examining room. He asks questions about her current situation and about her last appointment 5 months earlier. He takes blood pressure and heart rate readings, asks about current medications, and notes everything on a paper chart that Elena assumes is her medical record. Fran Martin, Elena's family doctor, appears a few minutes later, now 25 minutes since Elena's arrival.

Dr. Martin asks Elena about her symptoms and the reason for the visit, and listens to the account of the incident from the previous evening. Elena must admit to feeling well enough at the moment, having recovered her sense of normal health. Dr. Martin glances through Elena's chart, performs a brief physical examination, and asks about prior incidents, other symptoms, and her diet and health habits. She orders blood drawn for testing as well as cardiovascular tests. Suspecting metabolic syndrome and the onset of diabetes as a diagnostic hypothesis, Dr. Martin orders glycemic tests and gives Elena printed handouts to read. A nurse preps Elena with 12 electrodes and gives her a brief electrocardiograph test. Still, Elena leaves the center without further insight into her condition.

Elena experiences a nagging sense of frustration and incompleteness. Although she has been "cared for" institutionally, she still falls short of having resolved her health concerns. As a caregiver to her father, she knows firsthand how complicated medical processes can get. And she remains unsure about how she can personally take charge of improving her own health. As a patient, Elena's presence in the clinic signifies she has agreed to the social contract that confers rights on the physician and staff to examine and treat her under the customary conditions of healthcare. The professional arrangements, devices, measures, and controls at every step of the clinical process reinforce that she is "not in control." Yet Elena is uncertain what steps she can take to help herself, other than adhering to her doctor's orders. ■

Self-Care as Health Agency

Elena has an unknown and abnormal health condition, and like most patients, she agrees to follow the standard care path by assenting to the traditional patient relationship. As more individuals choose a path of agency and become the decision makers for their health, a sense of disruption will grow in the healthcare system. Physicians say they want patients to take control of their health, but that means accepting the higher risks of nonadherence to traditional medicine and use of alternative self-treatments. An uneasy balance between patient and agent is already happening, led by new patient advocates on social media facilitating the transition to individuals taking control of their health agency.

A health seeker may cycle between being agent and patient and may never resolve 100% to either pole. In a serious health situation, a person will take action (agency) on matters of their choice and will also accept and seek care from others (patiency). Seeing the dynamics of choice and care in health seeking enables innovators to recognize that different communications, values, and incentives are necessary to meet the needs at service touchpoints.

How do we help people to help themselves? Does constant or incremental innovation in the simple services—online health management resources, health IT, consumer websites—address the societal and trend-level problems in healthcare? Better information resources are necessary and socially useful, but most IT systems and the personal health-oriented Web and mobile applications referred to as Health 2.0 are aligned to serve a single IT vendor or provider's requirements. Health 2.0 and social websites may "scale" to serve any number of health seekers, but they do not scale systemically. Instead, they may lock in the prior commitments of the provider to a given strategy, preventing new systems from emerging.

The affordances of technology are a source for innovation. The trends in consumer healthcare innovation are driven by the increasing power and accessibility of cheap computing, and by ubiquitous wireless and mobile platforms. The health information ecology is constantly growing with a profusion of both professional content and low-cost, user-generated media. Yet two basic disconnects are exposed in Elena's scenario: She has mobile access to information about her appointments, but not to health goals, prescription history, or test outcomes. And the physicians have installed a new electronic medical records system, but have no easy way to exchange this information with patients. Among the many disconnects in US healthcare is patient connectivity with health information.

Elena's situation is typical—as people age, they often find themselves dealing with multiple interconnected chronic diseases, such as diabetes, obesity, and cardiovascular disease. Chronic disease situations are not cured, but are rather managed and "lived with." As a growing aging population adapts to chronic conditions over longer life spans, designers have a major role to play in creating new tools for self-regulation and personal health agency.

Agents of Future Healthcare

People are taking charge of their own health in the 21st century by becoming "ePatients." The ePatient movement was inspired by the realization among a growing number of activists that the digital information divide was an unethical institutional barrier to patients obtaining the most effective treatment. According to ePatients, the "e" not only stands for electronically enabled but empowered and engaged. ePatients are wired agents of their own care, and they represent the social future of healthcare service.

ePatiency started with the individual need for and right to medical information that might inform a person's health decisions. Access to reliable and actionable health information has always been necessary for practitioners, and it is now becoming the case for patients. Since the advent of the Web, people have taken direct action by searching for authoritative medical research information for second opinions, and even first opinions. One of the earliest reported health information actions occurred in 1994, when Edward Murphy, a New Jersey insurance agent with a chronic hip problem, impersonated his family physician on the phone to a medical librarian to acquire a recent authoritative review article covering the procedure recommended for his treatment. Because his own doctor would not provide the article that Murphy had requested, he used social engineering to reach into the walled garden of publisher-protected medical articles. Today's ePatients are just as provocative about patients' rights, access to medical charts and personal data, and the rationale for procedures and medications. Statistics show that 57% of adults in the United States (2009)[1] and 75% in Europe (2007)[2] went online to inform themselves about a health question. In 2000, only 25% of US adults indicated that they went online for health information.

Advocates for personal health agency empowered by Web-accessible information may call themselves ePatients, but it's not a *patiency* movement. If *patient* is a clinical designation for "healthcare user," the ePatients initiative demonstrates the informed public's frustration with the presumption of patiency—the expectation that people will take a passive and accommodating role under professional care. Activist and informed health seekers can, for the first time in history, collectively challenge the presumption of patient adherence to prescriptions, orders, and recommendations. Whereas physicians can research and inform themselves about one patient's situation for only a limited time, ePatients may invest dozens of hours into researching a condition that informs their own well-being. Although access to health information remains unequal—even university research libraries typically restrict access to their expensive online medical journal subscriptions—articles of interest are searchable via PubMed in the National Library of Medicine's abstracts.

Health Information as a Public Good

According to a 2009 Pew survey, half of all online health inquiries are intended to learn about a health situation for a person other than the information seeker.[3] Furthermore, people readily share what they have learned with a spouse or friends, so the quality of information becomes a critical issue. Consumers may not understand the differences between information sources, and although some have the time or background to conduct thorough research into a health condition online, most information behavior studies show people find information that *satisfices** their immediate question. Therefore, health seekers do not usually require original medical research articles, but prefer summarized information with sufficient guidance to inform personal action.

Satisficing enables people to make quick work of the Web's ubiquitous access to an overwhelming volume of sources and references.[4] It is the rapid sensemaking of information that helps people determine the criticality of a health situation. The slightest symptom sends people online in search of information—to distinguish between a cold and the flu, or to determine whether a brown spot on their back is a mole or a melanoma. The health seeker cannot be 100% certain, but can make a fuzzy distinction between the need to act or to wait out a physical process.

This type of fuzzy decision is characteristic of a sensemaking process (described later in this chapter as both a research method and a cognitive

---

* Cognitive scientist Herbert Simon coined the term *satisficing* to describe the behavior of *sufficient satisfaction* of a decision, where a workable threshold of acceptability is suitable. People satisfice as a way to make decisions with incomplete information and partial comprehension. As a rational response to complexity, humans trade off completeness for sufficiency and make do with the information they have at hand.

process). In sensemaking, the notion that people collect data, make clear decisions, and then act on them is exposed as a rationalist fantasy. In reality, people learn, struggle, and take actions oriented toward meeting personal goals. Those goals are not always rational and may be poorly formed, yet they initiate and bias information seeking and its use.

Scientists and intellectuals such as Harvard University Librarian Robert Darnton[5] have declared open access to health and scientific information as a public good. Science and health research funding agencies are establishing new models of open information access with publishers, and open access versions of research articles are more often available. In theory, there seems to be a clear moral argument for the value of "open knowledge." In practice, a vast ocean of poorly vetted, peer-written academic articles is not the best resource for public readers attempting to make sense of a health question. More is not always better, especially when the original information source was not composed for public use.

In activist discourses, the research articles are declared equivalent to "knowledge," as if content were a direct transmission of wisdom from the scientific lab. In reality, the extraction of usable knowledge from research materials is a difficult process requiring extensive training (and is the rationale behind the growing field of medical knowledge translation). The public is largely unable to vet these contributions, which are written as peer communications to scholars who are assumed to have a background understanding of the precedent literature.

This translation problem exists across all scientific literatures, but it becomes vital when individual lives may benefit from timely uptake of the research findings. The situation of a well-informed and motivated health seeker such as ePatient Zero Edward Murphy is the exception. If health knowledge is a public good, then a new literature or new genre (at least) might be created for the public that references current opinion and evidence, yet is readable by nonprofessionals. The frontier of applied public translation has not yet been opened, even in the Health 2.0 movement.

Inspiring Agency for Self-Care

When the general public considers health*care*, their frame of reference draws on the strong association with professional health services. Even the political language referring to healthcare coverage and insurance reform has damaged the notion of care as a human value in its own right. Consider then the design challenge of encouraging public and individual health by inspiring design interventions for care. The most powerful intervention is changing the paradigm or the rules of the game. The most fundamental intervention is individual health behavior change, which will allow the paradigm change to unfold.

Innovation research by designer Hugh Dubberly and his colleagues Rajiv Mehta, Shelly Evenson, and Paul Pangaro promotes a systemic cycle of self-care resulting in a model of the person as sole agent for health responsibility.[6] They radically repositioned patient-centered design (but not patient *experience*) by reframing the patient as agent. Responding to the growing problem that finds the vast majority of healthcare resources being consumed by chronic disease and later-life disease conditions, they identify a target outcome of shifting the system's chronic disease system from patients of care providers to individuals with care responsibility (Table 4.1).

TABLE 4.1 SHIFT IN FRAMING FROM TRADITIONAL HEALTHCARE PROVISION TO SELF-MANAGEMENT

	Traditional healthcare frame	Emerging self-management frame
Scope	Relieve acute condition	Maintain well-being
	Now	Over a lifetime
Approach	Intervention; treatment	Prevention; healthy living
	Expert-directed	Self-managed
	Apply standards of care	Measure, assess, and adjust; iterate
	Lengthy regulatory pre-approval	Learn and adapt as you go
Subject	Symptoms and test results	Whole person, seen in context
Response	Prescribe medication	Improve behavior and environment
Relies on	Medical establishment	Individual, family, and friends
		Social networks, others like me
HCP as	Authority, expert	Coach, assistant
	Dispensing knowledge	Learning from patients
Patient as	Helpless, childlike	Responsible adult
	Taking orders	Setting goals; testing hunches
Relationship	Asymmetric, one-way	Symmetric, reciprocal
	Command and control	Discussion and collaboration
Records	HCP's notes of visit	Patient's notes; data from sensors
	Sporadic	Continuously collected
	Dispersed between offices	Connected; aggregated
	Managed by HCP	Controlled by patient

HCP = healthcare provider.
Source: From H. Dubberly, R. Mehta, S. Evenson, & P. Pangaro. (2010).
Reframing health to embrace design of our own well-being. *Interactions, 17*, 56–63.

The traditional frame can be seen as *expert-managed* and the self-management frame as *patient-centered*. We can view these frames as not true opposites but as continua with several dimensions, reflecting proportions of expert/patient responsibility. Figure I.1 illustrates the various stages of identity, care, and service encountered by a given persona over an extended period. As a person moves from a consumer role into a patient role, his or her responsibility for health management becomes unevenly shared. Healthcare providers accept more responsibility for the (now) patient as illnesses become complicated or serious.

Today, family and primary care doctors are largely committed to the self-management model of healthcare. Doctors on the front lines treat patients as people with a complex mix of health and life conditions, and serve in advising capacities during their consults. The future of primary care is moving toward the expert-coach, whole-person model of engagement. Family practitioners (an ever-dwindling proportion of new physicians) are trained in the tenets of a patient-agency frame in current residency programs, even if their home institutions conform to the traditional model.

The expert model predominates in *acute care*, which constitutes the majority of healthcare for people under age 60. Broken bones, acute infections, and eye surgery require expert acute care. Yet as people age and become subject to chronic continuing conditions, the burden for self-care becomes higher.* The need for patient education increases, even if that burden is met with reluctance on the part of older adults seeking symptom relief.

A mix of modes is needed when dealing with complex health issues, multiple conditions, and complications. A diabetic or cardiovascular patient may need to assume a proportion of 70% self-care versus 30% expert care. A surgery patient might need the reverse proportion. A design opportunity exists to create a common language between practice and patients to help all stakeholders distinguish the different types and degrees of responsibility.

Managing Personal Health as a System

How do we shift the overall goal from healthcare as a *service* to personal management of one's state of well-being? Dubberly's model identifies an active cycle of *identify, measure, assess,* and *adapt* as a cyclic decision-management process (Figure 4.1). Health seekers inform themselves from sensor observations (feedback from devices and measures), information resources, and their social networks to assist in decision making.

---

* Design for graceful aging is a significant, growing innovation opportunity actively researched in labs such as the University of Toronto's TAGLab (http://taglab.utoronto.ca) and in health applications being designed by companies such as GE and Intel (http://careinnovations.com).

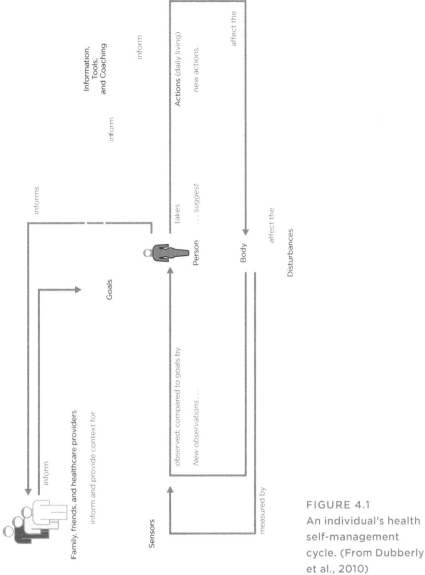

FIGURE 4.1
An individual's health
self-management
cycle. (From Dubberly
et al., 2010)

How feasible would this method be? Biofeedback systems have been available for decades and provide for easily measured indirect responses (heart rate, skin resistance, brain waves, and blood measures). But the portability of mobile platforms and built-in multifunction sensors enables designers to easily display the values from health-sensing devices as mobile functions. The major feedback loop involves the health seeker's body signals, sensors, and the change in state detected by senses or sensors.

Feedback cycles can be embodied in interactive artifacts (portable media and medical devices) and even electronic documents such as personal health records. Their self-management cycle is a continuous decision process, as Dubberly's suggests, like the W. Edwards Deming and Walter Shewhart PDCA (Plan, Do, Check, Act) cycle.[7] The PDCA cycle is a quality control practice often integrated into healthcare management processes at the macro level and is a key principle for service process design. Five steps are actually indicated:

- *Assess* a situation.

- *Plan* for change or adaptation by fact finding and identifying purposes and questions.

- *Do* the change or process intervention as planned.

- *Check* or study the analysis and summarize what was learned.

- *Act* or deploy the change or improvement (and plan for the next steps).

A wide range of PDCA resources are available on the Internet for health service applications, based on years of macro-level institutional applications.

PDCA is based on a management metaphor and does not translate well to the cognitive or decision-making level of activity. For everyday self-care management that requires less "planning and doing," the tactical fighter pilot's OODA loop (Colonel John Boyd's cycle of Observe, Orient, Decide, Act) may apply.[8] Drawn from a cognitive model of the situation awareness required for tactical air combat, OODA represents how one or more actors interpret and act upon a situation as it emerges. It defines a cycle of continuous observation and orienting to scan the environment and locate signals of importance. When signals (or bio-messages) are detected under the "orient" mode, a decision must be made. A decision is followed by action and then feedback about the effectiveness of the action. This loop cycle reinforces one's self-awareness of discrete behaviors and the impact of health decisions on differing conditions. For example, a diabetic observes a series of measures, adjusts (orients) based on a glycemic value, decides whether intervention is required, and if so, acts.

The service designer will find that PDCA supports the requirements for cyclic feedback in service processes. Interaction designers should look to the OODA loop to create UX drivers for observing and orienting self-awareness. Today, the OODA loop is emerging in mobile application design in diabetes monitoring and tools such as Massive Health's Eatery (https://eatery.massivehealth.com).

Mobile Personal Health

Although preventive health management is not a new trend, smartphone handsets and mobile interaction have given designers a new target. Health 2.0 technology is supplying tools to end-user health seekers that actively support general or disease-specific health awareness.

Consider how complicated everyday life is for the diabetic. Even with a state-of-the-art continuous glucose monitor and micropump, the diabetic must wrangle an assortment of products and tools needed throughout the week. In 2010, Italian designer Mauro Amoruso won the Diabetes Mine grand prize for Zero, his vision of a system that replaces the constant blood testing and injection ritual with a seamless wearable device communicating to a mobile display (Figure 4.2). Though not yet feasible, the concept represents an achievable target.

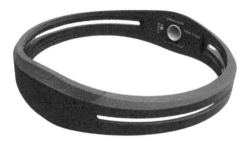

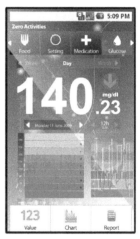

FIGURE 4.2a,b
The Zero concept includes an armband device (a) and personal information display (b) to replace the entire complicated mess of insulin management. (Courtesy of Mauro Amoruso)

The Zero armband is a refillable single-device concept that surpasses current technology and sets a target for industry to achieve. The smartphone display presents glucose levels and the ranges throughout a period of time, as well as insulin availability and dose, history, and expected impacts of food.

This interaction design concept accounts for several tasks associated with OODA. The graphical display allows a user to *observe* glucose levels (140 mg/dl) and *orient* by attending to the trend indicator (up arrow) and daily glucose measure graph. *Decide* (a cognitive step) and *act* are aided by the Zero's five control icons (Setting, Glucose, Food, Send, Bolus). This monitor displays feedback from sensors embedded in the armband unit, which continuously senses blood sugar (by built-in cannulation) and injects insulin from a small reservoir to balance the glycemic system. The Zero system exemplifies the ideal for continuous health management and decision making.

While the miniaturization and mobility of computing has enabled designers to pack more functionality into smaller handsets and tablets, consumer sensors and physical interfaces have lagged. Large healthcare concerns such as Medtronic have been working on less-invasive diabetes devices for years. The goal of the designer here may not be to ensure feasibility but to aim for a functional and aesthetic solution that can inspire engineering innovation.

These emerging tools and the associated cognitive models share an underlying design theory that people are willing and able to affirmatively manage their own health conditions. The biggest problem with health management has been (and will be) patient adherence for the people whose lives are less conducive to sustaining healthy habits. Helping the already healthy is easy. Helping people who are not so inclined, and who may be the majority of patients in some regions, is our real design challenge.

Reframing the Patient as Agent

Dubberly and colleagues model the stages, states, and transitions in moving from patiency to agency through self-care management (Figure 4.3):

- Forming an initial positive personal health loop (stages 1 and 2) with reconciliation and habituation

- Reinforcing self-care (stage 3)

- Sustainably managing one's health (stage 4)

- Participating in the contextual change that impacts larger social trends

Although the stages of self-care may appear to be a proposed "solution" to the wicked problem of improving healthcare for all, these are presented by the authors as scenarios for envisioning design proposals (the purpose of this book as well).

The first step of intervention in a complex problem is achieving understanding and reframing the problem. As a design thinking method, reframing creates a new problem frame and scope, an intentionality that establishes a new course of action. The intent guides new actions that route around the current problem system, rather than attempting to solve entrenched issues with insufficient scope and means.

Reframing creates a new context that can obviate the old way of viewing a problem. The context of the illegal practice of music downloading was reframed by the introduction of iTunes, a new service mechanism to encourage legal downloads at a pitch-perfect price point. Though stellar market success is not the intent of healthcare design, cultural change and new practices emerge in many cases from the reframing and the attempts to create new services that intersect and mitigate the existing problem system.

Consider reframing patients and users as *health seekers*. What system responses could be created to serve the needs of "people seeking health" as opposed to "patients under doctor's orders"? The three versions of the health-seeking journey in Figures I.1, II.1, and III.1 represent the different motives, drivers, and touchpoints for different framing contexts.

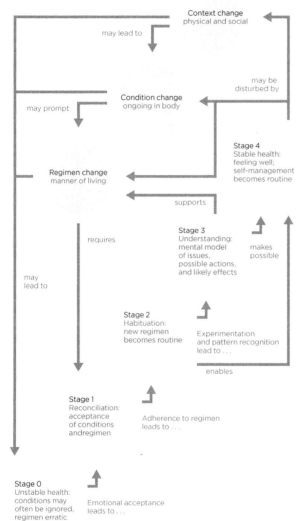

FIGURE 4.3
Stages from self-care
to agency. (From Dub-
berly et al., 2010)

Reframing lets designers focus on personal agency, with alternative scenarios of problem structure leading to vastly different approaches to
problem "solving." Scenarios are treated as design proposals, not as rigorous
experiments. Prototypes of services and processes, as well as systems and
interfaces, can be sanctioned and observed for systemic effects. Large-effect,
relative differences can be recognized and reinforced. Successful programs
can be scaled up to the next organizational level and evaluated with appropriate measures and techniques for the trial.

The staged process in Figure 4.3 is a macro-level scenario that, in some cases, may take years to accomplish. Dubberly's team suggests using versions of health "dashboards" to display continuously updated micro-health measures to facilitate personal awareness of health status and progress toward the next stage. They promote the idea of displaying an integrated view of sources (e.g., health records, prescription data, narratives) and sensors (noninvasive physical sampling).

Health 2.0: Everywhere and Empowering

The simplest path to transformation is to declare that a new era has arrived. After the first wave of Web services recovered and rebranded itself as Web 2.0, health services followed (at about 2006) with an active bevy of start-ups and Web products. The Web 2.0 movement embraces user interconnectivity, activity streams, and information feeds from multiple sources, user-generated content production, and lightweight applications with rich interfaces. Health 2.0 apps adapted Web 2.0 technologies and development approaches to health information resources. Medicine 2.0 followed as a research and practitioner conference. Both trends are rapidly evolving into new directions of technology development, healthcare business models, and informatics research on new media in medicine.

The mutually reciprocal goals of patient empowerment and Health 2.0 both converge on tools for health decision making, personal information management, and helping people orient to well-being. The Health 2.0 movement has inspired new applications for user-generated content across all healthcare niches. Start-up incubators envision "interactive health" as the next major trend, and portfolio development groups such as Rock Health are focused entirely on health applications.

ePatients were among the first to take advantage of the democratization of user engagement and production enabled by Web 2.0 tools. The expanded reach of communicating and sharing ideas (blogging), community discussions (wikis and social networks), and user classification (tagging and foldering) shifted users from passive searchers to active participants. ePatients created the first health and disease communities and activist blogs, and institutional and commercial healthcare services followed only later. Health 2.0 is creating new interfaces and robust applications to facilitate wider societal access to these tools.

The Reach of Health 2.0 for Broader Impact

Health 2.0 has launched several important trends toward responsible self-care, personal data management (the "quantified self" movement), and patient advocacy (the participatory medicine movement). Health 2.0 maintains a strong view of the role of technology in enabling health, and is largely technology driven. We cannot yet describe statistically or even qualitatively the reach of Health 2.0 into the health, lives, and values of everyday health seekers. There may be hundreds of small markets across the Web for different niche health products, but the connection of small health-related technology start-ups to mitigating long-term healthcare issues remains unclear.

According to a recent article, the Silicon Valley start-ups heading up Health 2.0 products are creating apps for small, self-referential markets of early adopting technophiles.[9] In other words, Health 2.0 trends like quantified self may largely be helping the already fit and healthy track their health, as part of the technology-obsessed 2.0 lifestyle. According to the article's author, Kanyi Maqubela, the weakness of the Silicon Valley approach to Health 2.0 may be the lack of diversity, access, and business models for attracting the unhealthy people who need better paths toward improved health: "The quantified self and accompanying mobile health revolution needs to puncture markets which are usually invited last to the party. If entrepreneurs in this space are serious about making a difference, and about staying relevant to an evolving population, they need to invite these demographics first."[10] Maqubela recommends that start-ups work with healthcare incumbents, including government, pharmaceutical companies, and hospital systems, to improve their productivity in the larger healthcare ecosystem.

There may be several routes to scale applications at a system-wide level. Connecting to incumbents may be the fastest path to reaching large markets, but effecting change may be limited by the existing behaviors and values in that channel. Connecting directly with health seekers through social networked communities may take longer, and the resulting community may not be as vulnerable to market intervention or regulation. Most Health 2.0 applications are not (yet) facilitating care through provider networks. Moreover, once a patient has committed to a platform, they will be less likely to expend resources interacting on other similar networks.

The highest-impact Health 2.0 application, PatientsLikeMe, creates social care by engaging qualified patients in peer exchange and the aggregation of personal data for evaluation and comparative analysis. PatientsLikeMe also helps organizations by making that data available for treatment and outcomes research. Yet it has only (roughly) 165,000 registered "patients," many of which are inactive. This is a huge membership for a Health 2.0 community, perhaps the largest. However, compared to the overall healthcare market, Health 2.0 reaches only a tiny proportion of possible patients. Kaiser Permanente's HealthConnect patient platform claims 8.6 million members.

Practitioner advocates view technology as secondary to the change in practice and patient engagement. Physician Scott Shreeve encourages practitioners to embrace the emerging opportunity to disrupt healthcare practice and policy by combining technology innovation with business and practice changes to create a virtuous cycle of innovation. Shreeve's definition of Health 2.0, although not universal, has broad acceptance in the United States: "A *new concept of healthcare* wherein all the constituents (patients, physicians, providers, and payers) focus on *healthcare value* (outcomes/price) and use *competition* at the medical condition level over the full cycle of care as the catalyst for *improving the safety, efficiency, and quality* of health care" (emphasis added).[11]

The most compelling thrust of Shreeve's orientation to Health 2.0 is to focus innovation on service system change, not applications. The technology marketplace has since aligned with the functional perspective of changing healthcare delivery and information by adapting tools and practices from Web 2.0. The technology view is gaining ground, supported by the annual Health 2.0 conference, through lionizing start-ups with incubators such as Rock Health, and even by trademarking the Health 2.0 label.

Practitioners and scholars working in the high-touch clinical field have assigned Medicine 2.0 to the practitioners, including the trademark and conference. The original definition of Medicine 2.0 is technology-focused and even identifies the constituents of the healthcare system as *user groups*:

> Medicine 2.0 applications, services, and tools are Web-based services for health care consumers, caregivers, patients, health professionals, and biomedical researchers, that use Web 2.0 technologies as well as semantic web and virtual reality tools, to enable and facilitate specifically social networking, participation, apomediation, collaboration, and openness within and between these user groups.[12]

A systematic review of the published and online (gray) literatures[13] reveals 46 unique definitions of Health 2.0 and Medicine 2.0, but says that the two schools seem to have converged around seven recurrent topics:

- Web 2.0/technology
- Patients
- Professionals
- Social networking
- Health information/content
- Collaboration
- Change of healthcare

The review authors concluded by fusing the two terms together as Health 2.0/Medicine 2.0 and declaring the field as a still-developing concept, which is strikingly similar to the narratives emerging from both camps.

Health 2.0 started with patients, not start-ups, adopting relatively simple Web tools—wikis, free blogs, video sharing, online community services—using off-the-shelf tools to build specialized portals for communicating with other patients and providers. Technology enablers preceded the "user need." The adoption of generic tools (such as WordPress, used for health blogs like

Diabetes Mine) preceded the development of the commercial services (such as Alliance Health) that often follow entrepreneurial innovators with sustainable support.

Online engagement is not health *care*. Scaling thousands of users online does not scale service for thousands of patients. Although patients can be superficially examined remotely, physical examinations are done in person. Medical advice must be given in a context of understanding.

Start ups are easy to launch but difficult to sustain. Hundreds of online healthcare products will consolidate to dozens (or fewer) sustainable ventures. Beyond Health 2.0, the next frontier will be transformation of practice and direct service models, driven by the largest-scale factors current generations have ever known:

- Population: aging demographics with complex chronic conditions

- Costs: rapidly increasing societal cost burden as demographics shift

- Technology: new biotechnologies, information technologies, and medications creating increased demand

- Life span: expansion of lifetime costs as global populations gain more access to healthcare and live longer

Health 3.0: Inclusive and Communicative

While Health 2.0 apps and Web services are being developed for consumer and business-to-business applications, the major health IT (HIT) vendors have delivered enterprise applications for hospital and healthcare systems of any size and scale. Chapter 7 presents cases and lessons from some of the largest implementations of electronic health and medical records (EMR) systems currently installed. A spectrum of thousands of software systems exists in the categories between the single-user Web app and the enterprise EMR. Information technology has become an active partner, even a team player, to support human care in the processes of care service delivery.

Even a quick sweep of the HIT landscape shows significant differences between the emerging Health 2.0 applications and enterprise vendors. Health 2.0 is almost entirely composed of Web-based or mobile applications, a bottom-up profusion of mainly single-purpose software applications without significant platform development. Their advantages of user focus, nimble adaptation, focusing on a single problem, and rapid iteration follow the disruptive innovation playbook. Their strategies work best with target markets of smaller enterprises, healthcare industry corporations, and individual users.

HIT systems are primary-vendor, platform-driven, large-scale software systems based on government and industry standards and designed for highly structured workflows. Nearly all primary vendors are providing for end-user interaction and distribution through Web (thin client) user interfaces. Most EMRs are currently providing interfaces for tablet and phone-based mobile apps, based more on industry trend than healthcare service need.

HIT services are becoming true platforms that allow organizations to capture patient and transaction data as enterprise assets. HIT enables distribution and exchange through critical standards such as HL7 (Health Level 7), an ANSI-certified standard for data exchange between vendor systems. HL7 provides a standard basis for defining and sharing any healthcare document, or any hospital, lab, or imaging report, using the Clinical Document Architecture (CDA) specification.

Consider the wide spectrum of healthcare practice and clinical applications in Figure 4.4, a framework that encompasses enterprise HIT, point of care decision support, practice management, patient engagement, and clinical references. A full range of clinical roles are shown, from administrators and clinicians (in care networks) to educators and researchers (learning networks), with "patients" located in the center.

The framework centers on patients (health seekers) as the purpose and intended outcome of most clinical applications. Clinicians (of all disciplines) and trainees are the professionals most closely engaged in patient care, and are included within the circle. HIT applications are aligned toward institutional applications (at right) or technological applications (at left). The exemplary services indicated are today's current leaders in those categories.

Patient-focused decision support (on the technological side) includes tools for health information and self-care, if not diagnosis. Patient communities (on the institutional side) create social networks for interpersonal exchange and support. These communities are starting to replace the institutional function for individuals, and institutions are in early stages of creating online and local communities for their own constituencies.

Today's patient-centric applications will inspire new forums for engagement and dialogue between the public and professionals, and the role of mediators will expand. *Apomediaries* are new roles for credible information brokers and participatory community managers. As identified by Gunther Eysenbach, founding editor of the *Journal of Internet Medical Research*, apomediaries are central to facilitating user engagement in the emerging interactive healthcare world.[14] Apomediaries serve as volunteer navigators for health and disease communities, such as the active mediators on the popular Diabetes Mine health blog. This extension of the coordinator role can be seen as the leading edge of an institutional innovation yet to be capitalized on or formalized.

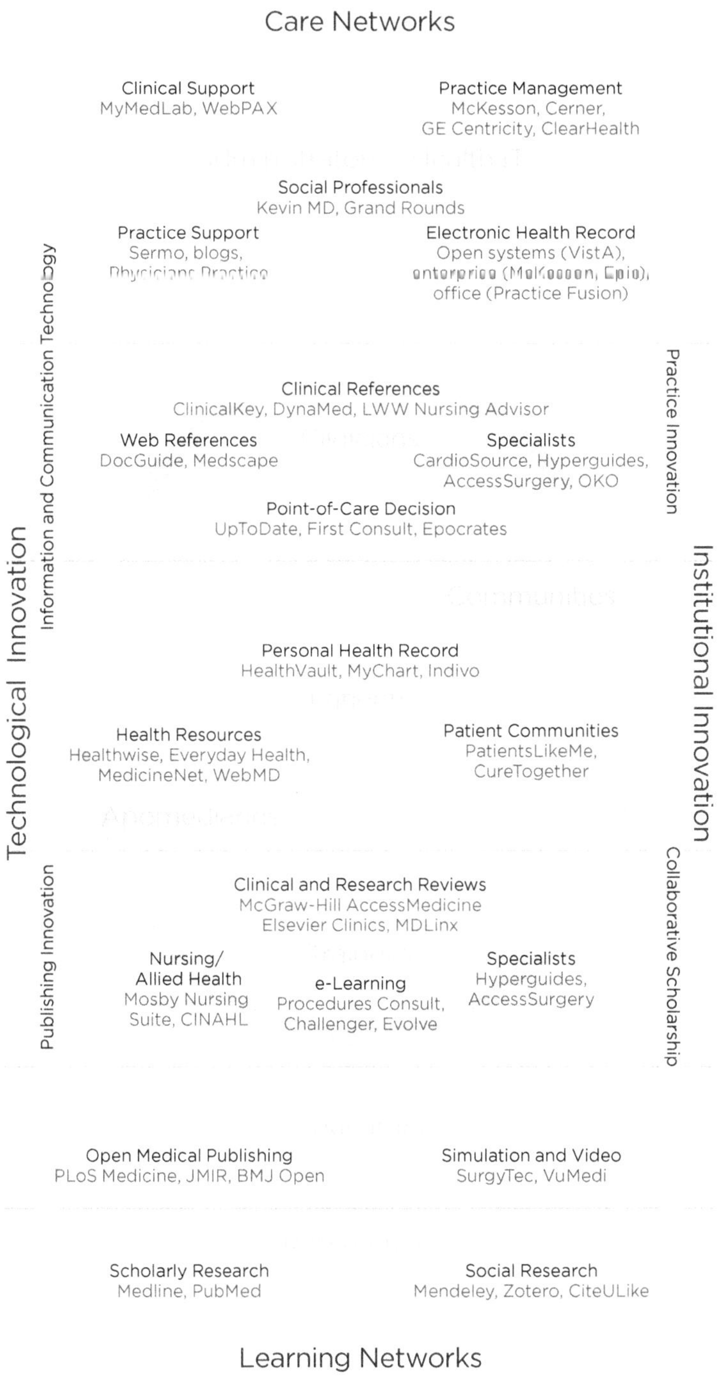

Care Networks

Clinical Support
MyMedLab, WebPAX

Practice Management
McKesson, Cerner,
GE Centricity, ClearHealth

Social Professionals
Kevin MD, Grand Rounds

Practice Support
Sermo, blogs,
Physicians Practice

Electronic Health Record
Open systems (VistA),
enterprise (McKesson, Epic),
office (Practice Fusion)

Clinical References
ClinicalKey, DynaMed, LWW Nursing Advisor

Web References
DocGuide, Medscape

Specialists
CardioSource, Hyperguides,
AccessSurgery, OKO

Point-of-Care Decision
UpToDate, First Consult, Epocrates

Personal Health Record
HealthVault, MyChart, Indivo

Health Resources
Healthwise, Everyday Health,
MedicineNet, WebMD

Patient Communities
PatientsLikeMe,
CureTogether

Clinical and Research Reviews
McGraw-Hill AccessMedicine
Elsevier Clinics, MDLinx

Nursing/
Allied Health
Mosby Nursing
Suite, CINAHL

e-Learning
Procedures Consult,
Challenger, Evolve

Specialists
Hyperguides,
AccessSurgery

Open Medical Publishing
PLoS Medicine, JMIR, BMJ Open

Simulation and Video
SurgyTec, VuMedi

Scholarly Research
Medline, PubMed

Social Research
Mendeley, Zotero, CiteULike

Learning Networks

Technological Innovation

Information and Communication Technology

Publishing Innovation

Institutional Innovation

Practice Innovation

Collaborative Scholarship

FIGURE 4.4
Health information technology spectrum.

Consider the impact interactive healthcare is already having in leading institutions. Mike Evans, medical director of the Health Design Lab at St. Michael's Hospital in Toronto, draws the comparison between changing healthcare practices and new management thinking: "If you make the analogy between Web 1.0 and Web 2.0, I think the system before has been very reactive, not interested in user experience. It's about putting out fires. And now in Health 2.0, we are seeing that we need to get out in front of these problems, we need to anticipate problems, with patients driving the bus."[15]

How do we get patients to "drive the bus"? Evans's vision of agency is one initiated by health seekers or patients themselves. It is a people-centered design movement in which human and community needs drive design, and technology is subsidiary to the values of care.

The Health 2.0 and HIT ecosystems fill hundreds of niches that reach beyond patient and professional services. However, in the evolution of patient-centered service, even purely administrative applications have to connect to patient needs at some point in the value chain.

DESIGN BEST PRACTICES

- Health is experienced individually but is managed socially. Health seekers are not isolated patients but community members. A traditional user-centered approach can overlook systemic relationships by overly focusing on a defined technology or a specific market segment.

- Design thinking is not a solution to every healthcare problem, but rather a perspective and set of guidelines for finding and framing the right problems where design practices can provide extraordinary value.

- There are a small number of universal information needs. As a starting point, design information to support the wayfinding of these needs for health seekers.

- Any design process requires trade-offs between providing a simple answer or the complexity of multiple options. Safety rules—the risk to a health seeker making the wrong choice should be the guiding principle.

- Health 2.0 is a transition phase, not to Health 3.0 but to a consolidation of information services integrated at the point of need. These will include patients, point of care, patient management, practice management, research, and education.

Case Study:
St. Michael's Health Design Lab—
Health Design for Self-Care

US healthcare providers are incentivized to compete with each other for patient and physician business, a situation that warps the service landscape and demands technology and institutional innovations to maintain competitiveness. Hospitals and group practices make strategic investments in specialized equipment and systems, affiliates for diagnostic imaging, and expensive physical plant renovations. In the smaller, publicly funded Canadian system, institutional networks find innovative ways to make an impact on healthcare at the point of *most leverage*—not always at the point of service but at the points of citizen learning and awareness.

This design case describes one of the projects of the Health Design Lab (HDL) at St. Michael's Hospital in Toronto, a patient-facing innovation group managed by a joint clinical, business, and designer team.

Mike Evans, a family physician and director of the HDL, stays connected to popular culture and media as a way to improve the public impact of health communication. Evans gives talks, broadcasts as the House Doctor on CBC Radio, and writes newspaper columns to further his goal of reinventing patient education. At the HDL, he and a team of healthcare innovators have been designing new approaches to education and public engagement with health issues. Evans and the HDL have created a true transdisciplinary design team—filmmakers, designers, marketers, researchers, clinicians, technologists, and patients—to create tailored media that speaks to people today. The HDL is creating virtual "knowledge buffets" for patients to interact with and to optimize their self-care, including mobile reminders, social networks for chronic disease patients, self-selecting videos (skills, inspiration, advice) with peers and experts, and comic book–style health books for children and patients with low literacy. Evans described the HDL team as collaborative solution finders:

> We are mostly patient facing. To be able to create the perfect solution, you need to be clinic facing, clinician facing, and patient facing. Our niche is definitely the patient. We have a couple of strategies within that. One is the collaboratory concept; most interdisciplinary healthcare means that a pharmacist, a nurse, and a doctor are working together. Almost all solutions in medicine are derived internally, from the people in the clinic. There is little user study and there is very little of bringing filmmakers, writers, MBAs, [and] technologists along with patients.[16]

For example, the HDL designed a series of colorful baseball card–style flash cards for diabetes medications. The cards reveal a seriously playful side of care design, presenting information in a way that engages patients and caregivers.

Innovation through Collaboration

In another project, the HDL joined a larger consortium, Toronto's University Health Network, to design systemic responses to cardiac care for chronic patients—in particular the wicked problem of atrial fibrillation (AF). A signal of more serious emerging disease conditions, AF is experienced as serious when it occurs and is difficult to identify and treat in isolation. It is a symptom of a bigger problem yet, disguised as a condition, requiring treatment and expensive continuity of follow-up.

The HDL team developed a series of patient communication resources to intervene in the "front end" of AF care. Know Your Colours is an assessment tool for patients designed to capture and utilize information on unplanned care, impact of symptoms on quality of life, stroke risk, and management to improve care. Results of the quiz are then classified as "green," "yellow," or "red," with specific advice provided for each (Figure 4.5). A physician-facing side of the tool provides straightforward direction to the physician. According to designer Heather McGaw, "We envision this tool as eventually becoming a stand-alone, available at multiple touchpoints (e.g., in waiting rooms and online) and through various mediums (e.g., paper, kiosk, tablet, online)."[17]

The tool is aimed at motivating patients to work with their healthcare team to make sure they are receiving optimal treatment to prevent stroke and manage their symptoms.

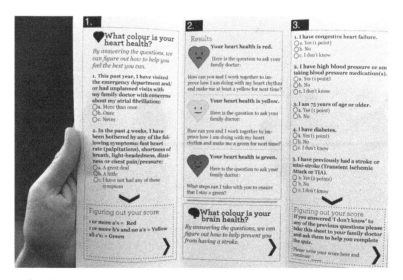

FIGURE 4.5

The Know Your Colours atrial fibrillation assessment tool (model). (Courtesy of Health Design Lab)

The HDL has adapted creative workshop processes for ideation and concept design. A cross-disciplinary brainstorming session was conducted for the patient-centered AF care problem. A team of clinicians—pharmacists, a family doctor, an emergency room physician, a nurse practitioner, and the HDL medical director—were engaged with three designers, with facilitation by clinical lead and designer McGaw.

Lori MacCallum, who is a pharmacist, assistant professor at the University of Toronto, and HDL clinical lead, produced the AF research and collaborated with McGaw on developing visually effective artifacts for the workshop and project. MacCallum's advance fact finding included a review of the medical literature and expert interviews. The findings were then distilled into key "care gaps" in the management of AF, defined as points in the patient journey where care delivery might break down or opportunities might be missed to effectively treat the person with AF. The workshop engaged clinicians in working with three key gaps:

1. Poor initial diagnostics in the emergency room for AF symptoms

2. Lack of standard process for routing AF conditions

3. Lack of consistent AF management

Personas were developed from the background research to represent each of the sub-populations of AF, such as Johnny Fit, Mary Multiple Chronic Disease, Caring Kristy, Frail Frank, and Tom, A Guy's Guy. One persona in particular was key to the process. Tom, A Guy's Guy was representative of a traditional and aging segment of the population who are not online, would never be online, and might distrust outreach programs (Figure 4.6). The program and artifact were designed to meet the most difficult of persona types, with the expectation that if persona Tom's needs could be met, the other types would be easier to meet.

The care gaps and personas provided clinical reality and structure to the brainstorming session and kept it focused on possible patient outcomes.

User segments were stuck to the wall and referred to throughout the session. The brainstorming generated roughly 100 ideas, which were reduced by group voting on concept strength and highest priority. Participants voted for their top two choices, and a consensus was reached on a starting point. The ideas were captured and displayed in a concept map and shared with participants to validate the starting point.

Based on the priorities and ideation, a self-identifying quiz was chosen as the initial HDL product for the Innovate Afib program. Various concepts were developed by the designer with content provided by the clinical team, following an iterative process of simultaneously creating and editing content while designing the information architecture. The initial version designed for patient use was defined as a paper instrument.

A Guy's Guy | Tom

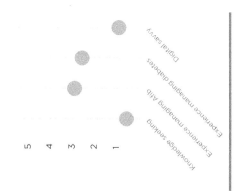

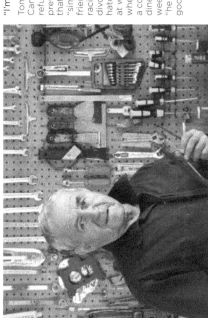

Profession: Mechanic Age: 62

"I'm not interested in taking rat poison"

Tom is a mechanic. He immigrated to Canada from Poland at age 30. Tom refuses to go on blood thinners for stroke prevention because he read somewhere that it is rat poison. He calls himself a "simple guy" and enjoys poker with his friends on the weekends, watching car racing on TV and 2 beers/night. He is divorced and does not have children. He hates technology and has been frustrated at work recently because of a new policy where he has to enter his work orders into a computer. He eats out at his favorite diner 4 nights a week, except for the weeks he sees his family doctor because "he wants his cholesterol number to be good when he does his bloodwork."

5			Knowledge seeking
4			Experience managing AFib
3			Experience managing diabetes
2			Digital savvy
1			

Key Characteristics

Identifies as a "simple guy"

Traditional

Divorced

Hates technology

Medical History

Type 2 DM

CAD

MI

AF

Medications

Atenolol 50mg OD

Metformin 1g BID

Ramipril 10mg OD

Atorvastatin 40mg OD

ASA 81mg OD

Influencers

Friends

Family doctor

Tradition

Frustrations & Pain Points

Hates technology

Resistant to blood thinners

Gets frustrated easily

FIGURE 4.6
Persona for Tom, A Guy's Guy. (Courtesy of Health Design Lab)

The HDL completed usability testing with patients in various stages of care (in-patient internal medicine, electrophysiology treatment, pain clinic treatment, and primary care). The paper version was evaluated and refined before it was designed and promoted into digital online channels (including a mobile app and online Web resource). The AF assessment tool is planned for wide use in family practices, and the HDL will continue to collect feedback and monitor its uptake.

Although baseball cards and short video documentaries may not seem like the stuff of Health 2.0, these communication tools use creative design to promote health in the larger community, simply and directly. Their lesson is to follow the needs of real people—to meet them where they live and to speak their language. This community focus does not inhibit the HDL from facilitating design for more complex, integrated healthcare issues.

Designing Healthcare Communications for All Communities

The HDL is designing tools for public use on the Web and has become far more accessible online. Evans says his patients typically see Dr. Google first and are somewhat informed when they visit his practice:

> The Health Design Lab was started to redesign the patient education experience, to make it richer, more effective. Right now, we give patients pamphlets, and that is the extent of the patient education. There is a large Dr. Google effect out there, and this marks a huge paradigm shift in medicine. Ten years ago, no one did that, and today 75% to 85% of people who visit me in the clinic are visiting Dr. Google.[18]

The resulting cultural change is that healthcare providers are now able to reach out to patients, online communities, and the public by adopting the media channels their patients and families use. If the goal is effective health communication, the means to communicate have become easier for producers and consumers, and technologies that enable sharing and listening fade into the background as human connection takes place. In fact, Evans points to the social technology of collaborative design as the most powerful tool in the HDL's work: "I would say our greatest achievements have come from the collaboratory, like partnering with a filmmaker to do digital storytelling. In Health 1.0, that might have been done with medical media, where a patient comes into the hospital and reads a script in a designed space."[19]

Produced as conventional media that is hosted online, the HDL designed videos to create a personal context for patient understanding and to help people communicate with family members or take action on their own health (Figure 4.7). The HDL recognizes that patient information seeking leads them to a wide range of information that is self-selected by the seekers. The more authentically compelling the media, the better the chance people will discover it and pay attention. According to Evans, "81% of people are going to the Web, but if you have chronic disease, it's down to 62%. The people who need it the most are not accessing the resources. Follow-up research shows that if you led them to the well, showed them how to use the resources, they were heavy users."[20]

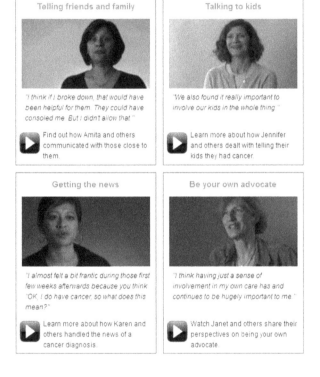

FIGURE 4.7
Health Design Lab's
"Truth of It" cancer
experience
documentaries.

To address the problem of public users finding relevant resources, the HDL's "Truth of It" series shows real people talking about their own cancer situations, empathically interviewed and presented with crisp, professional-quality video values. Viewers were found to identify with others with their condition, rather than a doctor or an actor, and personal relating was considered more likely to result in personal action. As more people discovered the series, the HDL expanded it, and it has become very popular. The videos have become embedded across multiple media channels (clinics, self-care sites, health websites) and in a variety of media modes (YouTube, Twitter, mobile apps), reflecting the different ways patients access information.

Although the HDL business model may seem uniquely Canadian, the "health design research" approach can be transferred to the United States and other locations in the form of regional health design networks and health design centers at the major research clinics. For example, Mayo Clinic's Center for Innovation operates under a mandate of enhancing care practice, redesigning medical services, and reducing process overhead through an internal core team and a large network of supporting organizations. Like the HDL, Mayo's focus is oriented to large community outreach. However, Mayo's organization has a dual mandate of internal process improvement, to which the Canadian groups are not especially dedicated. The Mayo model would be inappropriate for a hospital or regional system, but the HDL business model could be a shared-support, regional design center that assists multiple inpatient and outpatient clinics without competing between them.

The HDL and St. Michael's demonstrate that healthcare innovation can be initiated with a small group of dedicated clinical and design professionals. As their mandate has expanded, they have introduced designers from OCAD University, ethnographers and qualitative researchers from the Li Ka Shing Institute, and local design firms. As Evans explained,

> Our niche is . . . prototyping. We are not looking to become a WebMD and to have all the resources on our site to manage cancer care or diabetes care. We feel our role is more [about] bringing together the collaboratories—bringing together the different skill sets, applying a design process to that, and having an initial iterative process where we prototype a resource and then hand it back to the funder.[21]

Healthy people seek designed experiences and artifacts to enhance their appreciation of life. People facing an illness or a caregiving context may be so immersed in the constraints of the situation that their ability to recognize the possibility for a better experience may be dramatically curtailed. The provision of better experiences begins with those who deliver help and care, because they can communicate with hundreds of patients and have the chance to influence each one in a positive way. There are many opportunities for direct providers—physicians, nurses, staff—to recognize and innovate. However, clinicians have little time and no mandate for process innovation. Innovation will continue to lag efficiency and operational values unless the costs and value to practices can be credibly established. Organizations like the HDL can help build this case for the healthcare professional community by documenting applications and successes, and showing measures of improvement in treating patients earlier, good care management, and reducing return visits.

- The opportunities for healthcare service design often arise at the level of direct care, not from top-down strategy.

- Any organization serious about community outreach will benefit from design values that better leverage their investment. Even simple print and Web communications can be vastly improved to amplify their impact.

- Design teams connected to healthcare organizations are a very new trend, and there are no perfect operational models yet. The best examples are in-house designers who learn the field from within.

- The typical digital agency model is not recommended for care design because of the significant requirement to understand actual patient care and community needs.

- A vernacular design approach that communicates in plain words and simple visual communication may best reach patients and health seekers where they live and work.

- From a social perspective, underserved patients need more assistance than the well served and computer literate. A real design challenge is found in communicating simply across social and language barriers.

Methods: Tools for Agency

Three design and social research methods (among many) offer design tools for agency, practices that enable design researchers to elicit personal meaning from the perspective of the health seeker. Empathic methods aim to understand experience from a person's point of view and to relate the experience faithfully. Agentic methods dig deeply into a person's expression of meaning, their causes and passions, and may help them achieve or communicate large goals. Although these are not tools or methods for direct agency to effect change, they help researchers make an advocacy case for the agents of their studies. These approaches are inspired by social critic Ivan Illich's *Tools for Conviviality*, which advocated enabling people with "tools that guarantee their right to work with independent efficiency."[22] Video ethnography, design documentaries, and Dervin's Sense-Making Methodology return the primacy of communication to the person. While the designer organizes these methods on behalf of a project, the goal (at least directly) is not merely to optimize the system or service in which the person participates. These tools present a person's experience as closely as possible to the concerns in his or her worldview.

- **Ethnographic field observation** and contextual interviews are the fundamental basis for the following methods. Ethnography in clinical and patient settings has been covered deeply in the literature, ranging from design ethnography for patients to professional practice ethnography (including medical practice, education, and HIT).[23]

- **Video ethnography** allows the researcher to capture real-life activity with on-site interviews and recordings of everyday consumer behaviors.[24] This method allows the design and client team to construct interpretations with community participants beyond the typical recording of on-site observations.

- **Design documentaries** allow designers to create empathetic presentations of complex information scenarios as video storytelling. They are a powerful tool for attracting and educating the public about health and disease management, and they can educate and inspire large organizations to communicate compelling narratives to inspire action.

- **Dervin's Sense-Making Methodology** (SMM) is a deeply researched social sciences method for understanding human experience in learning, self-informing, and understanding another's lifeworld experience. SMM is unique in experience research because its research base supports both a methodology (the framework and philosophy) and a series of techniques for its implementation in the field.

Ethnographic Observation

Ethnography can be considered the basis for the following methods, and readers unfamiliar with ethnographic research methods might start with fundamental works[25] and apprenticing with experienced ethnographers. Skills in field research and observation must be developed with experience, and the clinical setting is no place to experiment. As a social science research method, ethnography investigates social behavior and human culture within specific settings. The traditional methods of cultural anthropology require the ethnographer to observe a culture for sufficient time to learn the norms and values of the people in that setting. For professional practice settings, or for practical design applications such as new service or IT design, more rapid and applied forms of ethnographic research have been validated.[26] Data collection is based on qualitative research practices—interviews, note taking, video, and photography. Ethnographic data is analyzed by open-ended discovery of patterns within discourses, and by mapping data to internal categories of theoretical interest to the study.

Ethnographies are often initiated by a series of observations in the setting using a framework such as POEMS, developed by Institute of Design professors Vijay Kumar and Patrick Whitney,[27] or the e-Lab's AEOUT, two well-known observation frames that guide the investigator toward meaningful and structured observations:

- POEMS (People, Objects, Environments, Messages, Services): This framework also serves as video observation tagging categories for video ethnography.

- AEOUT (Activity, Environment, Object, User, Time): The e-Lab framework provides a basis for journal recording of observations over extended periods. Entries can be categorized and mapped to any of the major category labels.

These frameworks are advance guidelines to orient observation in workplace settings, where long observation stints are often out of the question.

Video Ethnography

Video ethnography is often employed as an empathic method, lending immediacy and vivid narrative to healthcare product design by presenting the stories of real health seekers. Although video can be recorded in any situation deemed helpful for design, optimal applications involve situations where behaviors are hidden to product or clinical team members:

- A patient's experience at home, where clinicians have no access

- The experience of a person remembering and taking medications at home or work

- The experience of a diabetic managing tests and insulin kits

- The experience of a consumer in a store or clinic making choices among options, such as over-the-counter medications

Video allows a single ethnographer to document situations of use that capture the reality of everyday health concerns. Danish professor Jacob Buur's examples in *Designing with Video* show video employed as a tool for documenting experiences inaccessible to other means of research.[28] Jason Moore of Xinsight carried out a video documentary with Buur for Novo Nordisk, a Danish healthcare firm with a core business in diabetes care products. Moore reported how he was able to capture the private experiences of diabetics and share this human realism with a development team responsible for injection device design:

> As we were entering people's private lives, we decided to work through video recordings rather than bring people in direct collaboration with the design team. . . . The participants were mainly mechanical engineers who work with designing needles and injection devices. . . . The goal initially was to get to know the people in the video, and later to identify design opportunities and envision new products.[29]

Moore points out that video in itself is not sufficient. Client observers must be sensitized to understand the meaning of interactions and statements to their design decisions. A video card game was used to engage the design team in collaborating around the meaning and opportunities represented by the video experiences. Using index cards to record their own interpretations about segments of the observed video, the engineers, marketers, and other client team members contributed their ideas and concerns about the use of their products in these scenarios. This led to a more substantive anchoring of the video research than merely presenting and discussing the findings from the video ethnographer's perspective.

They noted several ways in which video ethnography informs design:

- It bridges the gap between people and patients and the designers.

- It enables designers to reconsider their view of "problems" and "solutions."

- It gives designers real-life support for design decisions.

- It provides a way to develop an ongoing story in the design process.

- It provides a clear artifact documenting the situation and its motives and relationship to the organization.

Design Documentaries

Data collected through traditional means are often dry, impersonal, uninspiring, and/or lacking context. Design documentaries are the manipulation of compiled research data, including text, video, audio, photographs, and illustrations, into a short-form video format used to inspire dialogue, locate possibilities for exploration, and further guide the design research process.[30] Their audience and use differentiate them from documentary films.

This method is useful for a discovery phase, research review, problem assessment, and early prototyping, and to instigate a deeper dive. The resulting production of design documentaries can be used as true-to-life personas and as public presentations of consumer and patient responses to new services, health practice changes, and so on.

Design documentaries were originally developed as a design research experiment by design anthropologist Bas Raijmakers,[31] but they were found useful as a method to help design teams:

- View their subjects as *people*, not just as customers (or patients).

- Better envision how their designs would impact people.

- Understand their emotional attachments to the people for whom they are designing.

- Obtain more information and details on a person's environment and on how certain events really play out in everyday life.

Design documentaries are best used when research material requires an emotional bridge between the subject and the designer. Although beneficial when presenting or reviewing research results with the design team, filmmaking preproduction considerations can help plan or strategize a user research design. (For examples, see www.designdocumentaries.com.)

Dervin's Sense-Making Methodology

Dervin's SMM comprises a meta-theory, methodology, and a series of research techniques developed by Brenda Dervin over a 30-year period of scholarly work and research development.[32] SMM affords design researchers a rigorous and descriptive method for interviewing and discerning experience patterns, while also mapping to a theoretical framework that guides analysis of participant data and assessment of its meaning.

Used correctly, the methodology provides a rich source of qualitative, experiential data. It leads to compelling understanding of the reality of human experience with technology and services, and the understanding of information behavior. SMM expands our capacity to reach deep insights from studying these experiences:

- Information seeking

- Online experiences

- The experience of learning and being a learner

- Living with difficult health situations

- Being a member of an organization or other social group

- Being a consumer of complicated services such as healthcare

Among the several schools of sensemaking theory and research, the SMM process is interpreted differently, even for similar problems. These approaches investigate how people pursue goals and make sense of events, develop mental models, and interpret data in problem solving, and how people in organizations form a collective understanding of situations.

Dervin's SMM is the only approach that integrates a method of experiential inquiry—an interview and analysis method that provides a research framework for addressing questions of the individual's encounter with resources and information in his or her negotiation of everyday complexity:

- What is the reality of people's experiences with information or systems?

- How do we interview people to understand their experience?

- How do we make critical assessments about how people make sense of and communicate their experience?

Figure 4.8 illustrates the experiential journey of a health seeker toward an intended outcome, adapted to Dervin's theory of user sensemaking. The unit of experience is the *situation*, represented by the person in her context (bubbles) and her situational starting point (represented by her position at the left, moving through life toward goals on the right). At all times she is experiencing a range of thoughts, emotions, anticipations, expectancies, urgings, and considerations. People are intentional, goal-driven actors, and Dervin's method recognizes that human experience is always in motion, and that sense is made through "verbings," or actions in the world, not by identifying information or goals as passive objects (nouns).

In line with the notion of verbing, the figure represents a person navigating the obstacles, gaps, and "muddling through" in interactions with things and resources and in pursuit of goals or outcomes. The outcome (on the right) may be one of many concurrent goals undertaken, as is typical in health seeking. Dervin's SMM examines every aspect of this journey.

Dervin describes the methodology as a way of inquiring into the authentic experience of informants from their perspective, in their own words, and related to their own purposes:

> The point is that Sense-Making aims to arrive at a useful understanding of human sense-making to be used in the design of information and communication systems and procedures. In method, then, Sense-Making asks actors if they bridged gaps and how. The how is not constrained: actors are explicitly asked what emotions they felt, what feelings they had, what ideas or conclusions they came to; and actors are asked how each of these helped and/or hindered.[33]

The neutral questioning or sensemaking interview is an empathic interview method that generates rich data for understanding individual goal-seeking, service experience, or information behavior.[34] The neutral interview is empathic in the sense that, with open and nondetermined questions, the participant is free to respond with his or her own narrative and personal context and is not constrained by the typical demands of a product-centric interview. Even in user experience, researchers typically establish a strong focus on *use* of interfaces or products, as opposed to genuine *experience* in the hermeneutic sense of personal meaning. This apparently simple set of questions probes the understanding of how an individual really thinks and responds to situations. Used correctly, it lends structure for a rigorous inquiry into the actual experience of a person in a situation.

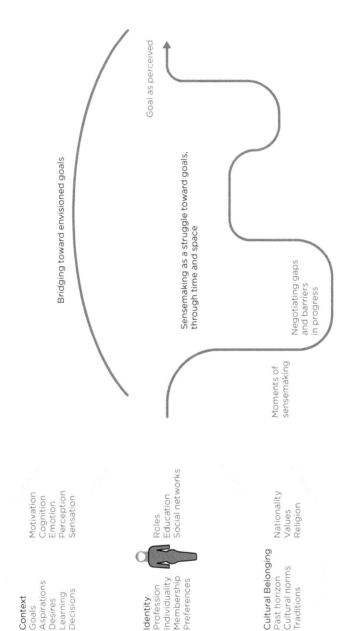

FIGURE 4.8

Sensemaking in the health-seeking context.

The interview process was designed as a neutral and general instrument, originally for librarians to interview participants (and patrons) about their information needs without biasing their responses in any way toward certain resources. These neutral questions are associated with three fields of experience of the user or participant: (1) the situation, (2) the gaps in experience, and (3) uses and helps for user intentions:

UNDERSTAND THE SITUATION

1. What brought you to this point?

2. What happened that stopped you?

3. What are you working on?

4. Where would you like to begin?

5. What aspect of this situation concerns you?

UNDERSTAND THE GAP

1. What seems to be missing for you in this situation?

2. What do you need that you do not have available?

3. What brought you to this point? What are you trying to understand?

4. What are you struggling with? How is this typical, or not?

WAYS OF SEEKING HELP

1. What services or tools are available?

2. What would help you?

3. What are you trying to do?

4. Where do you see yourself going?

5. If this could turn out any way, how would you want it?

6. How do you plan to use it?

- Situating agency is not just a social sciences approach to user research. As design researchers, we are responsible for presenting a person's life and choices in the context of their own experience and goals.

- In all contexts, method selection is critical to the research goals. Direct, in-depth, face-to-face interviews with patients help us to understand health seeking. Interviewing is the baseline method upon which others are combined.

- Video recording of (patient) health-seeking situations is not advised as a standard method. It applies when an ethnographer can gain access to real-world insights unavailable by other means. In a patient context, video recording can be experienced as intrusive and the data must be very carefully handled. Video data is typically viewed and interpreted at a later point, making it subject to meaning loss.

- Video interview methods must be reviewed for ethical concerns, presented to participants using informed consent, and the files protected by the researcher to ensure privacy agreements are met.

- A sensemaking interview approach can be integrated with formal evaluations or interactive usability sessions; however, the intentional sequence of questions should be maintained as a whole inquiry process and not intermixed at the question level.

CHAPTER 5

Patient-Centered Service Design

Elena's Story: Health Self-Service

Elena returns home to check on Ben before going back to work. Dr. Martin's office calls at 4:30 to report the lab results. Because she experienced only a "mild" faint, Elena did not get a full set of tests. Her bloodwork showed a borderline diabetes condition called prediabetes, with a fasting blood sugar level of 112 (mg sugar/per dl blood) and a glycosylated hemoglobin (A1c test) of 6%.

Her other scores are mixed, with an elevated blood pressure of 140/92 indicating hypertension, and a high TSH (thyroid-stimulating hormone) level of 6 suggesting hypothyroidism and an overworking pituitary. Dr. Martin asks her to monitor her blood pressure at home. The nurse contacts Elena's pharmacy to order the thyroid medication and a home blood pressure cuff. Elena schedules a follow-up visit in 1 month.

At home, Elena turns to websites such as Mayo Clinic and WebMD, as well as patient and health forums such as eHealthForum.com, to find information on hypertension, thyroid conditions, metabolic syndrome, and diabetes. Having multiple minor conditions troubles her, and she doesn't see a pattern. Discussions on the online communities help her understand how other people are coping with hypothyroid and what to expect of the medication. She finds wide-ranging ambiguity in interpreting the tests for thyroid conditions, but she also finds evidence from health social networks showing that people manage hypothyroid quite well with her medication.

Adding a few new health tasks to her daily routine is not a problem. As a caregiver, Elena has formed attentive daily habits while caring for her father and during the normal course of motherhood. She fills her prescription, takes her blood pressure daily, and as an outcome of her renewed attention to her health and symptoms, starts feeling better and more in control. ■

Patient Experience in Health Service

Elena assumes the identity of a patient as she accesses her right to healthcare. She has a diagnosis, medication therapy, clinical goals, and set appointments. To herself, she is not a patient, but a person seeking better health. Yet only patients have rights and legal options in the institutional system. *Patient* is a legal designation. From this point forward, Elena will be treated as a patient under care by the physician's office and by the hospital associated with her insurance policy in a health maintenance organization network.

A patient is not fully a true consumer or a "customer." Elena is not a medical market participant and is unlikely to seek another physician at this point or in future. She is expected to pursue health goals in the context of a patient and has little autonomy as a result. She could seek other treatment, end current treatment, or not follow doctor's orders, but the risks to her health and the associated risks of personal economics limit these choices. She and her physician have essentially entered a care relationship agreement. Dr. Martin is clinically responsible for Elena's physical care while under treatment, and Elena is expected to adhere to medication schedules.

These role designations are not just persona distinctions. The role makes a difference in nearly every design decision. Patients have rights to records, responses, and official communications, and to make their care decisions in clinical situations. Unfortunately, in the United States, people who self-manage their care outside the medical system have few rights to the resources of a healthcare "system." As people quickly discover, doctor's visits are often priced higher for uninsured patients than for insured patients with the same diagnosis, as offices are bound by system rules.

Cost-benefit decisions are not based on patient experience but on efficiencies and service delivery requirements. Patient *satisfaction* may be a critical measured criterion, but patient experience is not (yet) measured and integrated with service delivery.

Drivers for Service Innovation

Healthcare innovation is constrained by two structural drivers: (1) managing the *risks* of clinical services delivery for all types of patients, and (2) managing internal and network *costs*, as health services are delivered by highly regulated, shared service systems. These constraints maintain a focus on incremental, sustaining innovations at best, as opposed to radical (service) innovation. Regional healthcare systems cannot be disruptive in such an operating environment. They are the institutions that new services seek to disrupt.

With regulated or insurance-driven pricing, institutions are incentivized to grow large enough to distribute costs across their system and to raise sufficient capital for specialists and equipment. Hospitals invest in state-of-the-art facilities to attract practitioners and increase community visibility. But these drivers do not necessarily have a direct impact on the quality of care. Every institution claims a high quality of care. Yet quality of care can refer to many different measures. The Agency for Healthcare Research and Quality certifies four standards. The Joint Commission certifies 14 quality measures in its standards for National Hospital Inpatient Quality. These are outcome measures that reflect many different inputs. The measure of innovation is not as simple in healthcare as in other service industries. Successful innovation in mobile telephony can be measured by market share and adoption, as well as customer delight. Successful innovation in healthcare might actually be measured by improvements in critical safety and cost measures, as well as patient satisfaction. But the contribution of innovation is one of many factors in a complex sociotechnical system.

Many large US institutions innovate by acquisition. Large hospitals have the luxury of investing in differentiating equipment and facilities, such as the million-dollar da Vinci laparoscopic surgery system for minimally invasive surgeries. In clinics, acquisitions provide a path for innovating at the scale of service provision, allowing an institution to capture leadership in a service area. Acquisitions are "tangible," as are certain investments in health IT (HIT); electronic health records, patient portals, and customer-facing websites increase and enhance patient experience touchpoints.

Yet HIT, merely acquired and not effectively integrated with service, can backfire. Information and interfaces are integral parts of a sociotechnical system—the social system that organizes work and tools into a meaningful function in an organization. When technological systems are merely "installed" into complex operations, social practices change to adapt. If the systems are not integrated well, entire system installations can be rejected at great administrative cost. Health service design facilitates the effective synthesis of clinical practice and organizational routines with new technology to improve internal or customer-facing operations.

The concept of innovation is often introduced in the form of equipment, devices, and new medical techniques. The value of service innovation can be difficult for managers to quantify and visualize. Redesigning processes and practices to improve patient experience can be viewed as less tangible and harder to measure. Service-level innovations such as patient experience enhancements or even improved wayfinding are more difficult to quantify and justify using the standard metrics of cost accounting.

This leads us to patient experience. Healthcare systems have not had to innovate the provision of service as a competitive function because end customers (patients) have had little power of choice over hospitals or services in a referral-based care system. However, with US healthcare reform, patients will have more choice, and service innovation will become a significant driver. More recently, some hospitals have adopted a service design approach to the coordination of patients and care within the institution. More institutions are expressing interest in understanding and measuring factors of the patient experience.

In the United States, new organizational models such as the accountable care organization and patient-centered medical homes encourage providers to form sustainable and independent practices closer to their communities. Though these localized clinics may not be innovative at first, they have more incentive to create localized or personalized patient services for complex care. A decentralized organizational form enables an entirely new range of services. Providing a single patient concierge across specialty providers or creating cross-network care teams will be possible.

Improved organizational capacity is critical, as new roles will be integrated and perhaps led by service designers. Service innovation still requires clinical staff, IT, and project managers. But the processes and methods may be quite unfamiliar to clinicians and managers at first.

Making Healthcare Innovation Tangible

The right design can help heal. Architectural projects and physical environments are measurable, accountable as assets, and serve as focal points. Evidence-based architectural studies have demonstrated that simple design changes to buildings, rooms, and patient areas provide an immediate positive impact on patient health and family experience.

Clinical improvements may not be recognized by patients, even if care service is entirely patient focused. Medical environments are quite opaque. Patients receiving poor care or unnecessary but expensive procedures have a limited ability to compare. Respect for professionals keeps people from judging their own physicians negatively. In a recent case, investigators at St. Joseph's Medical Center in Towson, Maryland, discovered that the hospital's peer review process failed to uncover more than 150 unnecessary coronary stents implanted under direction of the chief of the cardiac catheterization unit. Even after more than 600 former patients of the cardiologist were notified of the problem, most patients tended to believe the physician had done nothing wrong, and many were convinced that the stent procedure had saved their lives. Although an objective review might suggest this case was a dangerous and unethical violation of good service, most of the patient customers did not recognize this, and many were unwilling to accept the truth. This case shows how healthcare services have become too complex for the patient to assess risk.

Patients face information asymmetry and cannot make free decisions about care alternatives. Patients are not expected to fully understand the different procedures that may be available for a treatment. Although statistical risks and possible outcomes can be explained to patients, clinics usually follow a standard set of procedures. Physicians may choose the techniques they know best and can perform reliably and safely. The design issue is to tangibly help patients get better, which involves a mix of directed activities. Physicians may advise qualitatively different treatments and tests, such as lifestyle remedies for sleep disorders instead of anti-insomnia drugs. The health outcomes of lifestyle changes depend entirely on health seeker choices, which places initiative on the patient. We would be too optimistic to think that people will self-manage effectively—most people need strong support, which is something we can design.

Personalized service will grow, funded at first by differential health plans. Personalizing clinical service means regular and personal communication, concierge-style management of referrals and tests, and personalized care approaches. Care plans and pathways for unique disease conditions may be supported by clear presentation and patient education. The case study in this chapter provides an example of tailoring care pathways to accommodate individual differences in complex care.

Good Care Is a Moral Issue

Healthcare is one of the largest service industries across the world's economies, but unlike most services, health *care* is an essential resource of modern life. It is institutionalized and in most nations managed as a public service, both as a public good and a natural monopoly. Health seekers are patients and not "care consumers" because they cannot self-inform sufficiently to make informed decisions among alternatives.

Cognitive science has argued and won this point. Humans are biased and irrational when making significant decisions, even when fully informed with the facts. Prospect theory, Daniel Kahneman and Amos Tversky's Nobel Prize–winning thesis, demonstrated how people consistently overweight the prospect of possible losses and undervalue potential gains in considering decision-making outcomes.[1] Called *loss aversion*, the theory shows that the emotional significance of a life or death decision, and the immediacy of the decision, place consumers in a weak position with respect to economic decisions that concern their health. Patients are likely to overweight the risks and undervalue potential alternatives. Because physicians are bound by the duty of care to recommend the safest effective treatment, patients may not hear about alternatives. Reconciling loss aversion into service design is a balancing act that challenges our ability to design better patient experiences. If we lived in a world of free economic choice and information equality, health seekers would be capable and confident of choosing nonmedical health alternatives, whether complementary or radical.

From a service perspective, patients are unique customers in this regard—they are discouraged from asserting agency. Patients are by definition subject to doctors' orders and are even more vulnerable to the market power of healthcare policy. When the means to deliver resources for health restoration are concentrated in commercial interests, the opportunity arises to exploit the dire need and motivation of patients. Physicians are expected to be trusted advocates for health seekers, and most by far are honest brokers. Yet physicians are targeted by commercial operators as spokespersons for new and profitable drugs or for tests and procedures that they have the singular power to order and potentially profit from.

The regulatory system and rules of engagement have been layered into existence by private providers and insurance regulations for more than 50 years. Makers of healthcare products are merely seeking return on investment as actors in a healthcare service market. At the national scale, however, selling biological human needs to benefit corporate interests creates an economic moral hazard. In more complicated health scenarios, a single patient may trigger payment events in every one of the many touchpoints in a health-seeking journey—for examinations, medications, tests, and procedures. Today it is only too easy to monetize each touchpoint.

Advocates for caring healthcare services find the entire private healthcare system model to be unavoidably unethical, as the goals of the service providers and their end customers are permanently in structural opposition. Individuals are unable to change the system or even their role; they can only choose to remain in the healthcare system or leave it.

A Systemic Design of Health Service

There is no single service line of business in healthcare, no true end-to-end service provision. Unlike in other service sectors, such as banking or travel, the customer–provider relationship is multistage and diffuse. Its customers have a special legal relationship as patients, a designation that enables access to multiple encounters within a system of services. There may be no *end point* of service fulfillment, because managing health is an iterative and ongoing process. The value proposition of medical care is the most compelling offer on the planet: Every human being seeks health. And human health is uniquely manifested in every person's experience and history, due to personal practice, history, environment, genetics, and interaction with infectious or viral agents.

The healthcare industry is widely diffused across business, government, and social sectors in the United States and Canada. An infinite expanse of touchpoints and interfaces can be identified or created for services innovation and improved design across the providers and networks for the different needs of care. For business and social service innovation, the opportunities are indeed endless. Yet these conditions also prevent innovations from scaling widely. There are no natural national populations of consumer service in healthcare, even in national healthcare systems such as Great Britain's National Health Service (NHS). Different age and social groups have very different needs, and not all health needs are served in the same way or equally across geographies and societies.

Public healthcare (e.g., the NHS and each Canadian province system) may enable more opportunities for *systemic innovation* than the sprawling network of providers and payers in privatized systems. Systemic institutional innovation has high social and commercial impact, as changes to processes can theoretically affect any patient and provider. A technological innovation may only impact its clinical users and the types of patients that benefit from its application.

In the loosely coupled private system, investments in institutional innovation will only pay off for the hospital or system. Among a growing number of other critical expenses to consider, service innovation experiments are difficult to justify, even in terms of patient experience. Patients do not have the explicit choice of selecting an inpatient care facility; their physicians and coverage determine their affiliated clinic.

In a publicly supported system, however, an effective service advance can be trialed and validated, migrated to other institutions, and scaled to the regional or national level. One popular service improvement is reducing wait times in emergency rooms or special clinics (e.g., dialysis treatment). Although these service experiments are also sponsored by and conducted at single institutions, in public systems there are no competitive barriers to the diffusion of effective practice innovations to other locations.

Public funding not only maintains a single regulation control for costs and quality, but establishes a common client and funding source for research and system improvements. Healthcare service innovations from other countries and systems, where public costs *must* be saved, have assessed and published solutions to many common problems, such as wait times and care pathways. However, innovations do not pass between systems well; they are often restricted or at least not promoted outside the system.

Sociotechnical Services

Healthcare service redesign is an institutional-level process, which affords some possibilities for change but limits many others. Institutions change slowly, and organizations within them tend to maintain routines until they are proven less effective than alternatives. Work practices coordinating professional care are complex, and knowledge becomes embedded in practice, which is not easily changed. IT is slowly adopted, and rapid or agile practices are not yet integrated into most institutional IT practices.

Designers have to become part of the system to effect lasting change. There will be a growing need for integrated services design as the new healthcare organization forms build out. Architects and planners are today's default design principals, but in the new organizations much more attention will be needed in organizational design, IT integration, and patient and community services. An entirely new type of design leader is called for.

These complex practices and institutions may require us to develop a different methodology for service design. Though we may treat healthcare as a service sector, the practices are sociotechnical systems, as found in education, energy, and security. The sociotechnical system is a social sciences perspective recognizing the interdependent organization of work practices, roles, tools, and technology. The goal of a sociotechnical system design is to integrate "the social requirements of people doing the work with the technical requirements needed to keep the work systems viable with regard to their environments."[2] As a whole social system, partial process solutions or policies can upset the optimal workflow established over time. Healthcare research and cases are rife with stories of disastrous IT installations that fail due to organizational practices and not usability.

Sociotechnical systems offer a research approach to the complex challenge of service redesign. Healthcare practices are seeking to integrate digital technologies and health records systems, and reduce cost overhead while providing better care to larger communities. Many so-called transformation programs have failed in the last decade because of the predictable systemic effects of social practices overcoming the best hopes of new technology or policy changes. In institutional healthcare (if not the consumer world), the service system is a sociotechnical system. Design proposals are supported and integrated by planned research cycles.

Sociotechnical systems in healthcare are organized at the topmost level by the common service delivery model of three clinical systems (in North America): inpatient, outpatient, and emergency. These are further organized by the functions provided by different clinical units or wards. Table 5.1 lists representative structures for three institutional types.

TABLE 5.1 THREE INSTITUTIONAL TYPES

Hospital	Hospital/office	Specialized center
Inpatient	Ambulatory/outpatient	Emergency; special; long-term
Acute and critical care	Examinations and tests	Long-term care facilities
Intensive care units	Chronic care	Ambulatory care
Elective surgery	Simple procedures	Pediatric care
Emergency	Outpatient surgery	Neighborhood clinics

Harvard professor and physician Richard Bohmer describes two basic healthcare "operating systems" that drive service and facility design models: the *sequential* and the *iterative* systems.[3] These models can be seen as the end points of a spectrum instead of two distinct operational models.

Two different sets of service conditions are organized: *sequential*, for efficiently delivering standard care services to a large volume of patients; and *iterative*, when an ideal care pathway may not be known for the condition or patient. The essential structural differences are listed in Table 5.2.

TABLE 5.2 SEQUENTIAL AND ITERATIVE SERVICES

	Sequential	Iterative
Mission	Efficient delivery of known solution	Evaluation and management of complex care for difficult problems
Beliefs and values	An ideal exists	Ideal state is unknowable
	Uncertainty is reduced before care	Uncertainty is reduced during care
Scope of service	Narrow	Diversified
	Higher capacity (throughput)	Lower capacity
Processes	Standardized	Nonstandard, or no protocols
	Assembly-line model	Job shop approach
Management policy	Centralized	Decentralized
	Broad span of control	Narrow span of control
	Reduced variation in performance	Improvements learned by variation
Human resources	Conforming, conservative employees	Problem-solving experimenters
	Repetitive tasks	Development of new variations
Technology	Specialized	General purpose

Adapted from R. M. J. Bohmer. (2009). *Designing care: Aligning the nature and management of health care.* Boston: Harvard Business Press.

The primary guideline is between the assembly-line efficiencies of routine care and "job shop" iterative processes for complex situations. Both of these modes call for different innovation models—incremental for sequential and exploratory for iterative. Sequential healthcare services can be improved incrementally, not radically, minimizing the risk in introducing variation to established organizational routines.

However, iterative healthcare is necessary for complex, multicondition, and unusual situations. Complex care requires multidisciplinary medical attention, rapid exploration and research, hypothesis testing, sensemaking, and multiple evaluations. If these activities seem to be defined as design process steps, this may reflect the underlying function of design and complex healthcare as logical problem-solving processes. In the same way that the scientific method supports deductive experimentation, the design process enables iterative problem solving with mixed reasoning strategies.

Due to the risks of coordination of procedures and communications, care innovations are designed as incremental innovations or changes within a well-understood sociotechnical system. Incremental innovation is not a bad thing. The goal of designing for care, especially in routine care, is to promote better health outcomes, not to improve business performance. Cost management is important, but managing complex patient care with safety and reliability is still the purpose, not creating new economic value.

Care Service Models

A practice can be designed to support a range of service types along the continuum from sequential to iterative, yet few facilities manage all types equally well. These service bundles represent different business models, as different value propositions are provided (primary purposes), and allocations of clinician roles, time, and shared services are needed for each variation. Cost and efficiency trade-offs must be made when integrating several models of care into the same facility, possibly with compromises in quality that would be unnoticed by patients. Simple examples of these types are shown in Table 5.3.

TABLE 5.3 MODES OF CARE IN THE SEQUENTIAL-ITERATIVE SPECTRUM

	Sequential	Sequential plus follow-up	Continuous	Iterative
Primary purposes	Screening Examinations	Single disease Well-known protocols and treatment	Multiple chronic diseases Common chronic "clusters"	Complex diseases Unusual protocols
Care mode examples	Flu shots	Type 2 diabetes with multiple therapies	Congestive heart failure, diabetes	Complex cancers
System mode	Primary care office	In-store clinic Urgent care center	Primary care Inpatient hospital care	Academic center Special clinic
Service design focus	Communications enhancement	Workflow and productivity	Treatment flow Care pathways	Personalized problem solving

Four service design approaches (bottom row) match the different mix of iterative/sequential care modalities. For sequential care such as public health outreach (flu shots) and conventional office visits, enhancing communications and access to care are typical design options.

Redesigning the provision of service is done incrementally. Service in the sequential care modes can be enhanced by direct *design* improvements, ranging from staff and patient workflow to specialized IT resources such as local electronic medical records and dictation transcription.

Continuous and iterative care demand a multidisciplinary innovation approach consistent with sociotechnical systems. Costs and errors increase with the complexity of multiple disease conditions and complications. Productive innovation opportunities are found in evaluating effective care pathways for complex care. Clinical care pathways are management guidelines for patient care for predictable, multidisciplinary clinical encounters wherein interventions are well defined and sequenced.

Care pathways are preferred organizational processes for care service, represented as flowcharts or decision trees indicating the different conditions, measures, referrals, and clinical choices available in a given disease scenario. These pathway models, or "algorithms," describe a preferred methodology for case services for a known disease condition. The most advanced example of a care pathway system is the Map of Medicine (www.mapofmedicine.com), currently used by NHS providers as a service redesign support tool. These maps are proprietary, but a representation of a common pathway application is depicted in Figure 5.1.

Customized and iterative care is expensive to carry out and difficult to justify in many institutions with factory health business models. Custom care pathways may require full-time, flexible professional staff not assigned to other services, and well-coordinated practices for optimizing patient situations and rapid clinical problem solving. Consider Elena's care pathway, which is unfolding as a conventional cardiac arrhythmia situation. But if her thyroid condition worsens and her metabolic syndrome intensifies into Type 2 diabetes, the convergence of multiple chronic conditions would escalate her risk, and these three (or more) disease processes would have interacting consequences. Without her taking personal agency to improve her well-being, her multiple conditions would trigger a customized care plan and specialized care team treatment.

These are not workflow situations but complex human system problems. Iterative care may require consults with specialists and multiple tests, running a risk of multiple interpretations and treatment trials. Practitioners also have access to specialized resources to help guide decisions. But the interaction of conditions requires research beyond the canonical cases, where expert intuition and experience make all the difference in decision making. As the developed world's population ages, cases of multiple chronic illnesses will become more common. To deal with the sheer volume, society will invest in a better approach—a sociotechnical services design.

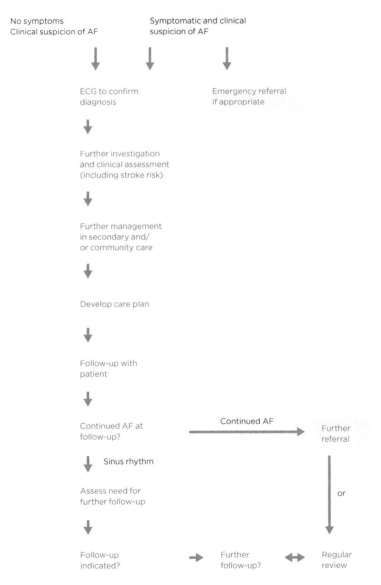

FIGURE 5.1
Care pathway for atrial fibrillation (AF).

Care delivery is not yet designed as a service offering, and there are no design practices yet for healthcare service systems. Care processes are first designed as clinical protocols, "designed" by specialized multidisciplinary clinician teams in committee processes. Clinical data tools and artifacts such as nursing shift change documentation, care plans, procedure protocols and checklists, patient data, and interview questionnaires are created by senior interprofessional teams, but without the benefit of visual design or sensemaking support.

There are significant opportunities for design thinking in this critical care process. Designers want to see iterative changes in the designed environment to sustain ideation and refine systems based on use feedback. Yet even so, prototyping and visualizing nonmedical services is quite simple compared with mapping clinical care pathways and medical decisions in a hospital or health system. Designers must acquire a much deeper level of domain knowledge to be effective than is expected in other service areas.

Evidence-Based Service Design

Inpatients spend most of their time during hospital treatment and recovery in a bed, often in a shared room. It might be obvious to anyone who has visited a hospital room that the experience of resting and waiting in this sterile, artificial environment could be greatly improved. The everyday experience of the inpatient constitutes encounters with the physical environment—from building architecture to room layout and furniture—and the presentation of services within a hospital and specialized clinics. Most of these environments leave a lot to be desired, and designed.

What if it could be proven that people heal demonstrably faster and better in beautiful, well cared for physical environments? Architecture professor Roger Ulrich's research into the direct beneficial health effects of natural and harmonious surroundings during care provides hard evidence to support this theory.

Ulrich's 1984 article "View through a Window May Influence Recovery from Surgery" was the first scientific recognition of the capacity of nature to accelerate healing in the clinical environment.[4] Taking a patient-centric perspective, Ulrich demonstrated that natural scenes and emotionally supportive artwork facilitate significantly faster recovery and shorter hospital stays. Living plants and natural scenery produced the best results. Artwork content, not quality, makes an empirical difference. Scenes of nature, placid landscapes, and animals measurably quickened the healing process.

Ulrich also formulated the theory of *supportive design*, proposing that healthcare environments can improve outcomes directly by promoting stress reduction, buffering, and coping.[5] Chronic stress severely limits the rate of recovery and delays the release of patients in acute and critical care. Supportive design focuses on the physical and interactive characteristics of the hospital to reduce the occurrence or impact of stressors such as intrusions, constant noise, loud or unwanted sounds, and cluttered or sterile visual fields. There are a multitude of passive service touchpoints for increasing comfort, ease, and even intimacy. The conventional models of systems workflow in service processes can be detailed to show anticipated patient sensitivity and responses to touchpoints (both figurative and literal points).

Evidence for Design

Ulrich's research originated evidence-based design (EBD) in the early 1980s, which started in hospital architecture and expanded to care processes, practice interventions, and device design. As in evidence-based medicine, the current "best evidence" in literature and practice is recruited to support decision making, with the explicit goal of optimizing defined health outcomes in measurable terms.

Evidence-based medicine relies on the highest appropriate standard of evidence for a clinical decision. The cultural and regulatory adoption of evidence-based medicine has created an environment of risk reduction that demands a similar clinical standard of evidence for any research-based decision, including IT or services. For well-known diseases, the randomized clinical trial (with blind control and experimental conditions) represents the "gold standard" of evidence. Needless to say, that standard does not apply in design research. But it conditions the culture in which design decisions are made.

What is the appropriate level of research rigor for design decisions for health? A major goal of EBD is to ensure research is transparent and replicable, so that other institutions can learn from the study. A secondary aim is that of communicating the effectiveness of service design and research methodologies through institutional research, demonstrating validity and appropriate applications in the professional literature.

The interface of a health records system could be measured not only through formative usability testing but for its actual performance in clinical service. Progressive hospitals with strong informatics departments, such as the Children's Hospital of Philadelphia, measure and track patient outcomes as a hard metric to determine the degree to which defined health measures are improved by their IT investment. If design research methods remain proprietary or applied only as commercial engagements, the value of design-led research will not be fulfilled on a wider scale.

EBD is not just the gathering of user research to inform design decisions, as in a user-centered design process. It is a rigorous equivalent to the careful application of scholarly evidence in informing care decisions, and generally includes the following activities:

- Reviewing current and retrospective research to identify precedents, mature findings, and prescriptive guidance from relevant studies

- Prioritizing and balancing the literature basis with primary data collected from actual patient data, subject matter experts, and professional observations

- Advancing theories and hypotheses to support observations, and structuring evaluations to test outcomes of design decisions

- Measuring outcomes after implementation, and assessing theory validity and any gap between observations and hypotheses

What Evidence Counts in User Experience?

Few design disciplines face the risk position of architecture and device design in health institutions. Devices must be approved by US Food and Drug Administration review committees, and architects certify their designs and are responsible for the plans followed by builders. Software user interfaces designed for standard operating systems are not subject to equivalent certification. Does it make sense for UX design to adopt evidence-based principles in healthcare?

Design trade publications and UX blogs show growing interest in EBD. The typical claims made for evidence (largely qualitative) do not build credibility when evidence is merely based on user observations. Usability testing is an essential evaluation method, and is especially useful when applied across the installation life cycle of HIT.[6] Yet usability testing cannot measure health outcomes, only user inputs and responses to interactive systems. In a sociotechnical context, it is supplemental but not sufficient evidence. The quality of evidence for assessing interaction design relies on the behavioral measures of task completion, error rates, and time on task. User satisfaction and, occasionally, learning rate measures are collected as evidence for design decision making. Yet no websites make the claim of improving one's life and health following the interaction.

Through iterative research on prototyped sociotechnical systems, better design can demonstrate outcomes based on measures of patient health. Measuring outcomes in response to service change requires longitudinal tracking of patients across cohorts large enough to measure an aggregate difference. This is unlike any process in Web or interaction design. It suggests a gap in health service design research methods. When lives, liability, and dollars are at risk, the due diligence of quantified evidence is necessary to ensure decisions are supportable across the organization.

Evidence for Design Outcomes

In medical practice, scholarship, care planning, and design decisions, "evidence" differs significantly—not only the types of evidence, but its definition and collection, quality evaluation, controls, presentation, and publication. For clinical decision making, typically accepted evidence ranges from randomized controlled trials (gold standard) to expert studies (weak), including a variety of types of evidence (observations, imaging, measured variables) relevant to diseases, biological responses, and applications to procedures, interventions, and public health.

Traditional operational studies rely on "outcome measures," but the measures taken often assume a causality between interventions and outcomes—a causality that may not always exist in a complex reality. Some clinics invest heavily in biostatistics research to infer outcomes associated with interventions, a complex but increasingly necessary undertaking. Evidence by type—from more to less rigorous—might include:

1. Controlled human interaction experiments; mixed-method studies (triangulated methods).

2. Patient observations; physiological measures; field experiment data (strong empirical).

3. Robust sampled ethnographic data; controlled usability interaction studies (empirical).

4. Small sample interviews; "hard" (rigorous, evidence-based) case study; extrapolations from field research.

5. Expert opinion; heuristic or multiperspective assessment.

With the growth of the Web and the number of people needed to build it, the UX field has expanded well beyond the original human factors community that started the field. The widespread adoption of "user experience" glossed over many of the original distinctive differences between practices. Although this merger has gained a broader acceptance of the practice, this general acceptance is less relevant in high-hazard, high-reliability settings. Today research professionals constitute an ever-shrinking proportion of the field. A different "standard of care" is necessary when designing a system for clinical professionals or patients rather than for consumers.

EBD established a rigorous research methodology for healthcare applications understood in principle by practitioners. But not every informatics user interface or health website requires strong EBD validation. An insistence on EBD standards in the early stages of a design program could significantly inhibit the innovation value from exploratory research. Allow formative design and organizational learning to at least reach a stage of development where summative evaluation on prototypes and service concepts makes sense.

Service Design for Care

Is the healthcare industry a pure service sector? Nearly every interaction—direct care, informatics, insurance processes—is part of a larger service system. Even clinical devices, ranging from medication infusion pumps to MRI scanners, exist within a high-touch service system with standard procedures. To be adopted or even meaningful, HIT innovations require integration into the context of a service system.

Almost any durable device or medical product is part of a procedure that delivers the product's value as a clinical or patient service. Every touchpoint in a clinical encounter represents a direct human service or a "surrogate" service. Hospital rooms, communications, nursing, treatment, even billing are services that can be improved by better design. Medications are not merely delivered to pharmacists and hospitals for patient use; they are highly staged services within an entire pharmaceutical industry ecosystem, physician understanding, and a prescription system.

Devices, medications, and even informatics systems attempt to disrupt service as minimally as possible in order to enhance adoption and minimize training, usage error, and liability. Changing routines in healthcare is not a trivial matter. The problem is not so much one of institutional barriers to improvement as it is one of committing a complex organization to a procedural change that risks new errors incurred by communication and coordination issues.

A Service Design Methodology for Healthcare

Can a service design methodology help clinical teams glue together fragmented experiences for a better healthcare experience? Design theorists John Rheinfrank and Shelley Evenson articulated how services were becoming experiences, and that design would evolve toward the flow of service experience. The aim of design for service was seen as "moving from 'user-centered' design of things to 'ability-centered' co-construction of meaningful experiences."[7] The foretold shift from a service to an experience economy will eventually inspire changes in healthcare. Children's hospitals are perhaps the current leaders in "staging experiences" for their patients, building colorful, fantasy-inspired atriums and play areas to create a fun and welcoming environment to distract from and offset the inpatient experience.

Modern service design offers a framework of methods for healthcare services, albeit one in which design is still seeking a perfect fit to practice. According to Birgit Mager, design professor and founder of the Service Design Network, service design thinking "addresses the functionality and form of services from the perspective of clients. It aims to ensure that service interfaces are useful, usable, and desirable from the client's point of view, and effective, efficient, and distinctive from the supplier's point of view."[8]

Dubberly and Evenson saw services design evolving into complex experiences and systems, beyond client and user-centeredness.[9] They propose *designing for services* by creating design languages for new service design. A design language provides a coordinating architecture for guiding the brand and process design and the ongoing evolution of a service project well beyond an immediate engagement. Design languages coordinate the provision of resources for co-creating value, the "staging of experiences," whereby services actually touch the human experience of their interaction.[10]

Service design has developed well beyond the baseline of UX methods to multipoint service offerings and the creation of intangible value, such as positive emotional experience. Published service methodologies lead with a wide array of UX and adapted design methods. Yet little consensus is found across design disciplines with respect to service models in healthcare and, in particular, evaluation methods and standards of evidence. This matters because service design recommends specific methodologies for redesign of service processes but is primarily design-led, not research-led, and breaks from evidence-based tradition. The new modes of service design could be problematic in healthcare, or at best may focus on ineffectual changes and potentially slow the opportunity for healthcare service design.

For the past 40 or 50 years, service industries have traditionally relied on strong analytical methods, systems analysis, and operations research to make business-led design decisions for complex services. Yet healthcare is too complex to rely on just one field or methodology exclusively. No single school of design thinking is sufficiently comprehensive to be effective in all complex situations.

Service design aims to both enhance a consumer's experience of the provider while also optimizing the design of service delivery and business transactions. But healthcare is neither transactional nor consumer-oriented, and the standard of evaluation (or care) is necessarily different than the standard for banking or travel planning. The rigorous research and evaluation of EBD might be considered the "standard of care" by which process changes are measured and claimed to be valid. UX and service design do not generally follow or publish scientific methodology in their delivery, as the risks for mistakes or system breakdown are not so hazardous in most domains.

Due to the high internal costs of clinical work, many of the technical efficiencies possible in clinical delivery have been identified, evaluated, and optimized. In clinical practice, the performance of a procedure is conducted thousands of times over, and technical inefficiencies have been driven out. This does not mean that the processes are perfected or even maximally effective, but more that the motivations for process change, being primarily regulatory or economic, have been satisfied or even optimized. Making further changes on behalf of patient experience is a new driver, and one with potential costs and risks. But these changes should not be merely branding or decorative in nature—positive health outcomes depend on deep knowledge of human physiology and behavior. Health services can link functions from the individual health seeker to the organizational level to radically improve service and the experience of care.

A Design Language for Care Service

A service is fulfilled when a change in condition is registered by the person receiving the output of an economic activity—a customer-supplier relationship. In designing for health, facilitating the effective change of a health condition is the primary goal. But no single design approach will serve and satisfy every service requirement. Not only are different methods necessary for the different types of healthcare modes and types of patients, but different philosophies, schools of methods, and consultation approaches are necessary for different service problems.

What is the target of service design? Is it the service clients expect? Is it a system platform for service delivery? The service systems view, according to IBM's Jim Spohrer and service theorist Paul Maglio, defines service systems as "dynamic value co-creation configurations of resources (people, technology, organizations, and shared information)."[11] These configurations create complex, nonlinear, socially organized processes. They are sociotechnical systems by another name. Service systems promote a strong focus on *value co-creation*, the proposition that value realized by the customer results from both the service offering and the customer's interaction and use. The customer (the health seeker) is considered the source of value, and the interface with the service offer is where most of the designable value occurs. This service-oriented logic has the potential to change the institutional model as new healthcare organization forms are planned and, yes, designed.

A design language for sociotechnical services design might be evolved for healthcare. The drivers for a language (or just as well, a process model) are clear—creating better patient experiences for lifelong health value, enhancing clinical coordination at the appropriate scales of organization, reducing medical errors, and saving costs. A design language would enable us to form new service ecologies, integrating environments, processes, clinical functions, and HIT, and to integrate the capabilities in design to align with the life cycle of the health seeker.

Table 5.4 suggests a design language framework based on the Rheinfrank and Evenson concept. A specific set of design options and placements would be constructed for a given service. Here the basis of a service design model for co-producing health value is expressed in terms of the sociotechnical system elements necessary in a clinical application.

TABLE 5.4 A SOCIOTECHNICAL SERVICE DESIGN LANGUAGE

Service levels	Design intent	Service design elements

Health seeker:
  Inpatient
  Outpatient
  Advocate
	Enable realization of health value proposition	Public and media awareness, communications
		
		On-site education
		
		Online content, video stories

Patient–communications interface	Enable awareness of health information	Online content resources Community media design
Patient–management interface	Enable enduring care relationship with organization	Direct correspondences Surrogate relationship tokens (e.g., free homecare kits)
Patient–clinical interface	Direct care service relationship	Health service experience Care planning Exam room and procedures Touchpoints: equipment, devices, tools, manner, process

Clinical care team:
  Primary physician
  Nurse lead
  Staff clinicians
  Pharmacist
  Residents, etc.
	Develop strategic and procedural clinical abilities and resources for care service	Socialization and team learning
		
		Continuing education
		
		Role development
		
		Personnel selection
		
		Care planning

Clinical–management interface	Enable design of resilient care services	Care planning Practice coordination Transparent accounting
Clinical–information interface	Enable effective clinical data, information, and knowledge management	Access and usability Function and fit to service Strategic fit to practice Clinicians and patients
Patient–life cycle interface	Enable lifelong health habits and care activities	Caring aftercare Ongoing relationship
Patient–care circle interface	Enable full life-cycle care after clinical services	Educating patients
Patient–payer interface	Enable seamless billing and coverage	Communication design

The service design language represents an initial formulation of what Richard Buchanan called *placements*, positions where designed artifacts or intangible services are located in the flow of use. The designer is left to choose how to best create the placement: whether to make self-health booklets, a website, a personal relationship, or an e-mail campaign. For clinical procedures, the practicing physician would set the constraints, but a service design might identify related "touchpoints," such as communications or room treatments, that facilitate a better experience.

Referring back to Figure II.1, we can map the design language elements as guides to placement along Elena's patient journey. Her health seeking proceeds from being a family caregiver to having her first incident and her navigation of the health system for diagnosis and treatment. Her first touchpoints (primary care) are the examination and first orders at her doctor's practice and her exchanges with friends about the hypothyroid medicine. As her awareness shifts to the need for self-care, her information seeking and communication paths become open to a wider range of information opportunities. Though conventional clinical processes would serve her well, the quality of care could be evaluated and enhanced along every dimension. This approach is defined by the Design 2.0 approach to service design—engaging clients and patients-as-users in rethinking care as a patient-centered service experience.

A Clinical Design 3.0 approach rethinks the patient experience as a continuity, integrated across organizations to facilitate full life-cycle care. Design 3.0 innovates by organizational transformation to plan changes in management, business models, and services to fulfill an envisioned value proposition. Whereas a single organization would improve care within its boundaries, an integrated practice can collaborate in a service system capable of integrating the primary, ambulatory, outpatient, and inpatient life cycle of Elena's health-seeking journey.

DESIGN BEST PRACTICES

- Patient-centered design attempts to address all the touchpoints health seekers encounter, from medical care and medications to management and communications.

- The most complex design challenge is configuring end-to-end service centered around the health seeker. Today care is treated as a series of discrete events managed by different clinical offices. Advising, diagnostics, treatment, medication, and preventive care are not integrated.

- Clinical service redesign today is led by practices. Service design provides a framework for full participation across roles in the design of better processes and patient touchpoints.

- Become familiar with (and know how to select) multiple methods to ensure the best fit to a client problem.

Case Study: Patient-Centered Care Innovation

Much good work in healthcare service design is being done in European and Canadian jurisdictions. But we cannot easily translate service design solutions developed for a given national system. Ontario is starting to adapt the accountable care organization model from the United States for community care practices. But could the United States adapt Canadian clinical service design?

The Canadian system has some advantages from a service design perspective. A superior process can be taken from prototype to scale at the provincial level by evaluating its validity and efficacy in a service setting. This would be a challenge in the United States, where each "system" or major medical center manages its own processes and is not beholden to a larger system.

Public health becomes "more public" when a single funder can take regulatory responsibility for local or regional public health emergencies, vaccination or flu shot campaigns, and public messages to help inhibit the spread of infectious diseases or airborne pathogens.

Center for Innovation in Complex Care

Toronto's Center for Innovation in Complex Care (CICC) is an institutional start-up, an innovation network formed among practitioners and researchers in Toronto's University Hospital Network, Canada's largest hospital center. The CICC operates as an open innovation group within the institutional structure, and organizes research projects with multifunction teams of physicians, nurses, pharmacists, industrial engineers, public health researchers, architects, residents, and designers. This diversity of knowledge and perspective gives the CICC an innovation advantage. Another significant factor in the CICC's success is its direct, immediate access to the hospital's internal medicine practice and patients. Barrier-free clinical access facilitates rapid testing of concepts and collection of data.

The CICC studies and enhances the entire process of complex care for patients with multiple disease conditions, which represents the largest burden on healthcare services. Physician and CICC medical director Dante Morra described its mission and approach to service innovation:

> People see healthcare as one thing, and it's not. There are three major streams of activity. The first one is the person going for an episodic treatment. For instance, they would need a hip replacement, and this can be done through one intense experience. This is like a manufacturing line, and it's not complex. It's one interaction, and if things go wrong there can be more interactions that follow. The second is the "well patient" in primary care. Sally is fine, but she is not feeling well, and she goes through the information and diagnosis phase. She goes back to her normal life.

The biggest mind-shift of healthcare happens when people start thinking beyond these two things. Most people have gone to their doctor with a flu, or they have had a major procedure done. When you look at the cost of healthcare, . . . if you look at the system, it's all chronic disease. The chronic disease vortex is chewing up resources. The system is not designed for this.

And the real problem is not providing diabetic care to Sally. The provision of specific care is easy. The real problem is how to provide care to a patient who has diabetes, kidney disease, and heart failure. And who is alone. That is where the opportunity for design lies. This is the level at which CICC is looking to address problems.[12]

Using a bottom-up identification and innovation process, Morra and his staff work with clinicians, stakeholders, and patients to map out problems with current healthcare practices and develop and test solutions. The team's direct access to the working clinical world allows for rapid observation, learning, and diffusion of knowledge.

The CICC created and follows an explicit, well-defined innovation strategy and a collaborative project management process. Handling more than a dozen clinical research and innovation projects at any given time, Morra and designer Leslie Beard coordinate weekly operational "rounds" to track and discuss the progress of projects. Just as in clinical education, the CICC staff refers to their weekly innovation project rounds as "bullet rounds," similar to the quick review of patient cases residents take part in before visiting the patients in the circulating rounds. The CICC staff also hold regular invitational lectures for research findings as a type of "grand rounds," the term for a prepared lecture based on the observations of a significant patient case in the clinic.

The innovation process draws from the everyday concerns raised by clinicians working in the University Hospital Network. As Morra explained,

We were formed to solve complicated problems. We started in the lean engineering methodology, value stream mapping with a heavy emphasis on process. But it stopped us solving the problems in this room. We may be able to solve the problem of how best to align the chairs in this room, but how do you align the chairs in the whole healthcare system? That's where you need the design middle layer. [13]

The Innovation Pyramid

The CICC relies on a well-defined innovation process to explicitly guide service innovations through a progression of stages so that efficiencies and economies of scale may be realized while accelerating learning and diffusion. Morra and Beard created the process with the CICC to provide a common language for practice innovation across projects, and Morra reinforces the progression "up" the scale for all projects. Morra often encourages research leads to consider how they might take a new process "to scale," meaning the higher stages of diffusion:

1. **Understand the issue and create a project.** Develop new understanding in order to disseminate new knowledge to improve processes with the goal of developing an intervention to change the existing system.

2. **Implement a pilot project.** Implement on a small scale to gain an understanding of the barriers to moving forward, and to develop an initial structure for system enhancement.

3. **Evaluate the project.** Determine the fit and feasibility of the process, and generate measures for full cycle review.

4. **Create a program.** Develop a program that can be implemented or expanded by other teams to drive large-scale systems improvement.

5. **Commercialize.** Disseminate the innovation into the marketplace and capture the value for society, the CICC, and/or the innovating team.

Even though the final phase is commercialization, the CICC is not structured to commercially develop innovations. Instead, the rationale of moving candidate projects from stage 1 to stage 5 is to diffuse innovations so they can have the maximum global system impact, a key mission of the CICC:

> Having commercialization at the top is meant to represent saturation and breadth of influence that transforms the system. It's not a higher order. The reason it's at the top is that the opportunity for disruptive massive system impacts is in the marketplace. . . . The ability to truly transform a global system increases as you go up the pyramid. So if I am working with the Canadian government, I can create a program that can affect Ontario. It may not be able to be copied anywhere. But if I create a new gadget, that becomes BlackBerry RIM, that goes international. . . . it's not more important, it's just about the volume and amplification.[14]

Innovate Afib

AF is the most common cardiac arrhythmia, the incidence of which is growing as the population ages. This disease is a cause of significant mortality and comorbidity—that is, it co-occurs with other related disease conditions with age. As such, it is a significant problem for healthcare systems everywhere because of the burden on clinical care resources, especially when considering the "total system" costs of the disease beyond just AF care (estimated at between $20,000 and $40,000 per patient per year). According to the 2010 whitepaper by Morra and colleagues, AF accounts for 15% of all strokes, and patients are at a significantly increased risk of death due to stroke and heart failure.[15]

AF has a significant negative impact on a patient's quality of life due to both its symptoms and the need for anticoagulation monitoring following diagnosis. AF frequently leads to palpitations, fatigue, heart failure, angina, and other conditions. The comorbidities of AF patients introduce complexity (interdependent relationships) into care decisions and disease management. Many patients suffer from diabetes, respiratory disease, and other chronic illnesses. They often see many specialists, take multiple medications, and interact with the healthcare sector at many points.

To better characterize and understand the nature of the challenges related to the disease, the CICC's Innovate Afib project employed a multimethod analysis approach that included interviews with clinicians across the spectrum of care for AF patients, a systematic review of current literature regarding the cost of AF care, and validation of the system (and map) with key stakeholders.

Interviews were conducted with 60 thought leaders selected for their discipline and perspectives, including cardiology, pharmacy, internal medicine, primary care, AF clinic, systems, and nursing. These yielded some common themes and challenges with AF care in the current system:

- Fragmented care delivery

- Poor communication between providers

- Lack of follow-up with patients

- Nonstandardized care

- Confusing guidelines and lack of consensus on quality indictors; no clear entry point to the system

- Operational issues (wait times, new therapies)

- Lack of patient education

- Difficulties with patient self-management

- Challenges with patient adherence to therapies

Associated with and resulting from these challenges, AF patients often experience a confusing care pathway, which may lead to (at best) basic symptom relief and prevention of further disease, or to deterioration (Figure 5.2). The way in which patients are managed in the existing system also results in increased utilization of resources, such as emergency room services, stroke rehabilitation services, and healthcare expenditures.

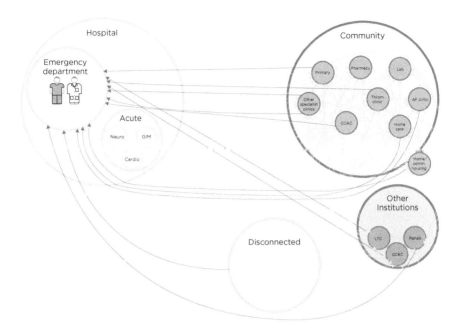

FIGURE 5.2

The existing network of disconnected atrial fibrillation (AF) services. AF patients flow chaotically among care providers. Disconnected patients are those who have been touched by the system but are now unaccounted for and may not be receiving proper care. This population is likely to end up in the emergency room. CCAC = Community Care Access Centres; GIM = general internal medicine; LTC = long-term care. (From Center for Innovation in Complex Care, Toronto)

An underlying assumption for the proposed new service process is the recognition that the healthcare system is in the midst of evolution—from delivery of episodic, fragmented care for individual conditions to multidisciplinary, team-based care of patients with multiple chronic medical conditions. As the general population ages, technologies change, and patients become more medically complex, taking a systems-based approach to managing this greater complexity will be the only way to provide comprehensive care that keeps people healthy and ensures that healthcare costs do not spiral out of control. Innovate Afib would reduce the system costs of the disease while simultaneously increasing the quality of care by reducing the complications of AF and improving efficiency and reducing redundancy.

Innovate Afib identified an "ideal care system" scenario (Figure 5.3) that would provide every AF patient with specialized anticoagulation management, around-the-clock patient access, follow-up within 1 week after any AF-related emergency room visit, access to specialist cardiologists when appropriate, and measured quality-of-care indicators. The diagram is read by observing the following six principles:

1. The patient is at the center of the system, not the disease.

2. Current referral patterns and existing infrastructures should be maintained and optimized.

3. A value-based care model will reduce costs and improve care.

4. Patient services should remain in their communities.

5. Knowledge translation for physicians and patient self-management is provided.

6. Communication is coordinated among all care providers.

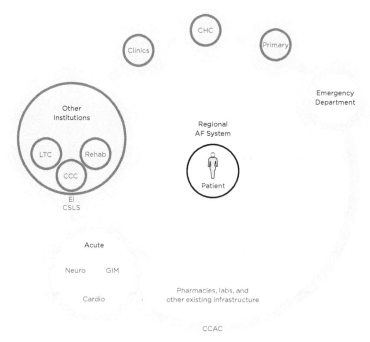

FIGURE 5.3
Proposed integrated service network for atrial fibrillation (AF).
CCAC = Community Care Access Centres (outer ring); CCC = Complex Continuing Care; CHC = Complex Health Centres; CSLS = customized supported local solutions; EI = existing infrastructure; GIM = general internal medicine; LTC = long-term care. Each of the bubbles can be customized per the CSLS model of local adaptation. (From Center for Innovation in Complex Care, Toronto)

At first glance, traditional designers and many readers may be unsure about where the possible design opportunities are found in this service scenario. Morra suggested that the best potential for high-impact innovations are in clinical and coordinated care processes: "Healthcare has been very innovative in creating new treatments, new drugs, new devices, new services . . . but not models and processes. What separates us from some of our colleagues is that they often try to create a product in one area. And if you want to create a product, you do not go into deep complexity. You carve out something small. But the problem is that products do not solve the true problems."[16]

LESSONS LEARNED

- Innovators in a hospital ecosystem must formulate practices in language appropriate to the current stakeholders and keep the vocabulary limited to essential terms (e.g., the CICC presenting its projects in "rounds").

- A well-defined innovation process helps clinical participants understand the common goals all share in the process.

- Service process design can advance the healthcare system toward its evolution from episodic, fragmented care for individual conditions to multidisciplinary, team-based care of patients with chronic conditions.

- Adapt a multimethod research approach, collecting traditional data (subjective report, measured observations) as evidence understood by sponsors. Clinical innovation benefits by publishing findings in medical journals, so a mix of EBD, design research, and clinical research methods can be used.

- Be prepared for clinical service design to take much longer than work in other domains. Agile processes are largely unknown in hospitals and are not recommended, as time to market is not a driver of innovation success. Effectiveness and risk/cost reduction are clinical goals, and quality and risk are compromised when optimizing for delivery time.

Methods: Design Research for Healthcare Services

Service design potentially represents a significant change and challenge to experience design and technology infrastructure design orientations. A comprehensive presentation of service-oriented design methods would fill another book.* Because the health sector is vast and by necessity conservative, a selection of methods for service innovation is meaningless without establishing a specific context. The integrated service design framework in Table 5.5 identifies the contexts in which the example methods stand.

TABLE 5.5 INTEGRATED SERVICE DESIGN FRAMEWORK

Design phases	Methods
Discovery/understanding	Participatory workshops Dialogic design Simplexity Stakeholder analysis/personas Customer journey mapping
Human-centered research	Ethnographic field research Sensemaking interviews Cognitive task analysis Values Sensitive Design (VSD) Empathic design research
Service concept design	Participatory workshops Simplexity Customer journey mapping Service touchpoint interaction Generative bodystorming Context mapping Service system maps
Process prototyping	Bodystorming (simulating use cases) Service blueprint Visual sensemaking Scenario storyboarding
Service process integration	Service blueprint Workflow analysis Developmental evaluation
Organizational readiness Service implementation	Service design plan Dialogic design Developmental evaluation

Note: Methods are coded by color: innovation method; experience design research; social science research; systems method; service design method.

---

* See A. Polaine, L. Løvlie, & B. Reason. (2013). *Service design.* Brooklyn, NY: Rosenfeld Media. www.rosenfeldmedia.com/books/service-design/.

Although many methods referred to in this book are applicable to a service design context, the methods in this chapter are uniquely so.

Participatory Scenario Design

The participatory scenario design process elicits multiple perspectives and experiential knowledge from people with a deep understanding of the field. Facilitating scenario development as a workshop process helps participants form shared mental models of user behavior associated with the product/service design context. By formulating scenarios as a collaborative process, people get the chance to share their own stories, wisdom, experience, and details helpful to the group's developing understanding. Such a shared understanding is more powerful than a set of storyboards developed in isolation by design researchers as a prepared deliverable. As a group's understanding evolves and their stories become embedded in scenarios, the resulting story lines of shared knowledge become a basis for future design decisions, many of which will occur as business or product development decisions well in the future. Scenario design can be viewed as an investment in the long-term process.

Guiding scenario design requires setting the context for the activity, typically as part of a series of design workshop processes. A sequence of activities may be structured along the following lines:

1. Review and discuss user and market research.

2. Articulate themes and priorities from research to carry forward into design.

3. Identify stakeholders and users from research and requirements.

4. Engage the team in defining personas as a small-group exercise.

5. Review personas and list relevant activities for each.

6. Identify common activities across personas, and cluster personas into sets where it makes sense.

7. Generate and sketch activity scenarios for high-priority persona activities.

Scenario creation starts at step 7. Participants generally start either by posting anticipated actions and events on sticky notes to generate a series of touchpoints and potential encounters, or by creating a timeline for the period of engagement and associating events with time dependencies. Figure 5.4 illustrates the scenario construction of the former.

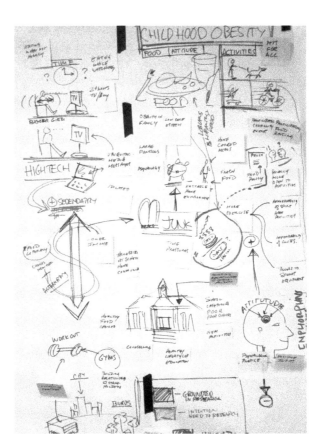

FIGURE 5.4
Creating a scenario of events and encounters for a health issue. (Sketch by George Shewchuk and Michi Komori)

Figure 5.5 illustrates the outcome of a timeline scenario. This shows the envisioned sequence of life events—from college to first job to middle age—to identify the points of intervention for health conversations. Although this is a much longer timeframe than a typical customer journey, the scenario process benefits from leaving the timeframe, experiences, and ideation open to the experience of participants.

Scenarios are generated for a set period (30 minutes is typical). A variation that is done within informed groups of varied roles or disciplines is to hold charettes of the first scenarios: A narrator stays with each team's scenario while all others circulate around the room and walk through and critique each of the scenarios. New sticky notes (of another color) can be added to annotate the sketches with additional events, touchpoints, or suggestions. Following the development of rough sketch scenarios in the workshop setting, the narratives can be integrated into design artifacts and shared with management and the development team.

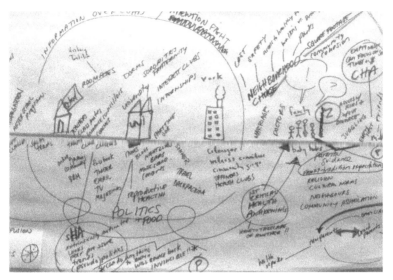

FIGURE 5.5
Timeline scenario for a health journey. (Timeline by Tai Huynh,
Jen Recknagel, and Jayar Lafontaine)

Generative Bodystorming

Bodystorming is a well-known method for simulating and designing action
sequences for services and interaction design. It allows the team and stakeholders to experience some of the functions and working relationships of
proposals, either during their formation or after prototyping. It has been
adopted and recommended in service design methods as a way to prototype
the experience of interacting with an envisioned new service both physically
and temporally. For healthcare services, which revolve around the physical performance of activities, bodystorming provides a way to run process
simulations with real people for innovative concepts that might otherwise
be prohibitive to prototype. Bodystorming identifies possibilities for innovation and tangible complications that would not be discovered in storyboards
or computer simulations.

Because many services are largely intangible products that deliver values
at points along the "service journey," the typical prototyping approach is
impoverished compared to interactive or industrial products. Very few services are fully tested as interactive prototypes with representative users,
unless they are largely interactive services. Even then, consider a patient
admissions process, for example. Although this is largely an online transaction for data entry, it also represents the patient's first engagement with the

healthcare center or system. The experience can be treated as businesslike and perfunctory, or as an opportunity to design a humane and orienting stage for a better experience. By default, if we let a critical process such as admissions follow the lead of an IT system, it promotes the worst aspects of the healthcare system in the patient's first encounter, reminding the patient that care is a bureaucratic and expensive process.

Bodystorming can smooth out the rough edges of a designed service scenario. It simulates the touchpoints and interactions in actually performing the service, and animates scenarios so that teams can uncover potential problems and reveal hidden assumptions embedded in the prototype. At least four bodystorming techniques have been documented for different purposes and different stages of a design engagement:

- **Designing in situ.** This is bodystorming with the development team working in the space or place in which the product being designed will ultimately be used. Although this could be a valuable experience for designers, it would be difficult to carry out in a working care setting.

- **Service simulation.** This is bodystorming as "strong prototyping" to represent the environment and local situations in which the product or service will be used. For example, a team has been hired to build a new handheld device for use on submarines, so they construct and model the hallways, spaces, and structures (out of cardboard perhaps) to simulate a submarine environment. It may not have all the properties of the actual field setting, but might appropriate the most salient objects. The team can change variables, such as lighting, or test how easy it is to walk through doorways and passageways of different sizes while trying to use the handheld.

- **Use case theater.** This classic bodystorming technique prototypes the space and place of service by using living personas, actors, and props.[17] In a wait time reduction scenario, a team might test their scenarios for improvement by simulating and timing the interactions of queues, entry and exit conditions, clinical procedure variances, and information collection. The design team would define service scenario scripts, rehearse the scripts so that performances were evenly conducted, and measure the time needed to service the queues under different test conditions. This technique is used more in an evaluative context, and is conducted in later stages of design.

- **Embodied storming.** This technique differs from the others in that the goal is to create embodied perceptions of use and interaction for a future service.[18] This approach is a *pre-ideation* technique, in which perceptions based on gut feeling precede the pursuit of perfect concepts. The design team improvises and learns from the observations of their experience in trying out the situation being designed for.

These techniques are not mutually exclusive, although they are almost never used together on a design project because they are useful at different times in the design process.

Embodied storming goes beyond just the creation of a "simulation" and allows the real-time generation of new scenarios that would not otherwise be considered. The technique is staged as a generative tool for creating insights that precede ideation and concept design. Early bodystorming also helps a team discover flaws and assumptions before brainstorming and concept development.

Embodied bodystorming requires people to act as physical actors in a situation, and not as conceptual designers distanced from things. Stakeholders and designers work in artificial situations when developing design concepts, becoming blind to perception (i.e., personal experience of an event) and instead focusing on the facts of representation (i.e., after the event). Bodystorming enables rapid communication between people, and the generation of unjudged, uncompromised proposals and scenarios. The performative mode tends to create sequences, themes, and conceptual continuity. They are like scenes composed by a "design troupe" rather than discrete ideas attributed to individuals. Ideas can be elicited from the scenario, but extracting them in isolation tends to disrupt the continuity of the scenario.

Generative bodystorming helps to create stories or themes from the service experience, based on the things and situations being perceived and observed. It enables translation of *tacit knowing* into rapid communication and generation of ideas contributing to the service scenario. By collaborating in tight generate/do/learn cycles, participants engage one another in simulating experiences and processes that are designed through joint acting and improvisation.

The distinctions between use case bodystorming and embodied storming listed in Table 5.6 show the value of this technique in service design.

Interaction design relies on personas as a way to represent users as the subjects for product design. Yet service scenarios represent dynamic coordinated activities, sometimes across a wide range of persona types. For example, a patient may only participate in the touchpoint of a tangible interaction with a service's delivery, such as a prescription being filled. Behind the scenes, the service involves multiple backstage actions with tangible items and intangible functions the patient never sees, such as physicians' orders, professional communications, computer entries, and movement of supplies and medications. These activities are not represented by persona types, and their service moments are not personalized—they are necessary interactions in a service workflow.

TABLE 5.6 USE CASE AND GENERATIVE BODYSTORMING

Use case bodystorming	Embodied storming
User-needs centered	Rapid communication and generation of ideas around an envisioned scenario
Product-design driven	Developing people and cultures through shared understanding
Creative problem solving/design thinking on site to enhance understanding of the problem domain	Rapid communication and generation of ideas around what the problem domain should be
Focus on physical problems	Problems are not always technological; sometimes they are sociopolitical or socioeconomic
Reenacting people's everyday performances and living with data in embodied ways by performance	Envisioning how people would respond to future scenarios that are presented without extra data
Quality of design ideas is heavily dependent on the quality of documents	Quality of the exercise is dependent on the quality of interactions and breakdown of cognitive and emotional barriers
Participants are researchers and industry representatives	Participants may not know anything about the subject area
Success is measured by the uptake of ideas by industry representatives	Success is measured by participants' willingness to explore together and build shared meaning around issues
Empathy toward users	Shared experiences and collective memory
Role-playing and following a script	Free flowing, not directed (aside from presented scenario)
Forced innovation of solutions	Exploratory but not solution driven

Personas can be a helpful tool for understanding the varying needs of different user archetypes, but they can be a crutch in service design situations.[19] Services must be designed and specified to enable an unforeseeable range of individuals to interact readily, easily, and fairly with a given service system. Focusing on personas too closely skews the consideration of *need states*— conditions of a situation that require satisfaction or reveal a breakdown. Although scenarios portray the interaction, information flows, and touchpoints of service, they do little to demonstrate the human responses to a service system design. The emotional and behavioral responses to a time-pressured, human-system need state can be played out as theater, with the impact of immediate and shared insights into the situation.

Generative bodystorming focuses on need states and can be applied as a design research method to help identify gaps and opportunities. A typical scenario finds design teams sitting around the table and talking about users as if they were segments "out there" waiting for us to discover their so-called needs. We classify customers by demographics such as age or gender, psychographics such as lifestyle, and behaviors such as purchasing patterns that we believe to be real enough to measure. If well funded, we go "out there" to conduct research on these different segments. Instead, or in addition, the projective role playing of embodied storming forces a team to attend to perceivable need states.

A single product or chain of service events might generate multiple need states. Because a product cannot serve all needs, we use embodied storming to focus on the needs that matter. If performed with a reasonably informed troupe, embodied storming will demonstrate the satisfaction of the conditions of these need states. An effective bodystorm is one that captures the need state, highlights the breakdowns, and shows how the change in process (the designed aspect) satisfies the problems as perceived. A good bodystorm has an immediacy and intimacy that engages clients and participants at a direct level of experience with respect to the real-world situation for which the team is designing.

We need to focus more on the different usage occasions with the product and service, and the needs that define them. This is exactly what bodystorming does. It goes even further because it allows us, both as designers and business owners, to see and understand what is and what is not working so that we can interpret design opportunities.

Guidelines for Generative Bodystorming

Guidelines for embodied storming are not rules because the technique is still exploratory and remains in continual practice.

1. Expect to spend 2 to 4 hours planning and designing the bodystorming scenarios, materials, instructions, and logistics. A series of bodystorms to evaluate different proposals requires more planning.

2. Assign five to eight participants per troupe. Larger groups can be split into two or more troupes that bodystorm the same scenario.

3. Every player must have a role; there are no background players.

4. Identify and create props for use in the scenarios. Props can have feelings and thoughts, and are interactive agents in the process.

5. Create large cards that identify the roles.

6. Create thought-bubble cards to show what a participant is thinking versus saying or doing.

7. Have a narrator or color commentator who explains things to observers. The narrator can stop the action, rewind, or fast-forward.

8. Approach the presentation of scenarios with the spirit of improv acting: "Yes, and..." rather than "No, but..."

9. Perform at least two skits, showing a before and after service scenario.

TIPS ON TECHNIQUES

- In the right context, any user-centered design method can be applied in healthcare service design. Sequence a series of research methods so they contribute significantly to each design decision.

- Participatory methods such as dialogic design and bodystorming are especially useful in co-creating and proposing new service interventions. Methods that result in consensus diagrams, such as challenge maps, enable collective understanding and enable managers to articulate clear proposals.

- Design research methods can blur the boundaries and nudge practitioners into making proposals for which their experience is inapplicable. Service designers without clinical experience should avoid advising on clinical content. Methodologies such as dialogic design and Simplexity make a clear separation between process facilitation and practitioner content.

- Generative techniques such as embodied storming provide an alternative to prototyping services. Because so many variations of possible activity are possible in a service available to all types of health seekers or professionals, the embodied methods allow designers to understand the complexities of an intangible service from a physical and temporal perspective.

PART III

Rethinking Care Systems

The final four chapters examine the human-centered and systemic design necessary for "backstage" processes of health services design and delivery. These focus on care practice and education, as professional practices and as human systems and services.

The Care Services Landscape

In developed economies, the services sector has surpassed the manufacturing and goods production sectors in terms of revenue size and employment numbers. Yet costs have significantly increased in service provision, especially in healthcare, affecting perception of value, consumer demand, and even employment. The increased costs in healthcare services have led to a societal contract in which health insurance is necessary to ensure even the possibility of adequate care. As service is decoupled from the reality of consumer affordability and coverage, however, this social contract will break down, even in countries with lower base costs than in the United States. When consumers have unequal access to healthcare services due to the unavailability or costs of insurance, then new service systems for healthcare must be designed, with some forms of healthcare service provided as public goods.

In any market, service providers often aim to dominate their service ecosystems with superior customer retention and perceived value in order to keep a sustainable advantage in their market. The healthcare sector is no different—health seekers (consumers) have choices, and large institutions are constantly seeking to differentiate their service offerings and quality. Yet the vision of *service* innovation has been slowly achieved in healthcare, especially when compared to the pace of technological innovation.

Services innovation aims for transformative changes in patient experience, business models, and the very role of the provider. Innovation produces change at the level of service or system management and embraces all types of creative resources, not just design-led processes. Experience design methods offer a design-led framework, but these are only half of the opportunity. System-level innovation requires stakeholder process design, service system design, new models of practice management, and community engagement.

The Health Seeking Journey in the Care System

In the shift "up-system" from the health seeker to the healthcare system, we encounter increased complexity. The human-centered design approach and user-oriented methods underserve this complexity because they design for optimal *individual* experience. A hybrid of systems and design methods are needed to achieve integration with health system touchpoints as suggested in the health-seeking journey in Figure III.1. This diagram interprets the primary patient encounter with these systems experienced by both patient and clinicians.

The backstage operations of a big box clinic may employ hundreds of people in specialized roles. Once Elena enters the hospital as a patient, she interacts with a handful of staff for a brief period. The service she enters at each stage represents a self-contained clinical encounter with different clinicians and locations for each appointment and procedure.

Here the touchpoints (in a health system context) indicate information collected for each encounter. Elena's scenarios in these chapters complete the journey through services—from the diagnosis of a major cardiac issue to living with and managing the complexity of her personal health condition—as she deals with:

- The changes in lifestyle and behavior required at each touchpoint.

- The contradictions between her health-seeking needs and the stress of adhering to medical orders.

- The contradiction between her shift from caregiver to family patient.

- The need to make choices of treatment and procedure that have significant life impact.

Even within many health networks today, patient information is not integrated across services, making a fragmented trail for patients in their clinical health-seeking journey. Each resource is an independent and often isolated data processor serving functions for that touchpoint only. Service continuity across clinical encounters remains a significant challenge, and one that may not improve as healthcare organizations transform into regional networks of smaller clinics with dedicated purposes.

Health Seeking | In Healthcare System

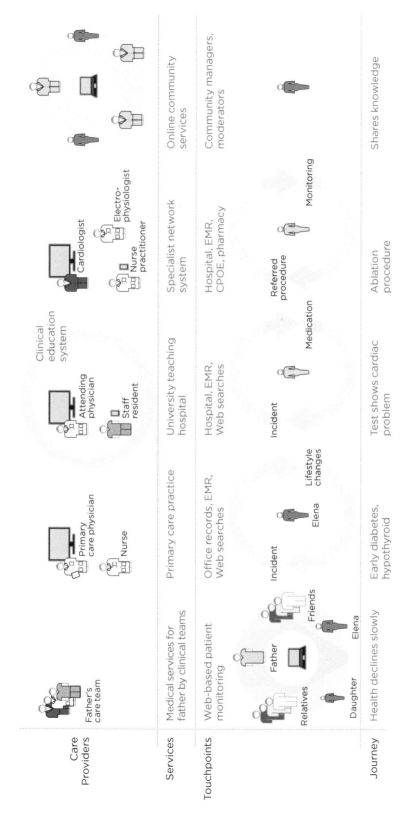

Care Providers	Father's care team	Primary care physician / Nurse	Attending physician / Staff resident	Cardiologist / Electro-physiologist / Nurse practitioner	
			Clinical education system		Online community services
Services	Medical services for father by clinical teams	Primary care practice	University teaching hospital	Specialist network system	Community managers, moderators
Touchpoints	Web-based patient monitoring	Office records, EMR, Web searches	Hospital, EMR, Web searches	Hospital, EMR, CPOE, pharmacy	
	Father / Relatives / Daughter / Elena / Friends	Incident / Elena / Lifestyle changes	Incident / Medication	Referred procedure / Monitoring	
Journey	Health declines slowly	Early diabetes, hypothyroid	Test shows cardiac problem	Ablation procedure	Shares knowledge

Design goals at the healthcare service system level include larger-scale interventions:

- Designing information system platforms as multifunction backbones to integrate multiple vendor applications in a common data model

- Designing health services as processes across departments within institutions to enable flexible workflow

- Redesigning information practices to coordinate patient health data, requests, feedback, and outcomes across clinical providers

- Co-design at the community level to mitigate chronic health problems through early intervention

- Providing integrated design, research, and human factors advising, communications, and workshops with clinicians and public health researchers to enable redesign of services and clinical work processes

FIGURE III.1
The health-seeking journey as navigating the care system.

CHAPTER 6

Design at the Point of Care

Elena's Story: Taking a Serious Turn

Elena's personal schedule gets the best of her. She continues to take her thyroid medicine, but her commitment to personal lifestyle changes falters less than a month after reasonable adherence. The stress in her life picks up, her diet remains uneven, and she is unable to keep a consistent exercise schedule.

Two months after the first incident, Elena finds her heartbeat racing, with the feeling of a flutter rather than a beat, and she faints again. When she comes to, she is lightheaded, dizzy, and pale, with a pounding and fast heartbeat. This time her daughter is at home to catch her swoon, and unsure why this has happened again, Andrea calls her grandfather for help. He shows up as quickly as he can, assesses that his daughter has suffered a serious spell, and the three of them hurry to the local hospital emergency room.

At the hospital, the admitting nurse asks Elena for the usual information: complaints, family doctor, insurance provider. Elena volunteers her prior incident, but the hospital does not have access to her records. Because the latest occurrence was clearly an acute episode with a prior history, more complete tests and procedures are called for.

Elena is given a full electrocardiogram (ECG) in an attempt to capture and isolate the pattern of the arrhythmia. She undergoes full blood tests for sugar, cell count, and cholesterol levels. Having caught the fainting incident quickly enough to detect the originating cycle this time, the ECG shows the telltale pattern of a heart condition known as supraventricular tachycardia (SVT), a regular but very rapid heartbeat originating "above the ventricles," resulting in dangerous heartbeat fluctuations that may occur acutely and without warning. Although SVT is not the first diagnosis for fainting, it finally explains why Elena fainted—the rapid arrhythmia, worsened by a blood sugar drop, led to a loss of consistent blood flow to the brain.

Elena's blood sugar levels now show the approach of Type 2 diabetes (at 120 mg/dl) and her blood pressure is again abnormally high. Her thyroid pill, though, has worked well—her TSH (thyroid-stimulating hormone) levels are normal. It remains unclear to Elena how her conditions are systemically related, and if they are. Every condition is treated as a separate issue, with different medications and advice. She cannot make sense of the diseases as a whole, making it harder to see how her life choices will improve her overall health.

Elena is started on blood pressure medication and is referred to a cardiologist. She is advised to return to her family doctor to address the possibility of diabetes. Back at home, she goes online to investigate the options suggested to her. The SVT diagnosis and cardiologist referral confirm that her situation is a serious one. She naturally wants to increase her understanding of the condition and to learn about the risks and effects of the possible treatment options. Elena follows up by scheduling a consultation at a cardiac care center. ■

Better Practice Is Better Service

From the clinical perspective, Elena's diagnosis and even her advanced treatment are routine. Dozens of patients a week are referred to hospitals and cardiac clinics with diagnosed arrhythmias. To the health seeker, the diagnosis may come as a shock and the treatments may seem exotic or risky. As always, a huge gap in knowledge, power, and comfort exists between specialists and their patients. These gaps seriously influence how health seekers experience their care.

The information gap of medical knowledge has narrowed with the ready accessibility of Web publications. The meaningful gap is the one between information and *knowledge*—knowing how to judge and act on the information.

A service experience gap also exists. The clinician retains the power to diagnose, prescribe, and deliver treatment. A typical patient possesses limited knowledge of what constitutes "good service" in totality. The threshold of "bad service" may come close to malpractice, but the range of a normal care standard is quite broad and experienced differently by individuals.

Will the future patient be treated as a customer to be satisfied at every step? A compelling candidate for future patient experience is found in personalized medicine, which is not personalized care, but rather technology-enabled personalized diagnostics. Based on sensor and genetic information gathered for an individual, early detection of emerging diseases and appropriate medication can be prescribed. The trade-off is that individual adherence and self-care will be expected. Although the medical technology may be manufacturable, personal behavior is not so controllable. Adherence will become more of a designed experience.

Comfortable care experiences cost more than do-it-yourself care. The direction of future policy is oriented toward compensating providers based on outcomes. The unforeseen effect could be that services become stripped down and efficient, aligning expected outcomes to the most efficient billable treatments. As clinicians are evaluated more on outcomes than on procedures, service quality *as experienced* could actually be perceived as worse than today.

How should established clinical practice models be changed to improve patient experience? Will improving experience at the patient touchpoints (appointments, reception, consult, preparation, treatment, recovery, follow-up) make a significant difference to the patient? Or done wrong, could it have a negative impact on provider efficiency?

Clinical care and care teams are not service industry employees. Hospitals cannot change service practices overnight. The regimes of primary care, emergency, acute, and critical care, surgery, and long-term care are taught and developed in education and certified in board exams and licensure. Very few services are as locked in to their educational processes as healthcare.

Business, law, and even engineering teach principles but not practice. Medical education requires that trainees spend more time in practice than in school. Changing healthcare service means changing training, and vice versa. This will be an evolutionary process, and many will call for rapid change. But medical education is already changing at a surprising rate.

A Design Opportunity in the Care Crisis

Primary care providers (primarily generalist physicians, but also now nurse practitioners and physician assistants) are essential to improving and sustaining good health at a community level. The primary practice is the first stop for any person with an undiagnosed illness or nonemergency condition. In the US healthcare system, primary care may be the only point in the health-seeking journey where a true patient-centered relationship can develop. Primary care physicians have the ability to integrate knowledge and experience of individuals and their histories and lifestyles. Although much of the emerging consensus in healthcare design focuses on patient behaviors and (rightfully) on prevention, primary is mainly where the care lives. Most people who become sick or injured show up first at primary care, regardless of their technological sophistication.

The societal need for primary care increases with an aging population, as multiple chronic diseases emerge, and older people are at risk for cancers and systemic diseases. The largest population cohort in history is now reaching that age, putting pressure on the system to adapt. A crisis is foreseeable, as fewer physicians have chosen family medicine or primary care after their education. Family doctors and pediatricians have increased caseloads over the years, resulting in greater numbers of episodic patients, more stress on the system, and unsustainable practices. The situation in the United States (and Canada) has reached the point of a declared crisis.

The developing crisis of not enough primary care providers for the population affects society on a large scale. The American Academy of Family Physicians estimates that by the year 2020, the United States will face a shortfall of 40,000 primary care physicians. This 51% shortage based on anticipated need will increase costs across the system and reinforce the existing trend toward specialization.

Higher salaries drive higher service and educational costs as a systemic effect, yet the onus is often placed on physician choices. But are there deeper causes? Has the fee-for-service business model and pay-per-procedure accounting of health insurance made primary care complicated and untenable? Are residents specializing because of their affinity for a specialty, or to afford more mobility and career choice?

Family doctors mitigate costs because they assess the whole person and take into account a wide range of life and personal options, recommending exotic procedures only as a last resort. They closely monitor possible medication problems. Family physicians promote whole family and community health by advising and facilitating personal lifestyle changes; simpler, lower-cost treatments; and prevention. Each step toward prevention saves costs incurred later by more serious problems and emergency room visits.

New primary care services are being designed and prototyped within the accountable care organization model, which brings a wider range of advanced and primary clinical services to smaller, distributed community care centers. Several early-stage organizations have formed (Kaiser Permanente, Mayo Clinic), and it is notable they are referred to as *prototypes*. That does not, however, suggest that these new practices have been *designed*. A design-led (D3.0) management process would facilitate integration of care and service systems, architecture and workflow, organizational resources, IT, public and patient communications, and the new business model.

Many of the incentives for change associated with the human dimensions of a service system (education, salary, workload, lifestyle, prestige) are not designable functions within the service. Education in particular has significant long-term influence on practice, as new entrants into any practice tend to bring techniques and new thinking to the field. But it is changed within its own system, renewed by integrating changes from practice trends, emerging societal needs, and new learning. Though highly standardized, clinical education is changing rapidly for a new generation of medicine, bringing with it the potential for system-wide change in healthcare.

Where and How to Innovate

Herbert Simon was an early proponent of treating medicine and management as *design* practices because they "change existing situations into preferred ones."[1] How is medicine like design practice? Medicine is a knowledge process that bases care decisions on information, technology, and resource availability. Doctors quickly research a patient's situation based on evidence, frame the problem state, and design care plans that facilitate preferred health outcomes. We might call this Clinical Design 1.0 (CD1.0).

Clinical Design 2.0 (CD2.0) redesigns care procedures and services that systematically improve outcomes. Medical researchers evaluate new surgical and intervention techniques in rigorous, controlled comparative trials to ensure that the procedure performs reliably, is repeatable, and is ultimately better for the patient. Medical device designers transfer emerging technologies—sensors, electronics, fabric and materials—into improved products for technical procedures. These may dramatically change the opportunities for future products and health management, such as the noninvasive skin sensor developed by C8 MediSensors that could replace the daily invasive ritual of blood sugar monitoring with a wearable device.

Though not defined as a *design* practice, Clinical Design 3.0 (CD3.0) transfers knowledge and practices from organizational design and sociotechnical systems toward high-performance care organizations. The initial toolkit of research methods and design processes deploys organizational innovation tools such as business and practice model design. CD3.0 generally covers the range of practices that involve all members of an organization, across services and departments. At this scale, stakeholder co-creation and innovation management guide organizational design, whereas CD1.0 and CD2.0 are driven by expert knowledge and user response data and can be considered more evidence-based.

Clinical Design 4.0 (CD4.0) co-creates practices of caring in a community or societal context. CD4.0 care is exemplified by the systematic design thinking being introduced into public health problems by innovative physicians such as Mike Evans and the Health Design Lab (see Chapter 4's case study). Large-scale public health initiatives (such as the successful Smoke Free Ontario program) are planned as multiyear research and intervention programs at the public system level. Reviewing each level of clinical design, we have:

- **CD1.0: Individual human use** of products and devices that meet a specific individual need, such as personal test kits with instructions, or insulin injection kits for diabetics. These are responses to conditions, with products designed by vendors and provided by physicians.

- **CD2.0: Healthcare services** provided by teams in clinics, institutions, and online. Care activities are provided as services to health seekers, but are performed as work activities by a service team.

- **CD3.0: Clinical and educational institutions**, including clinical education, organizational management, and service program development.

- **CD4.0: Social and policy design for the healthcare industry** includes health system planning, community and public health strategies, and national and regional systems.

Each level calls for different methods suitable to accomplish its use cases. Adapting product design methods to the organizational practice context (CD3.0) would fail because of a mismatch of method to desired outcome. Adapting systemic design to the individual (CD1.0) is overkill.

Medical practice has a deeply established culture and will have to change systemically to change substantively. But professional cultures resist intervention by foreign practices; design processes will prove themselves in the new world of outcome-driven healthcare.

Design education and design practices are not organized to serve healthcare today. Most large health systems are largely advised by the expert-led management consulting model that has been predominant in corporate cultures for more than two decades, and the recognition of value from design firms is negligible overall. Yes, large design firms may have dedicated healthcare practices, but there are *few clinically experienced designers*. Furthermore, in care organizations, unlike in product or service companies, designers do not yet have leadership or ownership of the design outcomes. In most cases (not all), their work conforms to the direct needs of organizational management as essentially "work for hire."

The integration of new disciplinary practices into a deeply set culture such as medicine can easily take a decade, but many institutions are clearly seeking the dramatic improvements in value of design to patients and healthcare business. The early adopters of design—clinical and management leaders—may initially see value in tactical improvements and may not recognize the possibilities for systemic change and inevitable barriers in staffing up to design better services and IT. A model such as the CD1.0–4.0 domains may enable better-informed strategic planning for the development of an integrated design research discipline in healthcare.

Different Design Modes of Care

A design process should match the level and variety of a context to accommodate its complexity, as shown in Figure 6.1. Each arc represents a different level in the sociotechnical system, and each requires a different design process with different stakeholders. Each corresponds to a *significantly* different context with differing systems, interests, and values.

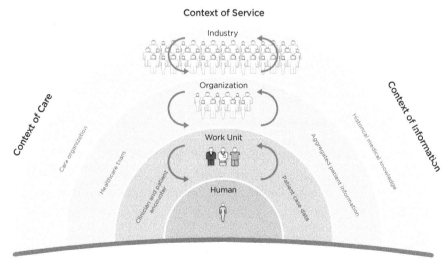

FIGURE 6.1
Contexts of service in care design.

Three contexts for *innovation* are shown: care, service, and information. Each context encompasses some services and excludes others. In any given project, care delivery, service provision, and IT might be interwoven. Yet one of these contexts will lead and define the purpose (e.g., IT) and another may be the internal client (e.g., pediatric care). Design and research methods selection and deliverables may differ significantly as a result.

What are the substantive differences among healthcare tasks, services, and the "system level"? The four dimensions of *service* in Figure 6.1 range from individual behavior to industry dynamics, aligned with the CD1.0–4.0 progression:

1. **Care design for the health seeker:** with the aim of fostering self-care and preventive awareness in individuals

2. **Clinician-patient encounter:** direct exam, diagnosis, and treatment of a health seeker by a care team

3. **Healthcare team:** care planning and role configuration for the healthcare professional teams and practice areas

4. **Care organization:** organizational strategy, business model design, and organizational development

Each level endorses a different concept of "care," a complex of values, orientations, delivery models, and motivations that currently do not map across these levels of activity. The care encounter and care organization encompass different functions of care.

The context of *care information* forms a hierarchy of data sources for service management and decision making. A series of transformations follow the Data-Information-Knowledge-Wisdom (DIKW) hierarchy. The DIKW schema was developed for management applications by systems theorist Russell Ackoff[2] and has been extended to knowledge management and, more recently, design research analysis.

- **Data:** Data acquired by sensors, self-documentation, and care practitioners, often recorded in discrete fields associated with a single record (e.g., a patient's record from a single appointment).

- **Information:** Patterned formulation of data that indicates semantic meaning. Information may range from documented content to medical articles to summarized patient narratives (e.g., a trend pattern distinguished across multiple data entries).

- **Knowledge:** Cognitive understanding of the meaning of information to relevant problems, sufficient for competent action. Knowledge can be represented as a verb, not a thing, as in *knowing how* (e.g., recognizing that a trend pattern of glucose levels signals the onset of Type 2 diabetes).

- **Wisdom:** The ability to act on information with an understanding of short- and long-term consequences (e.g., hypothesizing the source of a disease condition and recommending systematic changes instead of medication).

As innovators, we face the challenge of enabling outcomes of healthcare through a supportive, nondirective design context. In large institutions, in particular, a given "problem" will have multiple contexts, agents, communication technologies, and organizational requirements. Our role may be subsidiary, a frustrating place for those making change. Even recognizing the plurality of meanings of "care," designing for care is a new organizational role and there will be friction. Design research methodologies will also find resistance and need to adapt to context. It does not serve us well to declare that any preferred design methodology (e.g., experience design) is optimal for a given problem, because our methods may bias the solution toward only the outcomes the method enables.

Designing Health Education

Clinical education introduces long-term influences on the complex system of healthcare. Changes in practice and method consistently taught will propagate throughout a national healthcare system, but can also promote near-term shifts in clinical culture and practices.

Clinical practice is a Western cultural form with its roots in the initial successes of the adoption of scientific medicine in the early 20th century. Yet the way doctors (in particular) are educated for practice is by extended residency apprenticing with senior clinicians, similar to ancient guilds. Residency is a sophisticated immersion of learning in action, technical work, and scientific culture, a process not found in other professions.

Since the 1960s, articles in the medical literature have called for changes in the long-standing models of residency and medical education. Though not obvious to patients or others outside medical education, pedagogies and curricula have made huge changes in the last decade and are continuously moving toward student-centered education. Molly Cooke and a University of California, San Francisco team advocated new roles for promoting clinical teaching, a policy change they call "the Academy movement."[3] She identified the certification and development of education, the university model, and professional values as opportunities for change. Related concerns include the increasing numbers of complex and chronic patients and the need to focus on outpatient and community (and home) settings, rather than only on teaching hospitals. These are all rich opportunities for new design practice in healthcare.

Educating Designers to Educate Clinicians

Clinical education in all fields has only recently transformed after roughly 100 years of traditional science-based training and apprenticeship. Reforms in educational content, working conditions, and educational financing have shifted in just the last few years. Change may appear slow because clinical practice is highly constrained, the medical school and residency regimes are deeply ingrained, and clinicians are not faced with the institutional crises that necessitate change. Medical education has responded to demands from certifying bodies and clinical employers, and even to changes in culture and mindset from incoming students.

Consider the extraordinary range of information and services available in healthcare education. Everything from medical textbooks and e-learning systems to content delivery to research translation for practice can be considerably improved and integrated as D2.0 products. However, the educational process is not just a D3.0 institutional change; it is a socially transformational D4.0 process. Educational innovations affect all related institutions over time, so a significant design-led intervention can pay off.

Educational systems are notoriously difficult interventions—they are institutionalized, highly stable, and continuous yet complex. As with other social change problems, schools and educational services require a long period of adaptation for recommendations to show sustainable improvements.

Professionals do not generally like change when it happens to them. Designers might better understand why their contributions may be greeted with skepticism. Design interventions represent changes to careful daily routines, which require unlearning the old process and learning a new one. Even something as simple as a universal checklist can present a cognitive burden. Cognitive workload and technical work intensity are already at maximum levels for residents. So where might we find support for assisting clinical educators in rethinking the long-established order?

Service Design Issues in Clinical Education

Any educational system presents a complex challenge for service design. Learners are not customers, and education is not understood as a service by its administrators. Some educational processes—online resources, distance education, curriculum management—may be innovated as service concepts. But education is based on public service traditions. Conforming education to service methodologies could instill biases toward commercial values that might conflict with academic values. Many educators would argue that service design's pursuit of efficiency and value delivery are not suitable for educational practice and excellence in learning. Yet academic leaders have been calling for the redesign of clinical education for decades. How might we best approach this problem?

Services have been "designed" since the first modern service was created. Consider that Thomas Jefferson designed the US patent office in 1790, based on the British patent registry, and that the original criteria and even the legal process have changed little since then. Government services, such as the US Social Security program, were carefully conceived as standards across national or industry levels. Unlike products designed for sale through retail distribution networks, services are resource networks that can satisfy transaction requests from any customer through mediated channels. Successful services have always been designed and supported as social and technological systems, requiring sufficiently flexible standards decoupled from their technologies. Yet healthcare may be one of the last industries to adopt a designed regime to produce sociotechnical services.

Innovating Big Box Clinical Education

Hospitals have leveraged their "big box" administration to heavily invest in advanced medical and information technology. Hospital *services* have retained their essential patterns, however, and differ little in 2012 from 1982. In fact, a description of hospital organizations in 1888 is surprisingly similar to today's structure.

Hospitals are organized into separately staffed and managed departments that treat patients by acuteness and temporality. The introduction of associated outpatient or urgent care in the 1980s reduced the burden on emergency departments, but many service units have remained remarkably unchanged over the years. With the cost and societal pressures of various healthcare reforms, the basic model of the clinic has not yet been successfully challenged. Could the clinic be transformed by the newly educated clinical leaders entering hospital services, with support from their faculties? Should system-level change start with education? How could education drive institutional innovation? What if clinical education were reformulated as a service (D2.0), organized and led at the institutional level (D3.0), and transferred across the educational sector (D4.0)?

As both a local and transnational institution, medical education is complex and crosses levels of design process. For this reason, the "target level" of design method is the position that gives effective access to the adjacent two levels most crucial for the outcomes. Positioning education as a D3.0 project, we can inherit the service design methods of D2.0 and "reach up" to the adjacent strategic scale of D4.0. The rationale for this process is that an organizational leader can transfer practices across institutions (D4.0), but service-level projects (D2.0) may not reach across organizational boundaries.

The need for a new frame of design thinking and research is driven by the order of complexity. D2.0 is driven by *customers* (or users), and a D3.0 institutional context is driven by *organizations*, regulators, and patients.

The complexity (and risk of getting it wrong) in D3.0 increases by an order of magnitude.

The opportunities for designers to contribute to service transformation are enhanced and expanded when embracing the D3.0 perspective. Rather than merely producing visual and digital artifacts as end products enabling clinical activities, designers in the D3.0 context are involved in:

- Embracing organizational-level services design as a participatory process.

- Employing creative and analytical problem-solving tools with diverse multidisciplinary (clinical and staff) teams.

- Coordinating and facilitating innovation processes for organizational teams.

- Evaluating new service proposals and their fit to other services and systems in use.

- Facilitating visual integration of concepts and proposals to communicate design options.

Taking a D3.0 position sets priorities. Organizational outcomes take precedence over resident education, but there is no reason not to improve all touchpoints. As in any D3.0 project, the needs for change are apparent, so where do we invest? Today's clinical practice is the outcome of a long process of education, one that generates well-qualified specialists. But the traditional focus on technical practice and medical knowledge ignores emerging social and public aims for healthcare improvement and a healthy society.

Doctors can be forgiven for replicating the same educational system—after all, it produces clinical excellence and arguably achieves its primary objectives. Success makes any system more difficult to change. Also, the most difficult competencies to teach, if not to learn, are those that may change a practice that trainees have not even become competent at managing.

Contexts and Content of Clinical Education

Medical school is only the beginning of a lifelong career of learning and practice. Postgraduate education and residency establishes the physician in a career timeline that requires constant updating of knowledge and performance, from passing board exams to periodic maintenance of certification. The level of performance required to manage a concentrated workload of 80 to 100 patients a day is learned in a 3- to 5-year residency (7 years for surgery and some subspecialties), where 80-hour workweeks are typical.

Education is more complex than clinical practice because it has multiple foci and measures of success. It usually involves research, which practitioners do not do.

Clinical work involves much more *routine* than residency. Education places residents and faculty within the operational environment of live clinical practice, then layers multiple paths of learning and practice onto the routines. Residents learn in a high-tempo, high-risk mix of scheduled and improvised occasions. Education has multiple outcomes, whereas clinical encounters may have a single path from admission to discharge. Residency is mediated by multiple entities, ranging from the university and hospitals to the American Council of Graduate Medical Education and the academy boards that certify practitioners. Making simple changes to education does not necessarily scale beyond the institutional boundary.

Clinical work is technical and physical work. Not only is it not online, it is only peripherally enabled by information resources. Most of what we consider user experience is tangential to technical work. In fact, paper records (whether patient records or clinical notes) have been found in numerous studies to communicate more effectively and accurately within clinical teams than electronic records systems.[4] Information resources for clinical diagnostic and treatment decisions are common when learning in residency, but once in practice are used infrequently. No experienced doctors prepare to perform a common procedure by brushing up online first (although they may review the steps of a complicated technique to refresh their memory). Clinical work is not automated, nor should it be if the object is *care*.

The outcomes of clinical education (and all post-secondary learning) are social and public goods. Social goods include access to healthcare, public health and community care, the ethical use of appropriate technologies and procedures, and the movement toward a patient-centric vision of healthcare. These outcomes are associated with a shift from D3.0 to D4.0.

Design Strategies for Clinical Education

How do doctors do what they do every day? How do they acquire their extraordinary blend of human, physical, cognitive, and technical skills and manage to maintain superhuman schedules from medical school through practice? How is their training designed to develop these skills and mindset?

Medical practice has been based on craft skill since the founding of the clinical tradition, and long before as guilds of trained healers and surgeons. It is a sophisticated craft, but one of a tradition of independent practitioners with significant autonomy and professional prestige that lives in cultural conflict with the bureaucratic mode of the hospital.[5] Residents train in an apprenticeship to learn the hands-on work and manners of their attending physician mentors. Once accepted in a residency, doctors are *socialized* until they attain a defined level of skill and pass final board exams. That is, much of their training happens as a result of continual exposure to the culture of medicine. This cultural socialization forms the persistent mental models that maintain the profession and its practices.

Culture reproduces itself for our own survival, and it outlasts all of us and our interventions. An understanding of culture is necessary if we are to change it or propose service design models. Designed services can bring great productivity and enhance knowledge sharing and production, but interventions in process and technology have done little to change the essential routines of clinical training. As a stable, widely distributed, high-performance social system, clinical education is not easily changed by "design thinking." There are few entry points for designers to study, observe, define, and introduce prototypes. Changes to education take years for adoption, overcoming barriers to co-creating, evaluating, and diffusing new processes.

The progression of medical education (Table 6.1) indicates very different educational approaches (learning modes) and objectives for each stage of education or practice. These translate to differing information needs and resources used in each stage, and different service models.

TABLE 6.1 LEVELS AND MODES OF MEDICAL EDUCATION

Practice stage	Learning modes	Objectives
Medical school	Didactic, instructor-led courses in dedicated university programs; extensive reading and testing; problem-based small group learning; clinical practice training (third and fourth years)	Completion of program with high marks in courses; high scoring on board exams; learning practice of "doctoring"; licensure
Residency (dedicated training in elective specialty)	Apprenticeship by rounds (observations), doing procedures under guidance of attending, and teaching; typically includes a research rotation	Mastering procedures and clinical routines; passing specialty boards; acceptance into fellowships; entry into practice
Fellowship (subspecialty training and research)	Research, advanced procedures training, and clinical practice; often involves continuous teaching and practice in related specialties	Completion of program required for specialized practice or academic role
Practicing physician (private or group practice)	Learning in reflective practice on the job; learning how to manage a practice; logging clinical learning hours for continuing medical education	Growing a practice and maintaining currency in the field
Attending physician (medical faculty and practicing clinician)	As faculty, learning advanced clinical practice; clinical research; continuous learning in course development	Academic progression; senior staff roles; publication

Trends in clinical education change slowly because disrupting the education of doctors midstream may introduce unforeseeable risks that outweigh the value of innovation. Educational IT has always lagged practice and cannot be counted on to drive professional change. To be acceptable across institutional contexts, online resources must precisely represent acknowledged canons of education and the baseline of current knowledge, *not* the cutting edge of new procedures and devices.

Fundamental changes to education are formulated as top-down strategies. Yet innovations in *technique and technology* are often created as bottom-up practices that are advanced further in the training context. These are very different types of innovation.

Information Practices in Clinical Education

Medical, nursing, and other clinical education programs require intensive didactic learning, journal reading, anatomical dissection, patient interaction, hands-on procedure training, and technology-based simulations. Few educational experiences match the intensity and variety of teaching methods found in clinical education. It involves learning medical skills, technical and machine skills, communications practices, coordinated team activities, institutional rules, and industry regulations in a demanding institutional setting. Learning takes place across multiple knowledge domains—physical, biomedical, biological, technical, organizational, and informational. It demands full attention to the clinical tasks at hand, and optimal access to facts, formulas, lists, and techniques from memory. The trainee's information tasks cannot be separated from care practice or the learning process, and because medical research, knowledge sharing, and technology never go idle, these drivers continue throughout the entire life cycle of professional practice.

Clinical education is not yet directly delivered online to the extent we find in administration (trainee evaluations and logs), clinical data (health records), or clinical decision making (online research resources). But it is rapidly changing. Education is a complex multichannel activity, and not every task can be—or should be—automated or socialized online. Most medical schools video record all basic science lectures, and students download and watch them on their own time and often at rapid speed. Students now spend more time in small problem-solving teams than in lecture halls. These are contextual changes, not technologies. Allocating mere content and clinical media to the Web as if it were facilitating *education* would be a significant mistake.

Residents are both doctors and advanced students, and are constantly learning from experience with patients and colleagues in clinical situations. Although they have access to a wide range of resources to answer questions and concerns, many often start with Google, using specific terms to filter out nonclinical references. Residents report that they generally select only high-credibility site references (not Wikipedia).[6] They may start an information search on familiar sites, but then follow completely different information paths than nonprofessionals.

Residents show a different path through the information ecology than other clinicians. They navigate between resources located in *care networks* (electronic and social system networks supporting direct care services) and *learning networks* (networks and resources enabling tools for education and research) during their training. They may start and stay with learning networks in their internship and second year, then use care networks more often in their final years in residency as they learn the core curriculum and move fully into practice. When preparing for board examinations, residents cite a 3- to 6-month return to resources in learning networks.

Within a given day or week, residents may navigate among all the health IT (HIT) domains. Figure 6.2 shows the pathways among information resources followed by a typical resident during the course of a clinical day. In this scenario, a junior (first or second year) internal medicine resident may interact with seven different HIT resources during her first half-hour in the office:

1. She begins by reviewing the case schedule for the day to consider the treatments and procedures that will be needed and to prepare for questions that may come up during the rounds. She scans the patient list by unit in the Epic EMR. The EMR is efficient because the records of a given patient can be selected to view their current (or overnight) status and any updates to a condition or schedule.

2. An older inpatient being treated for liver complications from diabetes was to be discharged, and was observed with emergent vertigo. The case was moved to the top of the list, so the resident takes a few minutes to search the issue on UpToDate to help determine a care plan.

3. UpToDate does not help diagnose the causes of vertigo, so she scans for a clinical review article from recent research. Suspecting a drug interaction as the cause, she continues to research quickly for another 5 minutes, evaluating the scheduled medication.

4. A lung cancer patient requires a chest tube insertion to drain fluid accumulation. Although she has seen many of them performed, she is scheduled to perform the next one herself, so she scans the steps on Procedures Consult and watches the insertion steps on video. She prints the Quick Review as a checklist, just in case.

5. Reminders from the McKesson practice management system identify two patients to see before their release from the hospital.

6. Reminders from the hospital laboratory service indicate that new images and blood tests are available. She scans a blood workup and then consults UpToDate on the values.

7. She refers to Epocrates to determine medications and dosages.

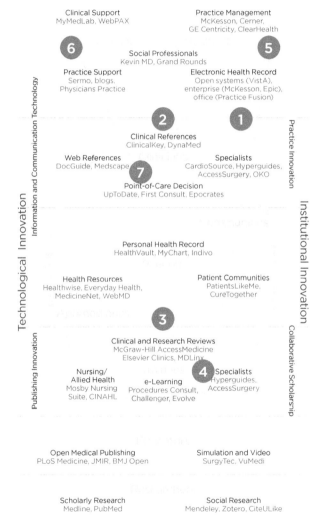

Care Networks

Clinical Support
MyMedLab, WebPAX

Practice Management
McKesson, Cerner,
GE Centricity, ClearHealth

6

Social Professionals
Kevin MD, Grand Rounds

5

Practice Support
Sermo, blogs,
Physicians Practice

Electronic Health Record
Open systems (VistA),
enterprise (McKesson, Epic),
office (Practice Fusion)

2   **1**

Clinical References
ClinicalKey, DynaMed

Web References
DocGuide, Medscape

7

Specialists
CardioSource, Hyperguides,
AccessSurgery, OKO

Point-of-Care Decision
UpToDate, First Consult, Epocrates

Personal Health Record
HealthVault, MyChart, Indivo

Health Resources
Healthwise, Everyday Health,
MedicineNet, WebMD

Patient Communities
PatientsLikeMe,
CureTogether

3

Clinical and Research Reviews
McGraw-Hill AccessMedicine
Elsevier Clinics, MDLinx

Nursing/
Allied Health
Mosby Nursing
Suite, CINAHL

e-Learning
Procedures Consult,
Challenger, Evolve

4 Specialists
Hyperguides,
AccessSurgery

Open Medical Publishing
PLoS Medicine, JMIR, BMJ Open

Simulation and Video
SurgyTec, VuMedi

Scholarly Research
Medline, PubMed

Social Research
Mendeley, Zotero, CiteULike

Learning Networks

Technological Innovation

Information and Communication Technology

Publishing Innovation

Practice Innovation

Institutional Innovation

Collaborative Scholarship

FIGURE 6.2
Pathways through the health information technology ecology.

There is no "one-stop shop" that integrates these resources, and as obvious as a single-source portal may seem, there have been no successful innovations of such a resource. Each is optimized for a specific information task, and that purpose may be incommensurate with even closely adjacent tasks. Billing and diagnostics are different use contexts, and superficial integration can be counterproductive. For example, attempts to integrate point-of-care information (e.g., UpToDate) with the EMR's diagnoses and lab results have not caught on. The assumption that patient condition data in the EMR might trigger a search is backward—the search for a *condition* at the point of care will assist in diagnosis, which would then be entered in the EMR.

Even if learned in coursework, clinical informatics are first used while on the job. Except for the EMR, only minimal training at best is expected or provided to busy doctors. The constant time pressure in a typical clinical day reveals the need for extremely concise information objects and minimal cognitive overhead. UX and information design enhancements can make a significant difference in "time yield," and saving a clinician a few seconds in a page view or navigation will be noticed and immensely appreciated.

Practice Research for Institutional Innovation

Practice-based clinical research is conducted to improve health outcomes by evaluating new routines based on empirical evidence from practice. Simple yet high-impact studies have led to better infection prevention, procedural error reduction through checklists, or better patient care flow to reduce wait times. Practice research can make a more significant and immediate contribution to patient health than traditional biomedical research, although disease research and drug trials make news and get funding. Practice studies are often overlooked as boring and administrative, yet recommendations can be applied generally and immediately.

Practice research can have a direct impact on individual patients' lives. The current mandate toward adopting preprocedure and patient checklists in hospital care is the result of practice research on the clinical effectiveness of checklists in preventing iatrogenic infections. The simple "undesigned" checklist reminds residents and surgeons of basic steps in both complex and simple tasks. Physician and author Atul Gawande attests to the impact of this simple solution in his popular book *The Checklist Manifesto*.[7]

Gawande reports on the adoption problems associated with the very introduction of checklists into the work ecology. Checklists are generally associated in clinical culture with nurses and management, and doctors resist the idea of using checklists on a clipboard to remind them of the most basic steps in a process. Yet, studies performed by Peter Provonost at Johns Hopkins demonstrated that a basic infection-control checklist reduced deadly complications with central venous catheters, a common infection vector.[8] In the initial experiment, the 10-day infection rate dropped from 11% to zero. In a 15-month trial, only two infections were reported. The study indicated that the checklists prevented up to 43 infections and eight deaths and saved at least $2 million in associated costs.

The institutional checklist is typically a printed form with a single page of brief items to check and perhaps sign as an accountability routine for clinical care teams. Checklists are provided for both standard patient protocols and procedures. Checklists are starting to appear in online form as a guideline or reminder. A standardized protocol for basic procedure safety and accountability is shown (in part) in Figure 6.3.

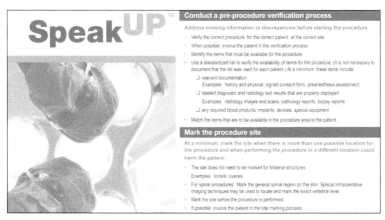

FIGURE 6.3
Universal protocol for procedure safety. (From the Joint Commission, http://jointcommission.org/standards_information/up.aspx)

Why do such obviously beneficial instruments find resistance in the regulated, risk-averse hospital environment? Two cultural factors work against the acceptance of checklists: clinical culture and research reputational culture. Senior residents often admit that they would not personally use (visibly) a universal protocol checklist, online or printed, of the type deployed in these studies. Universal protocol checklists cover patient identification, informed consent, marking the right site, sterile hygiene, and a "time out" to ensure general clinician situation awareness. Where an institutional mandate exists to use checklists, nurses or first-year interns typically follow the resident's procedure against the checklist as a delegated duty.

Practice research is also overlooked due to reputation factors. Although major published studies have demonstrated the efficacy and significant cost savings for guiding technical work with simple checklists, this practice research is often treated as second class by the scholarly world. As professor of dermatology Jonathan Rees pointed out, the funding and status bias of medical research relegates practice to scholarly irrelevance:

> Most medical researchers rarely, if ever, see patients. . . . However, many of the major discoveries that have had a direct impact on clinical practice arose from clinical disciplines rather than from generic biomedical approaches—consider hip replacements, cataract surgery, the importance of *Helicobacter pylori*, phototherapy, in vitro fertilisation, and minimally invasive surgery. In the biomedical model, these successes are brushed aside as being of historical interest only. From finding genes to gene therapy and stem cell therapy, both the public and research community itself are fed a biased view of medical advances. Cancer cured (in mice) again.[9]

Innovations Emerge from Practice Needs

High-impact innovations are more likely to originate from observing common situations in everyday practice. Many of the popular clinical information resources originated as simple content services created by a physician who saw a need in everyday practice or learning (including UpToDate, the Wheeless and OrthoBullets services for orthopedics, and the VuMedi surgical video–sharing service).

Sermo, a specialized physician networking service, was started as a way for doctors to exchange answers and ideas, and to replace the collegiality that doctors miss from their residency days. Sermo also originated from observations of a practice need, as founder Daniel Palestrant recognized that small-practice physicians have few ways to ask questions and exchange information with other doctors in an environment of trust and privacy.

These products all followed the essential Christensen model of disruptive innovation in their respective markets.[10] Harvard professor Clayton Christensen famously established the pattern of disruptive innovation, where the entry of a noncompetitive new product, serving an emerging market niche, can rapidly grow by increasing technology performance to overtake existing markets. The theory distinguished disruptive from *sustaining* innovations, which can be significant developments in their own right (e.g., new EMR systems that replace outdated products), but do not form new markets.

Each of these services started as a niche product in the physician marketplace, originally envisioned by a fellow doctor who observed a need from his or her own practice. Most of these introduced alternatives to long-standing practices, where a different approach was not yet obvious. An emerging innovation will be ignored by competitors because it focuses on an unprofitable and small market and poses no threat to their share. But some of these local solutions could grow quickly into popular platforms and replace current paradigms entirely. UpToDate has grown with the widespread use of the

Web and has replaced the reference books and literature searches prevalent before its success. As an early innovator, it was able to enter and capture the emerging market.

Given the sheer size of the healthcare market, it is telling that the disruptive innovation model has *not* been widely successful. Few sustainable successful digital innovations or online resources have been developed from the findings of clinical research. There are no successful health records platforms developed as disruptive innovations. Several well-funded, high-profile innovations (such as Google Health and Revolution Health) did not capture markets as expected. Cost savings and user experience are also not (yet) the significant drivers they are in other markets, so designing a better user experience is not necessarily a sustainable advantage. The healthcare sector is different.

Improving Clinical Decision Making

Clinical point-of-care and clinical decision reference systems are ubiquitous in residency. Interns now carry smartphones loaded with Epocrates and eMedicine. Today's residents are digital natives, having grown up with the Web, and are now the first cohorts of e-doctors. Since the early 2000s, hospitals have placed networked desktop computers in every ward, meeting room, and common area. Many clinics have switched their staff from pagers to smartphones. Physicians have access to high-quality online clinical references and research at any location or time, from the desktop or mobile devices.

As institutions implemented enterprise EMRs, one of the attempts at integration was to directly augment clinical interaction associated with patient records.[11] Available for over a decade in Web and handheld formats, clinical references are being integrated with patient records as EMR assistants. This HIT integration leverages the idea of actuating information in context, enabling the clinician instant access to drug or diagnostic test information from a preferred clinical reference database when a question arises or when prompted by values in the patient record. It is presumed this functionality will increase practitioner satisfaction with and use of the EMR as well.

There are two problems with this idea: the assumption that the EMR is actually *at* the doctor's point of care, and that the EMR displays terms that may require clarification by a reference search. These problems can be resolved by reframing how decisions are actually made.

The literature is inconsistent regarding the true effectiveness and appreciation of clinical decision support systems (CDSS) at the point of care.[12] In most cases, these studies should be considered a snapshot of the state of the art of the time. Though the trend 5 years ago was to integrate information at the point of the EMR patient record, the main users of the clinical reference at the EMR would be junior staff, as they would have both the need (based on less experience) and inclination. Experienced physicians are not inclined to use these resources when at the EMR. This attempt at integration may only be adding cognitive complexity to an already overloaded interface and task.

Experts and Clinical Information Practices

How do clinicians mobilize information at the point of care to form diagnoses, determine treatments, or make patient care decisions? My research on clinical information practices explained the differences in information drivers and online practices between residents and senior clinicians, all with access to the same HIT resources.[13] Differences are found in the intended clinical uses of information, but these applications also reveal differences in decision-making style associated with experience. Junior residents deal with relatively common, everyday situations that they might be able to resolve from clinical references such as UpToDate. Less experienced doctors need to understand the current state of the practice, any controversies regarding treatments, and pitfalls in therapies they may consider. These are issues well covered by online references.

Expert clinicians refer to different sources and content types than residents, and read them differently. Senior clinicians (5 or more years postresidency) may be both teaching faculty and practitioners. The more experience clinicians have, the less need they have to refer to a common condition. They are also less likely to see routine cases that residents can handle, so they do not require access to a comprehensive database of medical conditions outside their specialization. Because senior clinicians see the tough cases, they refer to primary journal sources, using searches in PubMed or Medline. There they are confronted by the problem of searching a vast biomedical literature that is not indexed by diagnosis or clinical condition but by research topic.

All doctors are time limited. Senior physicians may have much less time available than a resident for problem solving, and they deal with more complex cases. Senior practitioners (in an inpatient setting) have less need to look up general points of clarification for symptoms or diagnoses because they have a broad personal repertoire that surpasses the simplified outlines in the references. They may also specialize (if in a group practice) and can refer to another specialist for a unique problem they may encounter, again more reliably and probably more quickly than with online research. Practitioners usually develop expertise in an area and are known for and relied upon for complex or exceptional situations.

These findings are consistent with cognitive scientist Gary Klein's view of expert reasoning, known as recognition-primed decision making.[14] Physicians' decisions for complex and ambiguous clinical situations appear to be intuitive and personal, not rote or formulaic. Intuitive mastery comes from the ability to adapt deep patterns developed in the clinician's experience. This reasoning has been discovered across domains of expertise.

Clinical Sensemaking

We can observe two cognitive modes of information behavior—clinical *decision making* (a task supported by online resources) and clinical *sensemaking* for complex cases (a problem-solving characteristic of experts).

Decision making selects an optimal choice from options presented in response to a case. Because trainees do not yet have a deep repertoire (1,000 or more cases) from which to make self-informed judgments, they are obligated by training and liability to formulate decisions supported by evidence, rules, and best practices as documented in current informatics resources.

Open-ended navigation of a difficult problem based on limited information and an unknown content base is a classic sensemaking situation. If clinicians analyzed complex cases (such as rare diseases or odd symptom patterns) using a process of elimination or exhaustive search strategies, their solution-finding process could take longer than a patient might live! Sensemaking involves the assimilation of multiple streams of information and observations, testing hypotheses drawn from experience, using intuition to resolve gaps in knowledge, and accommodating (not necessarily resolving) ambiguity.

The *New York Times Magazine*'s "Diagnosis" column presents true stories of people dealing with complicated health conditions. These diagnostic puzzles are not easily solvable by logical analysis and are often resolved by an individual with unique prior experience with the exact condition. The column reveals the power of *recognition* as opposed to analysis. Some nonphysicians are able to correctly identify a rare disease from a brief narrative because they have personally encountered the disease and relied on pattern recognition of the symptoms and unique characteristics.

A clinician faced with a complex disease presentation, such as an unforeseeable complication, has the goal of resolving the patient's source condition. A truly complex situation involves not just information and a course of action and observation, but might entail patient culture and family conditions, personal history, unique biochemistry and medications, prior diseases, and unknown allergic responses.

Gary Klein takes expert sensemaking further toward decision making. Sensemaking is not a set of discrete steps, but rather a continuous process of testing the data of reality against different frames or models that the clinician poses to the data. Klein's *data-frame* sensemaking presents the mental construct of the frame guiding the interpretation of data (symptoms, signs, signals, information) to achieve an outcome or resolution to a problem.[15] Think of a frame as a mental model about a problem area populated with known facts, opinions, and memories from personal experience. A frame selects the perception of cues in the data and environment, enabling the efficient selection of possible meanings. Experts "make sense" by preselecting information that counts, rapidly sifted by their frames.

Unlike trainees, experts exhibit confidence in their frames and are willing to commit to them sufficiently to explore hypotheses available within the frame. They serve as filters or assessments to test how well a situation matches the frame. Sensemaking pulls together plausible narratives from the data that enable the expert to present a coherent "answer" rapidly.

No checklist is thorough enough to document and resolve the unique challenges of the human body in its environments. Many diseases behave as wicked problems, with multiple interacting sources and the inability to clearly determine an effective course. And each decision counts, as the opportunity cost of inappropriate treatment can be the loss of health or life.

How do we best design information tools to assist experts in sensemaking—in recognizing problems—when few have the experience to identify these unique conditions?

Fitting Informatics to Workflow

Practitioners often report that their use of online information tools declined throughout and after residency. As clinicians progress in a career, they have less need for information support at the point of care. They learn from their own case experience, establish a repertoire, and keep current using more advanced resources such as journals and review articles. This shift in information practices is consistent with recent experiments showing that senior clinicians use a "conscious reasoning" style for complex diagnostic problems, a process of supplementing or activating the scaffolds of long-term memory patterns.[16] Junior doctors have not constructed deep enough experience (or frames) to pursue conscious reasoning, so tend to follow the published guidelines or procedures for an identified condition.

Other studies have found that clinical references can improve performance but are rarely used by clinicians at the point of care or with the EMR. This variance is explained by suggesting that use of references is not yet established within the clinical workflow, or that interfaces are insufficiently easy to use. It is more likely that the EMR itself is not a conducive context for information for clinical problem solving, even if helpful patient data is provided at the point of care. Enhancements in usability and content may not result in increased adoption, as we would expect in other fields. In the institutional context, clinical need, habit, and ease of access are bigger factors than interaction usability.

Well-designed information resources and EMR interfaces present information aids following a temporal clinical workflow—the series of tasks performed in their standard sequence in the clinical setting. A standard workflow starts with patient presentation and delivers information aiding for some configuration of the following standard tasks:

- **Presentation:** the patient's signs and symptoms as observed
- **Diagnosis:** identifying and testing possible conditions that match the symptomology
- **Indications and contraindications:** the guidelines for treatment or avoiding certain treatments
- **Treatment:** therapies appropriate for the various diagnoses associated with the condition
- **Procedures/techniques:** steps to perform procedures to deliver treatment
- **Prognosis:** expectations for patient recovery or clinical outcomes
- **Aftercare:** guidelines for postprocedure recovery or home care
- **Patient education:** guidelines presented to the patient about the condition or treatment

Explicit workflow provides temporal bookmarking, giving a clinical user confidence in the regularity of content organization, which aids findability. But residents and attendings often see patients for just a single step in the workflow. They are picking up where other doctors left off, and are literally "thrown" into acting without having the ability to step back, reflect, and research. Assumptions of a primary disease and prior history precede the encounter. Other disease conditions may muddle the diagnostics, and medications may be potentially conflicting.

The conventional EMR, with its static patient record and incomplete history, cannot advise the clinician on real, implicit patient needs. If it attempted to do so, there would be little trust in the advice. The accuracy and context would be thought questionable, even if the advice was correct. One poor-fitting recommendation would doom such a feature forever. Instead, the closest approximation employed in practice is the *clinical alert*, the reminders and suggestions from the EMR rules database to prompt care teams to review possible conflicts or harmful outcomes from prescriptions or orders placed through the system. EMRs have been designed with a bias to push alerts to responsible caregivers, resulting in too many alerts and alert fatigue.

Several reasons for alert fatigue have been empirically discovered, but the primary reason appears to be that the vast majority of alerts are for possible drug interactions. In 2009 Harvard's Beth Israel Deaconess Medical Center analyzed a collection of more than 233,000 alerts and discovered that 98% warned of drug interactions, and that 90% of these were overridden. At this level of irrelevance, physicians likely override or tune out other alerts as well.

One solution to this informatics problem has been to encourage smarter *asynchronous alerts*—the updates sent to the caregiver's activity stream at a later point to indicate possible outcomes as a patient's physical status changes. Not only were these overridden less often, but they were found to be more relevant because of their responsiveness to changing contexts that the clinician could not have observed.

Cognitive Aiding of Team Care

Are new types of clinical information aids needed? Do experts only need clues and tips for unusual situations to act as a nudge in the right direction? How can a caregiver's always partial knowledge best be supplemented?

For decision aids to be effective, the information presented must be associated as specifically as possible with the context of a care situation. Yet these situations differ by specialty, clinic type, stage of care or treatment, and so on. The point of care is really a different point for every type of clinician.

The points where care occurs are spread out across clinicians and over time. Complex care is often performed by a clinical team, not by individuals working alone. Yet medical training emphasizes (and certifies) the performance and knowledge of individual physicians. Some residency education programs have reoriented their training toward team care, but these approaches are necessarily incomplete. Every residency trains doctors for a particular specialty. Coordinating team training across clinical specialties confronts a complex organizational environment that few (if any) institutions have resolved sufficiently.

Research and best practices are showing the value of developing explicit team practices in healthcare. Teamwork as a guiding process helps reduce individual and technology-induced errors, improves the coordination of care, and builds a culture of collaborative work in the clinical environment. Team-based care practices have not propagated widely in US healthcare, though they have been shown to improve patient outcomes. Healthcare management has yet to develop team approaches to process and workflow improvement, and team models have only recently been introduced into medical training. Several approaches to team development in 21st-century healthcare are recommended:

- Training team approaches in real-world settings

- Debriefing and solicitation of feedback from team members

- Including all team members in patient care planning and service decisions

- Creating processes of collaborative care as continuous improvement[17]

Field studies of clinical team performance in acute care,[18] emergency room, and critical care operations[19] reveal how complex operations and procedures are performed as integrated team practices. Technical clinical work is distributed across physicians, nurses, pharmacists, and anesthesiologists, all working on different requirements for an inpatient situation. For coordinated procedures such as surgeries and intensive care management (e.g., cardiac or respiratory incidents), standard teams of specialized clinicians are assembled as transient crews, performing roles according to expectations for well-trained situations. Teams are created and dispersed as needed, demanding a skill set of flexible collaboration by role, clear communication across roles, and giving and receiving feedback to improve collaboration.

In large hospitals, individual roles are trained by constant performance, and clinical teams conduct complex operations together with minimal planning and guidance. A visiting surgeon may work with surgical nurses and an anesthesiologist who have never met one another before the case. A well-known point for the universal checklist protocol includes a step to ensure each member of the surgical team knows everyone's names, to promote trust and coordination. The surgeon may provide directions and exceptions to standard protocols, but for standard procedures, strict role coordination has passed as teamwork for many years.

Each member of a clinical team performs technical work assigned to their role, communicates as needed with specific team members, and uses information and cognitive artifacts pertinent to their role. Yet the true collaborative teams envisioned by progressive institutions have not emerged. The efficiency, accuracy, and completeness demanded in acute care and clinical procedures sets boundaries on the ability of clinical team members to exchange roles or collaborate. There are no agreed processes for collaboration beyond the strict assigned roles in care planning. Today's clinical teams may believe they are working together in teams as effectively as possible. Yet a barrier to change or innovation is the belief that a current process has been optimized.

Design Sensemaking

A comprehensive picture of clinical IT domains for point-of-care, administrative, and specialist services was shown in Figure 4.4. Many of these tools help guide and educate the clinician to make better care decisions, and so should be evaluated by their effect on patient outcomes. This turns out to be a difficult result to measure.

Studies of CDSS over the last decade revealed high user satisfaction with these tools over time, but this finding may also reflect several known biases in sampling. Study participants are mostly residents, who as trainees appreciate having any information resource that helps their learning and performance. Early technology adopters (e.g., younger doctors) also are able to cognitively adapt their decision-making style to new tools and tend to be less critical of the tools' shortcomings because they have probably not used the many alternatives. In other words, CDSS resources could be much better, and the sample has insufficient experience to make the demand. They also do not usually pay for apps and information resources, so are not behaving as vigilant *customers*.

In contrast, clinicians in practice are much more deliberate in adopting information technologies, whether an EMR or clinical reference. As found in studies of other professional practices, doctors become highly skilled in resources learned in graduate education, and they maintain facility with those tools that were learned in their generational period. Learning new HIT requires commitment—not just the time to learn but the cognitive burden of learning to use a resource that may be used infrequently or that may require changing a stable set of known routines.

How well do clinical references like UpToDate or Epocrates fit the clinician's work ecology or decision making? Even though these tools may be commonly used and accessible through a university library subscription or hospital intranets, their use is always *discretionary*. Many different resources could be substituted for the same information need, and few institutions narrow their options to just a single provider.

Discretionary resources are third-party products that present content with no relationship to the decision context in which they will be used. For example, WebMD may provide useful (if nonexclusive) content, but the interface is overloaded with links, categories, and advertising, all of which bias the user experience as a commercial product (see Figure 2.1). The assumption is made that WebMD is being searched and read just like any other website, but the health seeker might be in a critical or compromised situation and not have the luxury of navigating the complicated interface. Health information needs, unlike most other information tasks, may indeed be urgent.

The risks of designing clinical informatics as end-user products is that the vendor can make design and content decisions without regard to the actual clinical task needs. Design decisions are often and effectively made based on inferences from a small number of observations, but the more distant these observations are from the front lines of practice, the higher the risk of irrelevance or commercial bias. The deciding factor for clinical resources should be whether the content design and user experience enhances or augments care practice and patient outcomes.

- Good CD2.0 opportunities include interaction design of clinical information resources, procedure simulation devices, and inter-active learning environments. These contribute to the overall redesign of healthcare education and practice.

- Educational service design needs a flexible strategy, a scalable service, and an organizational mindset. A CD3.0 strategy may integrate existing educational services (CD2.0) to adapt new resources to organizational strategy (CD3.0) and scale across the healthcare education sector (CD4.0).

- Advanced service design can provide multilayered support systems: training to support end-to-end guidance for complex procedures, scaffolding for quickly learning manual skills, and ambient and portable displays to enable distributed cognition and collaboration.

- A vast range of clinical and reference knowledge is employed in medical curricula. E-learning platforms have recently shown promise, if designed well, to improve curriculum management.

- Institutional drivers such as a certification or standards push, or even an organization-wide campaign such as an infection control strategy, may have key touchpoints with your service concept and will pull it through the organization. By aligning service enhancements to anticipated or new institutional re-quirements, the service changes will be accommodated as part of the expected change.

- Designers should not aim to reinvent clinical practice or work-flow (not yet). Clinical work is taught and deeply ingrained, and innovations that attempt to change labels or paradigms may just be rejected as poorly adapted to clinical reality.

- An iterative and perhaps lengthy process of service prototyp-ing is necessary for any clinical education or practice work-flow redesign. Iterations should be used as opportunities for increasing the circle of stakeholders involved in evaluating the process redesign.

Case Study: IDEO Continuity of Care

The California HealthCare Foundation (CHCF) sponsored a unique design challenge, led by the global design firm IDEO, to innovate the process for managing a patient's continuity of care. Collaborating as a team with CHCF, IDEO brought representatives together from the largest US organizations managing health information, including the US Department of Veterans Affairs and EMR system vendors Epic, Cerner, McKesson, and others, to uncover new possibilities for improving patient opportunities in the process.

The design study focused on the expressed need to improve the continuity-of-care document (CCD), which communicates and updates a patient's medical status and complex health concerns between clinicians over the duration of their care. Physicians and staff record and transfer patient information from diagnoses and tests, from primary care to specialist referrals, and between electronic health records.

Two major design opportunities were discovered in the continuity-of-care process: the inclusion of patients in communicating their own continuity, and the enhancement of EMR systems to enable patient collaboration with their care. IDEO's Abbe Don led the joint team's co-creation and design process to resolve health information and sensemaking concerns from patients, caregivers, and physicians. Four care challenges were discovered:

- Patients feel they are left on their own to figure out next steps.

- Patients with serious health issues work around the system to get the best care.

- Episodic and disjointed care hides valuable connections.

- Both patients and physicians doubt the reliability of (reported) health data.

These were translated into four physician needs and seven patient drivers for continuity of care. These were considered novel because the patient is not a user of the document but is rather a real life carrier of the data. In more patient-centered terms, these issues were expressed as:

- Represent what I truly care about.

- Present information in a way I can relate to.

- Help me cross-check my facts.

- Help me close communication loops among my care team.

- Set me up to have clarifying and guiding conversations.

- Clearly lay out the next steps.

- Show my trajectory over time.

The participatory workshop drew out compelling insights for future alternatives:

- The CCD process is not patient-centered because it is a document shared between physicians. It was never designed to be a patient instrument, so these emerging patient requirements are novel.

- Patients are starting to see the need for a secure and persistent location for their health data. A simple data storage solution ("Personal Health Record 2.0") was considered a design concept to pursue.

The research and workshop led to two design concepts and several future scenarios. Figure 6.4 shows a single page of the concept wireframe reflecting the design of patient-centered CCD data for a shared context. Patient and physician information needs (as shown above) are checked off for their relevance to the concept. Patient questions and concerns guiding the need for this view are shown in the page.

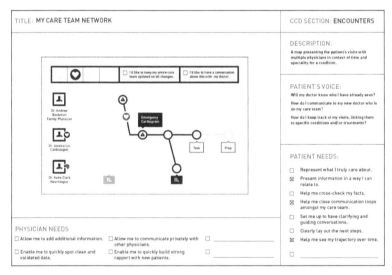

FIGURE 6.4

IDEO Continuity of Care: Project Synapse concept. (Courtesy of IDEO)

Two prototypes were prepared to reflect two modes of patient-centric CCD data presentation. The Timeline Meets Accordion concept (Figure 6.5) connected critical data elements that are today separated by multiple encounters and reports. The "accordion" view displays a section for each dimension of continuity, here shown in a website or tablet view, allowing the patient or physician to update and follow the history and current status of the healthcare journey.

A second "collage" concept presents a visual dashboard in a series of labeled visual boxes highlighting the current status or prominent data by selection. This concept suggests a future representation of patient care data in a mobile-friendly iconic display, integrated with calendar scheduling, communications, and patient health records.

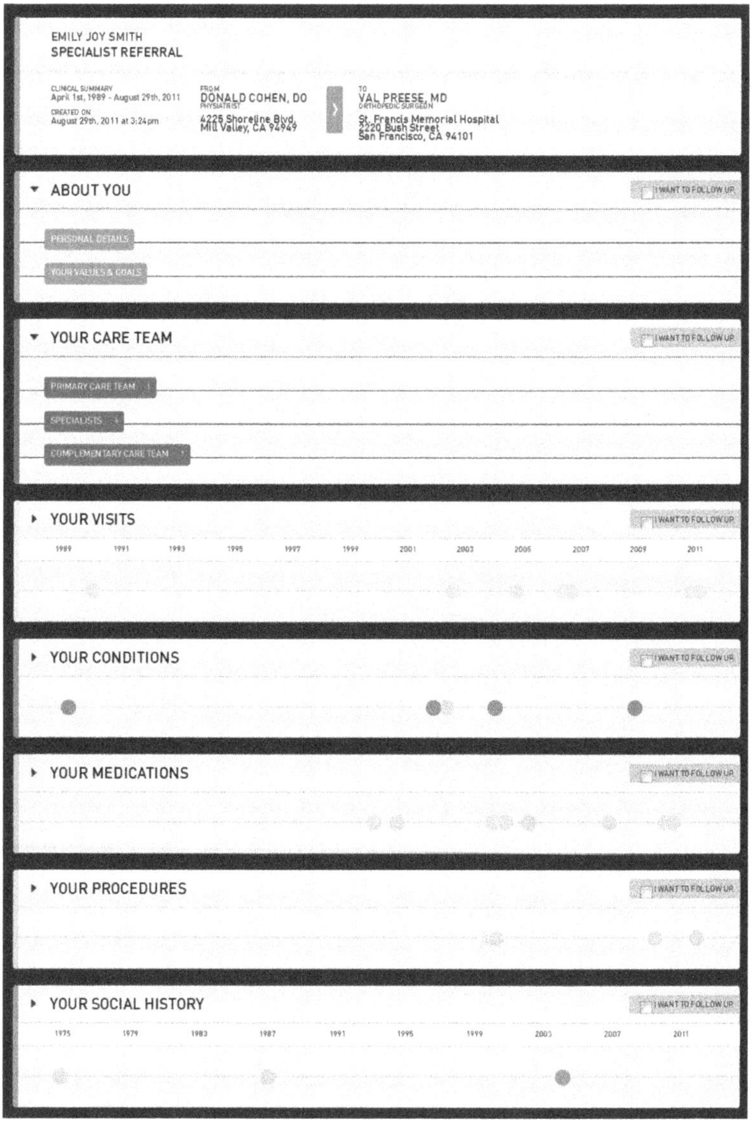

FIGURE 6.5
IDEO Continuity of Care: Timeline Meets Accordion. (Courtesy of IDEO)

These concepts support at least two scenarios or directions. One notion was a dynamic care plan process where the CCD served as an action plan for patients and a way to mutually align patient-centered goals with clinical team care and treatment schedules. Another scenario envisions an advanced EMR interface that summarizes patient data ("at a glance" summary) to create a mutual care plan. In both scenarios, the CCD process has been transformed from a passive data presentation to a patient-centered, active planning tool.

Project Synapse is presented online at CHCF (www.chcf.org/projects/2012/project-synapse-ccd-design).

LESSONS LEARNED

- Complex healthcare information problems can be simplified by articulating a new process that provides value to both providers and patients, rather than compromising on a format that serves only one or the other.

- The CCD case presents a fairly universal problem area, where many patient types might be expected to have similar information and navigation needs. A small-sample, rapid-research process was sufficient to develop the initial concepts due to the universal context of continuity of care.

- Nonprofit or agency sponsorship (such as CHCF) can support system-level design by engaging multiple vendors in the early design process, enabling all to respond to and benefit from the finding of a common research program.

- The CCD project also led to continuing universal design in the form of the patient record, with an open design contest sponsored by stakeholders from the Synapse project to solicit concepts for electronic health record design. See Blue Button: Challenge at http://blue-button.github.com/challenge/.

Methods: Stakeholder Co-creation

The Basadur Simplexity process is employed in a service design context as a powerful methodology for engaging stakeholders directly in co-creating their service concept. The second stakeholder design method relevant in the larger service context is Positive Deviance, one of a family of methods for organizational engagement. Both of these methodologies have widespread application and can be employed in other D3.0 and D4.0 contexts, such as management, customer-facing services, and information systems.

Simplexity Thinking

Min Basadur's Simplexity process has been in continual use and development since its inception in the 1980s as a creative problem-solving technique.[20] *Simplexity thinking* harnesses a group's ideation to generate a series of responses to successive levels of problem inquiry, resulting in a challenge map that serves as a road map to strategic design.

- **Applications:** The Simplexity process is used for strategic planning, ideation workshops, collaborative innovation, and participatory design workshops with clients and stakeholders. Because of the time necessary to conduct a full session, it is not generally employed with user participants as a *user-centered* design method. It is effective for identifying true priorities and mapping design proposals. It can be used as a macro-design structure for other methods and for project planning.

- **Requirements:** Simplexity workshops can be conducted with almost any group size, from 5 to 50 participants. Multiple facilitators are required for larger groups, but even with a small group, assigning a lead facilitator and a recorder/assistant is helpful. Breakout groups are typically most effective with five to seven people.

- **Workshop structure:** A full workshop requires an all-day commitment, or up to 2 days for larger groups or more complex problems. Planners should count on taking 30 minutes to introduce the session and orient participants, and up to an hour or more for each stage in the eight-stage process.

- **Preparation:** Simplexity is a sophisticated design process that requires training or experience to perform well. Trained Simplexity facilitators may require 4 to 6 hours of planning to design the sessions and organize the materials and logistics.

Simplexity guides practitioners through a series of progressive transformations of group idea generation and consensus selection. The entire process moves from generative problem formulation (A) through solution formulation (B) and implementation (C) in three phases and eight steps (Figure 6.6). This process can be followed for narrowly focused problems, such as identifying the best new features for a successful software product, or it can scale sufficiently to empower executives and stakeholders to formulate an entire business strategy and action plans.

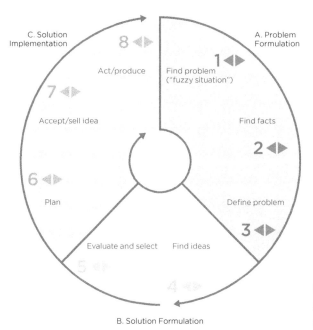

FIGURE 6.6
Simplexity method
phases and steps.

Creativity is maximized by constraining the process and allowing participants to focus on content. The eight steps follow a necessary sequence to ensure that prerequisites to each step are co-created. Fact finding is enhanced by achieving a powerfully framed problem. Clarification of the elements of the problem enable problem definition, which helps people find ideas that suggest solutions. Solutions are formulated in a two-phase dialogic process (Figure 6.7), moving from divergence (the goal being quantity and a wide range of ideas) to convergence (the goal being quality and selecting consensus ideas) as final solutions are selected in a rapid evaluative process.

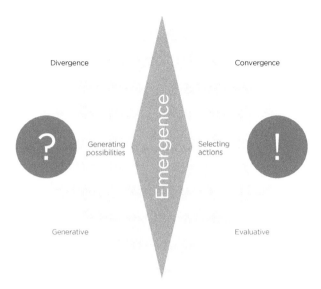

FIGURE 6.7
Dialogic process
language.

The best ideas are meaningless in innovation unless they are packaged for the audience, owners, or customers of the proposed solution. Simplexity takes a group of participants through a collaborative thinking process documented by sticky notes on boards organized to represent individual contributions for each of the eight steps. Each step is characterized by a common process of divergence and convergence, represented by the "<" and ">" symbols, respectively.

The process is not analytical and reductive in any stage, but instead reaches "convergence" of selected ideas by group progression. It organizes group participation around a central challenge, formulated as a focus question. Used as a facilitated and consultative method, the Simplexity process enables groups to generate highly readable problem maps and consensus solution scenarios based on a high variety of scenario alternatives.

Overview of Simplexity

Simplexity begins with a *fuzzy situation*, a deliberately undefined problem. Viewing the fuzzy situation from a neutral position, Simplexity guides a group of stakeholders from problem formulation to solution implementation. In each step, a process leader facilitates divergence, and participants generate ideas without judging or analyzing them. After a broad range of possibilities have been generated through divergence, participants converge to select the options that will be brought forward to the next step.

The three-stage implementation process ensures that the design team's momentum carries to the planning and promotion of the selected solution as the way forward.

A. PROBLEM FORMULATION

Step 1: Problem finding consists of anticipating and framing issues of importance. The result is a continuous flow of new, present, and future situations, changes, and opportunities for improvement for an organization.

Step 2: Fact finding is a rapid research stage of gathering information considered pertinent to the fuzzy situation. Observations are *then* evaluated and selected from those considered most helpful toward the next step.

Step 3: Problem definition converts the facts and elements a group selected into a wide variety of creative challenges. Participants select those that offer the most innovation opportunity. This step ensures that the selected problem definition represents the most effective presentation of the challenge tested by the process.

B. SOLUTION FORMULATION

Step 4: Idea finding creates a number of wide-ranging potential solutions to the target problem definition. As in each stage, a divergence generative step is followed by converging on a small number of preferred possible solutions.

Step 5: Evaluation and selection generates a variety of selection criteria potentially useful for making an unbiased and accurate evaluation of the potential solutions. Participants select from the field of possible criteria and select those measures most pertinent to qualifying the solutions to take forward into implementation.

C. SOLUTION IMPLEMENTATION

Step 6: Action planning generates specific actions envisioned to lead to a successful installation of the solution.

Step 7: Gaining acceptance considers the ways solution ownership can be generated. This is both management and stakeholder planning, a framing process that identifies value propositions for solution benefits and risk mitigation.

Step 8: Action/production assigns individuals and fixes commitments to the actual activities for each action, defining responsible individuals, milestones and dates, and clear deliverables for each action.

As simple as the process appears, the power of the innovation method is in organizing ideas so that collective wisdom is generated in the process. Participants recognize the emergence of transformative patterns of ideas as they work through each phase. The continuous "testing" of group ideation through multiple cycles ensures that ideas found to be sufficiently effective and wise are raised and refined through iterations and dialogue.

The Simplexity process model draws on inductive reasoning, synthesis, and abductive reasoning. Inductive reasoning is involved in the divergent steps in each phase, wherein participants generate ideas that answer the question. In the convergence step, participants label and select appropriate example ideas.

Synthesis is involved in each phase as participants align a set of concepts with the problem carried forward into each step and fuse related ideas together in new forms.

Abduction is the style of iterative reasoning used in effective problem solving, even if we do not consciously recognize it. Abduction occurs when we reason between inductive particulars and deductive explanations and find new formulations. By associating and comparing concepts in a structured network (such as the challenge map), people can explore meaning in the relationships between items and derive net new concepts.

A challenge map represents the set of challenges identified by participants and is a dynamic mapping of the sequence of ideas generated from problem solving to solution finding. It is generated collaboratively by positioning ideas from stakeholders in a network, displaying them from specific tactical needs (at the bottom) to strategic and desired outcomes (at the top).

Simplexity is structurally similar to other systems-thinking methods. The challenge map process is analogous to the abstraction hierarchy (Chapter 7) and problematique (Chapter 8). It aligns with other design and system-thinking models that leverage multiple modes of reasoning and cyclic structures to model human systems.

Positive Deviance

Positive Deviance (PD) is a stakeholder innovation practice that guides organizations to discover native solutions to difficult problems in processes or operations. Homegrown innovations can be located by scanning the organization for effective (or positive) deviances from the standard operating procedures. Healthcare and hospitals are often managed very closely to their established standards to ensure a consistent level of performance and to mitigate risk. However, innovative problem solving that is initiated at the front lines is often overlooked because, although not harmful, the "deviant" processes are considered contrary to accepted practices.

PD is based on the recognition that in every organization a small number of individuals demonstrate uncommon behaviors and strategies that represent possibly better solutions to problems than the mainstream practices. PD originated in the health field in 1976 and became widely followed after Tufts professor Marian Zeitlin compiled surveys that revealed how "positive deviant" children in poor communities were found to be better nourished than others due to their own independent resources.[21] The core goal of PD was to address childhood malnutrition at the grassroots level by identifying positive behaviors that worked well, and to reinforce the effective minority behaviors as opposed to focusing on critique and fixes. PD was further institutionalized as a process for social change, expanding to difficult problems in diverse areas such as public health, education, and healthcare.

A recent significant and successful PD application was conducted at six Canadian hospitals over an 18-month period in 2009–10. Physician Michael Gardam, director of Infection Prevention and Control, took on the seemingly intractable problem of the growth of "superbugs" that challenge hospital infection management.[22] By coordinating a continuing series of open dialogues and informational workshops, Gardam was able to build awareness of the ability to significantly mitigate the hospital-based sources of antibiotic-resistant bacterial infections. Many of these infections arise from irregular and insufficient hygiene practices, such as hand washing. Other vectors, such as patient transportation and ambient surfaces and fabrics in wards, are contributing factors.

Hospitals are covered with reminders about hand hygiene, but the notorious fact is that busy healthcare workers often get caught up in their routines and fail to wash between patients or even procedures. Gardam found that peer pressure and regular routines could be initiated in places where compliance was low by following practices discovered using PD. The PD practice is not a set of techniques but rather more of a systematic management process whereby opportunities are investigated to discover and learn from local solutions to difficult problems of this kind.

PD is a bottom-up strategy. Rather than defining the problem and drawing solutions from experts, the PD approach recognizes that the best solutions are discovered by those working closest to the problem. The process starts by actively requesting the assistance and participation of people from across all levels of an organization, so that a more open culture can be cultivated to better support the emergence of effective solutions. Multiple open dialogues and facilitated sessions are scheduled, using facilitated practices such as discovery and action dialogues and improvisational theater. Eventually (in a large organization), people with insight into effective local practices are found and encouraged to contribute their own experiences and observations. High-potential actions are identified from these conversations and new practices are presented to the organization that encourage others to try the activity found successful in the "deviant" outlier.

- Stakeholder engagement methods are necessary for system-level service design. Service changes require organizational agreement and consensus for adoption, so stakeholders should be drawn from all levels in the organization.

- Multistakeholder design methods are powerful techniques for mobilizing proposals in large organizations, but their effectiveness is highly dependent on the skill and practiced ability of the facilitator. Hire an experienced practitioner or get well trained.

- Stakeholder design is a CD3.0 management care practice. Any management practices can be configured by multistakeholder design, but not all are feasible design-led projects. A good sponsor is essential.

- Simplexity and Positive Deviance have uniquely successful applications in healthcare service design and problem solving. Other facilitated methods may be compatible with these practices. Art of Hosting (Integrating Open Space and World Café) and Appreciative Inquiry also provide effective stakeholder design processes for organizational innovation.

CHAPTER 7

Designing Healthy Information Technology

Elena's Story: Learning to Live With

At only 42, Elena is already facing a possible future of managing several chronic diseases. None of these common health conditions are complex in isolation, and they all can easily be managed once routines are established. However, each condition is systemic—the cardiac arrhythmia affects circulatory functions, diabetes affects metabolic functions, and hypothyroid affects hormonal regulation. They all affect daily life. The symptoms of one condition can interact with and feel like another. As her conditions and symptoms unfold, her emerging health situation becomes complicated. Elena must take several medications a day, perhaps from this point forward.

Elena keeps her scheduled appointment at a regional cardiac care center, where she first meets with a nurse practitioner to coordinate her assessment and treatment scheduling. With a supraventricular tachycardia (SVT) diagnosis, Elena waits to meet with an electrophysiologist, who will present a menu of options for her situation depending on her disease process severity and overall physical condition. She meets with Dr. Audrey Chen, one of the staff electrophysiologists, to review her electrocardiograms and other hospital tests. A cardiac scan is indicated to identify any possible complications.

Elena follows a nurse to the imaging center, where she meets with a staff radiologist. A 3D scan is necessary to identify the locus of the problem and guide the procedure. Given her age and good health, a 3D gadolinium-enhanced magnetic resonance angiograph is recommended. She accepts the injection, gets the scan, and then waits for processing and the resulting discussion.

Meeting with the cardiologist after the procedure, Elena is given several options, including an ablation, an implant, or continual medications. The clinician recommends a radiofrequency catheter ablation over the medication or implant alternatives, and provides patient education materials on each procedure. Elena is unable to decide on the best approach. Fear of a future complicated by chronic disease erodes her positive outlook, and her concern about the ablation procedure and its potential complications further burden her recovering health with anxiety. When back home again, she pursues the fourth patient information need: *Understand the processes and likely outcomes of possible tests and treatments.* Her searches, now sprinkled with technical terms such as SVT and ablation, yield more professional-leaning resources, such as Medscape and the HealthKnowledge community.

She finds online discussions by people with similar situations. She realizes that to improve her long-term health, she must exercise, improve her diet, and maintain her medication regime. It dawns on her that an SVT episode could occur when she starts to exercise, or that she may faint and seriously injure herself. So she goes back to the electrophysiologist, now determined to have an ablation. ■

Critical Design Opportunities

Electronic medical (or health) record (EMR or EHR) systems are being rapidly deployed in US medical clinics following the financial incentives in the 2009 HITECH Act. Because the incentives expire in 2014, most US hospitals and health systems will have installed some type of EMR system and will document their application based on "meaningful use" criteria. The rush to EMR deployment is positioned by industry analysts as an inevitable process that will provide wide economic benefit. Yet these systems are expensive undertakings with formidable multiyear phased deployments. In a typical large hospital, the installation of a full inpatient EMR system (and the conversion of patient records) can run to $100 million or more over a period of development and installation lasting 2 years or longer. Government incentives are not the sole cost driver in the near term, as vendors promote additional savings of tens of millions of dollars a year on unnecessary drugs, staff hours, and other resources managed by the systems.

An extremely wide range of systems and competing technologies are available in the US market. By some counts, there are well over 350 EMR vendors and as many as 600 unique systems. If these were all widely deployed, there would be little possibility of a shared standard and data interoperability. Data sharing between vendor platforms would be impossible. Such a large number of EMR systems suggests that a significant industry consolidation will take place as large institutions settle on a smaller set of reliable and sustainable systems. In the meantime, chaos will reign for some time before institutions themselves eventually consolidate as the healthcare industry changes. Given the typical life cycle of a major IT system (8 to 10 years plus the payback period), it is more likely that significant institutional change will occur before major EMR systems are replaced.

The major benefits of EMRs include the reduction of bulky and inefficient paper records, data sharing between clinical and administrative functions, and complete and consistent records of patient data. Although clinical benefits have been presented as co-equal to administrative efficiencies, field and survey evidence suggest that clinician needs are not well met or elicited in the design and implementation of these systems. Authors of the 2009 usability report across the EMR sector reinforced this finding: "EMR adoption rates have been slower than expected in the United States, especially in comparison to other industry sectors and other developed countries. A key reason, aside from initial costs and lost productivity during EMR implementation, is lack of efficiency and usability of EMRs currently available."[1]

Owing to a constellation of unique factors—healthcare is different, behind the times, and served by specialized IT—EMR systems show few of the contemporary trends in UX and interface design evident in other sectors. This would not be a problem if the systems were highly usable. But the basic human factors of EMR systems are often insensitive or hostile to the needs of clinical work, forcing users to work around clinically dumb lists and entries, requiring complicated navigation, and inducing dangerous error rates.

Risks in Automating Clinical Care

EMR systems are a permanent feature of the large clinical organization. Within 5 years, all institutions and most group practices will integrate patient records with an EMR. They support conventional clinical tasks as defined by the Agency for Healthcare Research and Quality: reviewing patient history, conducting patient assessment, determining clinical decisions, developing and distributing care plans, ordering clinical services, prescribing medications, and documenting patient visits.[2]

The EMR extends the clinic's capacity to perform medical work efficiently, sustainably, and safely. At best, the EMR could be designed and integrated as a reliable actor (literally a cognitive function) in the clinical network. The organizational roles of the EMR also extend cognitive tasks from the human to the system: managing memory (documentation as memory), performing medical calculations, and displaying relevant data for care decisions.

For all their medical sophistication, EMR systems are based on outdated IT and introduce significant interruptions to workflow relative to nonclinical systems. A cursory evaluation of any of major EMR reveals critical interface design and clinical workflow challenges. Most systems have employed rigid system architectures that cannot be changed or improved by institutional IT due to contractual service terms and proprietary code. EMRs can trigger potentially hazardous situations at every level of function:

- Clinical users learning complicated user interfaces

- Opaque and rigidly automated business and clinical tasks (lack of local flexibility)

- Relegation of patient information to a proprietary vendor database (constraints on display and management)

- Long-term lock-in of these systems by data usage, training, habit, and contract, preventing future conversion

Human factors studies within clinics suggest that EMR systems present significant design and usability challenges. It is not only possible but ethical to redesign EMR interfaces to support the information needs of clinical staff and patients to improve clinical work.

The oncoming wave of EMRs in clinics, hospitals, and entire healthcare systems presents an extraordinary window of near-term innovation opportunity. The initial installation and deployment period of an enterprise EMR often takes well over 2 years. This phase reveals disconnects with preferred practices, leading to identifying objective deficiencies (and buyer's remorse) that may trigger funding for design and user studies. Designers from information architecture to human factors are challenged to collaborate with clinical leadership to ensure EMRs can better support clinical work, task flow, and rapid information sensemaking.

A survey of EMR research reported on 24 systematic reviews and 94 research articles on patient record systems.[3] The study found that, regardless of the point of view, problems with clinical work were foreseeable in all cases, widespread, and unavoidable. The conclusion was that study design and control should be improved, and that patient outcomes were rarely considered in research, only clinician-perceived satisfaction or decision outcomes.

Presentations at human factors and healthcare conferences have demonstrated EMR design concerns and invoked the scenario of long-term lock-in of an installed base. Presenters have asked designers to join forces to address the possible wave of "information malpractice" as errors and oversights issue from poor EMR interaction design. A small core group of informatics professionals have argued for multidisciplinary advocacy to mitigate the known risks in current EMR design. Human Computer Interaction Lab director Ben Shneiderman has advocated for affirmative changes in the industry, following the successes of prior movements to ensure public safety by government certification of high-risk products such as medications and aircraft. He suggests designers and researchers start by "reducing medical errors of commission and omission," such as incorrect patient or treatment actions and medication events, delay in treatment, unintended or improper care, and sequence errors.[4]

Several high-profile incidents have occurred in which EMR data display errors have led to overmedication and reported patient deaths, but these have not affected the willingness of administrators to invest in enterprise EMR systems, especially given time-bound financial incentives.

The Usability of Meaningful Use

As EMRs are rushed into operation, the problems of poor interaction design collide with economic incentives and complicated business models. In hopes of obtaining the cost savings claimed by vendors and some healthcare economists, the HITECH Act is designed to establish consistent information management and data exchange processes for patient health and insurance information. In 2010, at least $34 billion was allocated to facilitate institutional adoption of EMR systems. Incentives aim to encourage appropriate adoption by providing base incentives of up to $2 million, as determined by a complex methodology for calculating payments based on the number of Medicare patient discharges over the first 4 years of the program (fiscal years 2011–15).

Enrolled hospitals must have claimed the achievement of initial "meaningful use" by FY2012. Meaningful use requires the provider to employ the EMR system optimally to achieve improvements in clinical outcomes, which are measured and claimed for incentive funding. A clear example of meaningful use was an award-winning project sponsored by the Institute for Family Health (IFH) using the Epic EMR.[5] Neil Calman, IFH's chief executive, reported that their initial EMR installation (2002) demonstrated no real improvements in their institutional health campaigns, such as pneumonia vaccination. However, IFH installed an electronic reminder system the next year, which resulted in an 18-fold increase in vaccination rates, which continue at around 80%.

Meaningful use has been carefully defined by policy, with billions in healthcare IT investment staked to that definition. Calman suggests that if a "meaningfully used" EMR could prevent errors in care, in effect a higher standard of care would be established to which all providers would be held accountable. For design purposes, the five key areas of meaningful use might be articulated toward care design, so that we better know "meaningful use to whom." For each category we might identify the "meaningful users" for defined outcomes, which are added to the list of criteria (Table 7.1).

Stage 1 meaningful use has recently transitioned to stage 2, which (according to foreword author John Halamka) will be "a natural evolutionary step that requires data sharing, patient/family engagement, and decision support." He notes that stage 2 will promote the integration of multiple data sources for clinician and patient/family access for shared decision making, or "patient/family mediated data reconciliation."[6]

TABLE 7.1 MEANINGFUL USERS OF USE CRITERIA

Meaningful use criteria	Meaningful users
Improve quality, safety, and efficiency	Will these values extend to include *all* users (administrative, clinical, patients, service providers)? Are there indirect stakeholders for these values (community, volunteers)?
Engage patients and families	Will patients and their families have access to records, bills, and clinical information? How will patient engagement be defined and measured so that their value can be realized?
Improve care coordination	Will the uses include all clinicians and staff in all services? Are clinical staff effectively supported in task coordination? How will the concept of *care* evolve with the automation of workflow?
Improve population and public health	Will EMR outputs support public health and public (noninstitutional) users? How exactly? Will there be public reports and transparent metrics of care delivery and problematic events?
Ensure privacy and security protections	Beyond regulations such as HIPAA, how will the EMR manage privacy? Will there be specific user and patient protections?

User experience is constrained by how "meaningful use" is defined and tested across the industry. Meaningful use requires institutions to justify EMR acquisition by assessing the value to care and patients, not just operational efficiency or cost management. Justifying meaningful use (in stage 1) does not require clinical evaluations or even usability testing to determine the fit of an EMR to processes. Instead, nearly any EMR on the certified list of almost 250 EMR vendors would meet the meaningful use criteria if a hospital merely documented how their expected uses planned to meet five high-level criteria. Usability is deferred to the system vendor, not the buying customer, and many EMRs have demonstrated complicated interaction and dangerously poor clinical usability. The fact that the EMR industry has protected itself with "hold harmless" clauses in their service contracts indicates that interaction, use, and information problems are known to exist in these systems. There are no safety guarantees in health information management. Interaction design is pushed down to local staff taking responsibility for the deployment of an enterprise EMR.

Major EMR vendors hold user organizations to nondisclosure, and even the most generic screenshots are withheld from the public. Any well-designed system would promote its user interface as a selling point; this is a sure tell that the interface will be negatively assessed under informed scrutiny. EMR interface specifications are not available to researchers or conferences, making it difficult for informatics professionals to conduct comparative analyses. When thousands of patient lives are at stake in the future deployment of an EMR, the industry-wide tendency to withhold user interface examples violates social, business, and care ethics.

Although clinicians may be concerned and skeptical about the complicated interactions, questionable search results, and navigability issues inherent in a new EMR system, they also recognize that the purchase decision is not a democratic one. But online discussions and reports indicate most clinicians are willing to defer judgment until after training and initial use. However, UX designers and informatics researchers know better. On first glance, many EMRs fail known heuristics of navigability, information density, nested and hidden data, misleading data sorting, and fit to practice and language. Further internal tests or even casual usability evaluations prove them right.

Meaningful Use to Users

An enterprise EMR imposes significant design trade-offs. By default it configures and restructures the hospital's patient and clinical management, coordination, and workflow according to the vendor's processes and data models. These systems establish a new and permanent information infrastructure in the host organization, and can be inflexible to the adaptations necessary to ensure effective fit to practice. The EMR industry is not promising future technologies or versions that will evolve to enable process adaptation and improve user interface interaction.

Furthermore, the meaningful use guidelines do not recommend specific UX enhancements to improve EMR integration with clinical tasks. Meaningful use is designed to help institutions coordinate and reinforce anticipated outcomes for a larger (organizational) system. Yet the primary values of quality, safety, and efficiency do not include user experience or organizational usability, or require the EMR to adapt to current best care practices. Because the criteria for acceptance do not define user-centric values, institutions are not (yet) advocating UX guidelines for EMRs. Except for the more progressive institutions, designers working with enterprise EMR are left with the unenviable task of defining very minor changes allowable within a tightly defined range of features in a locked-down user interface.

Evidence-based guidelines and standards for effective human use establish a basis for trade-offs among functions by criticality, cost, and design. Guidelines help coordinate the effective use of any new technology in a large institution. Even the apparently simple mobile phone requires a protocol for appropriate calling periods, coordinating communications among team members, and ensuring access for emergency and interruption. Toronto's Center for Innovation in Complex Care even published a research study evaluating the most effective communications methods for coordinating clinical care using the standard-issue BlackBerry smartphones.[7]

In this case, the meaningful use criteria give a starting point for an institutional dialogue on the criteria that matter. Table 7.2 indicates questions for each of the criteria that suggest ways to raise awareness of preferred values and the systemic effects possible with EMR adoption.

TABLE 7.2 MEANINGFUL USE TO END USERS

Meaningful use criteria	Meaningful use to users
Improve quality, safety, and efficiency	Consider the quality of *data*, *care*, or *interaction*? How exactly is *safety* understood or measured? Efficiency of what activity? What efficiencies do different users care about?
Engage patients and families	What is meaningful engagement? Merely using the billing record as a medical chart? Can the record be used to communicate?
Improve care coordination	How is care coordination defined? Is mere electronic communication assumed to be workflow improvement?
Improve population and public health	How are public research and reporting enabled? Are there plans for collecting and analyzing health demographics?
Ensure privacy and security protections	Will patients be disadvantaged by protections? Will patients as users be able to download and synch with a public health record?

Human Factors across the Healthcare Enterprise

As EMR systems are being widely deployed, a critical need for clinically focused interface design is apparent. This opportunity for multidisciplinary development will accelerate the inclusion of design and human factors professionals in healthcare.

The opportunity may also seem like losing a decade of progress in the UX field. In consulting and design agencies, the UX role has transformed into a hybrid design position, a creative mix of multimethod design research, strategic ideation, prototyping, visual and Web design, and design facilitation. The clinical organization is generally not prepared for this role, and its true design needs are likely to be too domain-specific for most generalist UX designers. Strong skills in application design, qualitative research, and human factors knowledge are needed to address the interface-induced errors and patient safety concerns of EMR systems. These roles may fall under human factors design and not user experience as we have come to know it, with research-informed practices such as usability engineering, cognitive systems, and work analysis, and activity-centered design.

Designing interfaces and experiences for institutional systems requires a different mindset from the safe, external world of Web product design and Health 2.0 services. Strong analytic, social sciences research, conceptual, and evaluative skills are needed, as well as healthcare industry experience.

Systemic and Situational Risks

Systemic risks are threats and problematic outcomes that propagate from a source throughout an organization or community. For example, infections that spread within a hospital (such as the MRSA superbug or an unexpected emergence such as SARS) may start from a specific source and become systemic, with many points of management. Situational risks are hazards or error-prone interactions caused by a unique or repeating situation, but are normally contained and have little system-wide impact. Data displays that can cause foreseeable errors (such as leading or trailing zeros in drug dosing) may be discovered as a situational risk and then determined to have systemic effects. Human factors analyses of the data design, cognitive tasks, and their interactions are called for to evaluate and ameliorate these risks.

Serious errors are directly incurred by known display and work practice interactions. Yet without a coordinated process for workflow design, assessment, and testing, normal human interaction can be expected to result in a high proportion of resolvable conditions. Data input, interpretation, and task coordination errors arise in the transition to any large-scale system deployment, but EMRs incur special problems and risks:

- Errors and inconsistencies involved in comprehensive process change to clinical departments

- Institution-wide transition from paper and mixed automation to full EMR use

- Risks due to inconsistent quality and uptake of training, as well as the reliance on training to compensate for poor interface design

- Breakdown of information flow between services as new electronic communications replace long-standing interprofessional routines

- Coordination problems as systems are rolled out in multiple stages of deployment

Furthermore, the availability of patient information from EMRs at the point of care does not directly contribute to improving patient health outcomes. If the purpose of EMRs is to directly support clinicians in improving patients' health, current research studies are not finding support for this claim. The simple but shocking conclusion of a 2011 study makes the case that EMRs do nothing to improve outpatient healthcare: "Our findings indicate no consistent association between EMRs and [clinical decision support] and better quality. These results raise concerns about the ability of health IT to fundamentally alter outpatient care quality."[8]

This study also revealed little impact of clinical decision support (CDS) on patient outcomes, except in one quality measure (avoidance of unnecessary electrocardiography). Several randomized controlled trials cited by the authors suggest a positive impact of CDS resources on asthma, hypertension, and angina. But notably these studies are dated between 2000 and 2005, a generation or two behind the current CDS interfaces and the current content of resources such as UpToDate, Clinical Key, and DynaMed.

Multiple observations across even similar hospitals (e.g., large urban pediatric hospitals) reveal differences in clinical processes and the adoption of IT as an enabler of technical work. For those able to conduct ethnographic observations and contextual research in the working clinical setting, each institution is found to have a distinct operational attitude, a unique organizational culture, and its own ways of organizing care practices.

We may discover in testing the resulting projects that our products do not fit every clinical organization. We may design a perfect Clinical Design 2.0 solution (e.g., a better EMR) for a Design 3.0 (organizational) problem that fails in transition to another institution's practice. The best practices from one clinical system may not directly transfer to another organization without transition and training support.

Further, introducing Web 2.0 interface genres, social network integration, and superficially improved visual design may distract or confuse clinicians focused on professional routines and everyday patient care. Clinical information interfaces are minimalist to ensure that content is observed precisely and can be acted upon quickly and unambiguously. In my experience, attempts to enhance the visual richness of clinical products can draw a critical reception from professionals. There is little latitude for advertising, promotion, or even salient images that highlight your content.

EMR Error Profile Risks

Inaccurate or misinterpreted data can harm a patient. In a paper-based process, physician order entries and prescriptions are cross-checked by several agents viewing a patient chart, order set, or prescriptions. Data displayed in an EMR transaction are perceived as accurate, legitimate, and complete. Precise data values must be entered and interpreted for diagnoses, treatment, medications and dosage, and the ordering of standard clinical procedures.

Well-known examples from clinical ethnographic studies on computerized physician order entry (CPOE), a core function integrated in EMRs, illustrate the point. CPOE systems are widely held as the best solution for medication-prescribing errors, perhaps the most easily preventable hospital medical error. Some studies report CPOE reducing medication errors by as much as 81%.

Professor and medical sociologist Ross Koppel and his University of Pennsylvania team discovered how automated CPOE systems induce errors that may be even more difficult to trap and recover in practice.[9] These types of errors are indicative of the data quality and perception problems that will plague EMRs throughout their maturing phases in institutional use. These were (1) information errors caused by fragmentation of data across automated systems, and (2) user interface design flaws reflecting automated rules that failed to correspond to clinical practice. The study found 22 situations in which CPOE increased the probability of prescribing errors. Although clinical staff are able to individually predict and work around these forced errors to perform safely and continuously, Koppel emphasizes that these errors are systemic and arise from the failure to integrate technology with actual work practices. These are not technical system design issues but work practice and even implementation process problems.

Koppel noted seven "fragmentation" errors where disconnects occur between user expectations and data display, triggering serious, potentially harmful responses:

- Selecting the wrong patient
- Selecting the wrong specific medication
- Medication update or cancellation linked to clinical events
- Computer management (downtime) problems
- Inflexible ordering interfaces
- Update delays on medication allergies
- Conflicting medications

Credible studies argue against the claims for administrative management and overhead savings expected from EMR and CPOE systems. A 2010 report reviewed roughly 4,000 hospitals from 2003 to 2007 and found that although many institutions had migrated from paper-based patient records to EMRs, the administrative costs actually rose, even among the most high-tech-enabled hospitals. According to lead author David Himmelstein, who oversees clinical computing at Cambridge Hospital, "Our study finds that hospital computerization hasn't saved a dime, nor has it improved administrative efficiency. Claims that health IT will slash costs and help pay for the reforms being debated in Congress are wishful thinking."[10]

Furthermore, the researchers claim that these hidden-cost problems and false solutions are endemic across healthcare systems and policy. Himmelstein's co-author, Steffie Woolhandler, stated in 2009, "The [US Veterans Health Administration] system now has our nation's highest quality and patient approval ratings. Congress should take note: To get the most benefit from our healthcare dollars and from health IT, we should adopt a single-payer, Medicare-for-all program. Nothing short of that will allow us to reap the full potential of computerization or to provide comprehensive, quality and affordable care to all."[11]

These research reports are not isolated. Journalists' reports have pointed to the problems of blind acceptance of EMR systems without considering the real-world clinical consequences, and both patient data errors and administrative problems have emerged in all types of institutions. A 2009 *Washington Post* article reported that "bipartisan enthusiasm has obscured questions about the effectiveness of health information technology products. . . . Interviews with more than two dozen doctors, academics, patients and computer programmers suggest that computer systems can increase errors, add hours to doctors' workloads and compromise patient care."[12]

How to Innovate the EMR?

Enterprise EMRs are becoming permanent infrastructure, and it is possible the major vendors will be locked in for a generation—permanent enough over a career's life span. At the current pace of adoption, the top vendors (e.g., Epic, McKesson, GE, Cerner, Eclipsys) will consolidate the field within 5 years. Especially after the HITECH Act stimulus subsides, purchasing boards will bet on sustainable EMR vendors, and those companies without sizable market share may be acquired or consolidated.

EMRs based on new technology (e.g., not based on the aging MUMPS architecture) may be excluded within the adoption timeframe. The largest costs that would restrain a replacement purchase are not the initial or annual software licensing fees, but the actual installation and management costs:

paper records conversion, staff training, support and internal promotion, and the organizational habits of use.

Industry incentives may have created an unintentionally static marketplace. The major EMR vendors are not motivated to innovate beyond their competitors' product or pace because once a large medical institution has committed to a vendor, the costs to switch to another are prohibitive. This leaves vendors with no incentive to innovate, as a creative upstart has little chance of threatening their market share within a foreseeable timeframe. With this EMR cartel guiding future development, some institutions will have to endure a glacial rate of upgrades.

Regional medical centers will also consolidate as leading hospitals continue to build on established centers and satellite facilities. The winning institutions will be those that manage costs, facilities, and clinical staff most effectively. These winners will also have settled on the major EMR vendors. They will not be using WorldVistA or smaller vendors whose system might not scale. Due to the long-term investment represented by these systems, many institutions will be locked in to their EMR for up to 10 years.

Evolving Health IT Design Capacity

Design thinking has arrived late, if at all, to the EMR and the IT departments responsible for their deployment. Data-driven infrastructure favors function over form, and data over human engineering. Most reported EMR innovations are those developed by healthcare institutional insiders designing localized "bolt-on" applications adapted to their EMR systems. The EMR vendors are not yet demonstrating a staffing commitment to improved human factors and user experience (traditional usability evaluation is a barely sufficient starting point).

We face real hurdles in attempting to design better EMRs. Most clinical institutions do not keep UX designers on their IT staff. Traditional development methods are used because a UX life cycle—user research, prototyping, iterating, user testing—is not yet supported by the skill base.

Criticizing a new enterprise-scale EMR system can be politically infeasible during initial deployment because the enormous expense and commitment to a particular vendor system was not made lightly. The industry shows evidence that usability is not a driving decision factor, so we might wait before charging a UX task force with an immediate interface redesign. In most healthcare organizations, the interface design and usability skill base will be technically too immature to consult effectively on strategic design.

By now, however, most industry sectors have experience developing user-centered design programs in large organizations. Healthcare, while lagging, can borrow from organizational practices in other sectors. Although most organizational capabilities in healthcare institutions are highly structured and tightly planned, innovation processes do not evolve well in top-down management. Establishing a vice president of innovation or even an internal innovation group does not ensure a sustainable practice. Most care organizations will be unable to recognize the value within the expected adoption period, and it may take a year or two before the group's talent can be utilized effectively. The proposed value will not pay off immediately.

A validated method for managing strategic innovation, known as socialization, counters the tendency toward top-down innovation in large organizations.[13] Socialization establishes new competencies such as UX design or customer experience by supporting a single project, with external consulting expertise and just-in-time training. As a new skill base is formed, the group employs new talent to meet the demand at the department level, but evangelizes the practices and advises projects in the larger organization. Taking a distributed and lateral approach to participation and cooperation, it generates demand from peripheral departments or service in the network. The network effect of peer-to-peer communications across functions creates new channels for cooperation. These practices are most commonly formed, redesigned, and re-formed in boundary-spanning business functions such as research and development, user experience, innovation management, or market research.

User experience can also be seen as a short-term research and development process assigned to the IT department that provides early concepts and field testing and adapts new products to defined user needs. User experience, as with any knowledge practice, contributes most effectively when it becomes a dedicated resource responsive to demand and emerging opportunity. To accomplish this, managers often attempt to "institutionalize" new practices as a route to defining (and owning) a stable organizational process. From a knowledge-creation perspective, however, a new or emerging business function should not be jump-started with a project that establishes its presence on the organization chart. Instead, an organic demand for its value can be developed over time with a smaller pilot team, allowing the organization to discover its successes and pull it into new programs by peer-to-peer collaboration.

Socialization flows from the bottom up, whereas institutionalization is top down. Rather than "importing" industry best practices into an intact organization, socialization creates demand from internal customers and quickly adapts necessary skill sets in accord with the current needs of stakeholders and users.

UX design represents a new practice in most healthcare organizations. It will take time to build a sustainable skill base, show results in projects, and socialize the value across departments. Four to five years can be required to establish a viable UX/human factors or design group if starting from scratch, due to associated challenges of integrating new functions across the organization. But the socialization model delivers immediate value within well-chosen pilot projects.

Organizational leadership requires proving value in the most critical and immediate needs, such as usability. The fastest path to organizational integration may be through a clinical informatics group rather than an IT or staff-level group. The UX design process employed by a group at Children's Hospital of Philadelphia (see "EMR Design Process" on page 240) reveals a successful model of skill deployment. The human factors design competency was developed hand in hand with publishable research in clinical informatics, giving it substantial credibility. Yet even this hospital does not support a design group; only a handful of clinics in the United States have established full-fledged innovation or design departments.

EMR Design Imperatives

UX designers may wonder how to best get involved in envisioning and building better EMR interfaces in advance of system-wide lock-in. The immediate imperative is ensuring that EMRs do not unintentionally harm patients.

If EMRs continue to cause "unintended" information conflicts in clinical use, even their "hold harmless" legal clauses may not save them from all liabilities.[14] In general, EMRs have not yet reached broader industry standard levels of human factors.

Remarkably and uniquely, user experience is not yet a significant business driver for EMR innovation. There are several independent reasons for this. User interface designers do not hold significant positions within EMR vendor organizations, and their influence may remain weak within the business, as they were over a decade ago in most industry sectors.

Second, user interfaces of enterprise EMRs are lagging up to 10 years behind the software industry. Interaction designers in the EMR field make similar critiques about their antiquated interface modes. But that does not necessarily mean that visual interface design per se makes a clinical difference. And third, once an EMR is installed, the ability to modify its interfaces may be severely limited by the institution, constrained by IT or practice controls.

The Right Design, or Designing It Right?

When hundreds or thousands of staff have learned to use a fully integrated system for computer-supported work operations, the highest-impact interface design will result from rethinking *functional* features that enhance work itself. Effective EMR design requires data entry and data display, forms and fields, and labels and language to align perfectly with clinical work. The perceived speed of task completion is much more important than engagement or satisfaction, as clinical staff use systems intermittently and in rapid bursts, and "good experience" is measured by the time *not* spent on a task.

At the point of care, computer task performance is specialized by division of labor, with specific tasks allocated to physicians, nurses, staff, and data clerks. Changing computer-based tasks and the divisions of labor can introduce risky changes in operation and training, potentially interfering with established role expectations, team communications that rely on task knowledge, and therefore ongoing patient care. Clinicians may now be required to use the EMR for specific regulated tasks, and soon EMR usage will be expected everywhere. However, many doctors may continue to learn only those transactions directly required for their job, such as scheduling, online orders, and entering procedure codes for billing. Printed patient charts will continue to be used for years. These sociotechnical constraints suggest internal service design (D3.0), not just UX design (D2.0), that may require incremental updates for years to align to practice.

Smart institutions will build a dedicated EMR staff and customize EMR interfaces for specialized clinical routines, reminders, test data calculators, and patient record viewers. The emerging opportunities for experience design innovators will be found in designing modular EMR applications with customized interfaces for clinical teams and medical specialties. Product ecosystems will form around those EMRs that maintain open application programming interfaces (APIs) or provide good development kits, allowing their customers and small software firms to build specialized modules for emerging needs. New tools are product inspirations for innovators:

- Dedicated mobile and tablet interfaces and data readers

- Specialized imaging viewers for radiologists, physician views, patient viewers

- Multiple database integration for epidemiology studies and clinical quality management

- Diagnostic decision support utilizing guideline translation and/or actuarial data

- Automatic assessment of patient history

- Educational content for both patients and clinicians

- Automation of mundane EMR tasks

- Clinical calculators and specialized reminders

EMR Design for Clinical Work

Introducing an enterprise EMR into an existing clinical environment will produce unintended consequences. It requires the redesign of everyday clinical practices, as an enterprise system becomes infrastructure that shapes human tasks by its new capabilities.

Clinicians are accountable for health outcomes, and the introduction of a clinical information system mediates responsibilities between human and automated roles. We can draw a direct line of responsibility from the physician, to an information service, to its ability to facilitate the outcomes intended by clinical staff.

Doctors may see up to 100 patients a day. The few seconds of time saved to locate an effective answer or use it in context matter, a lot. But how interface time-saving translates to practice is not a simple matter of designing for efficiency. In fact, manual tasks and paper artifacts that appear inefficient to designers or observers are often inherently faster and better coordinated than their automated counterparts. This is partly due to habit, a factor that should not be discounted. This is also due to team effectiveness—many professionals work as teams to manage patients with complex conditions, and paper displays provide a tangible, visible common ground when multiple clinicians work together.

Systemic Task Design

What are we actually designing—applications, user interfaces, or *clinical tasks*? The user interface and application are the abstracted representations of the clinical functions they are designed to facilitate. Defined tasks are always primary, but clinical work is increasingly supported by data capture, documentation, and coordination.

What level of analysis is the most effective for designing in the EMR context? A cognitive task perspective advances the view that information activity must be integrated as closely as possible into the sociotechnical system, which in the EMR context is generally bounded by the work unit, not by the patient per se. A unit and its staff are responsible for the patients under their care, and the unit specializes in certain clinical tasks intended to coordinate care for accountable outcomes.

Cognitive tasks are the essential procedures, problem-solving activities, informed decisions, and actions taken in the clinical setting. They are intellectual determinations and procedural actions performed in service of the clinical needs and are not necessarily information based. They are goal-driven decisions or actions triggered by the demands of the work setting, ranging from examinations and injections done on rounds to scheduled operations, and from nursing routines to clinical team care planning.

All clinical tasks follow a rationale of serving patient care, and most are well-structured repeatable procedures.

Cognitive scientist Chris Nemeth designs for the often-overlooked *technical work*, the essential activities needed to carry out clinical care, such as resource availability (What rooms are available?), resource and staff allocation, workload anticipation and prediction, trade-off decisions, speculation, and negotiation between clinical and administration staff.[15] Many consider technical work as merely the "background noise" of the clinical work ecology. When asked about technical tasks, clinicians say these functions are merely "the way we do things around here." Yet technical work is tightly coupled to clinical care, and the ability to perform these cognitive tasks determines how work is done and how patients ultimately experience care.

Clinical functions and technical work are both essential to managing care service. As discussed in Chapter 6, ecological interfaces supporting cognition are designed to be as transparent as possible. They must enable the *essential* task to be performed without interfering with the requirements for complex clinical workflow. Ecological interfaces are designed to enable the cognitive tasks supported by software. This involves designing to meet specific outcomes of goals that may be triggered by different events in the work ecology. Figure 7.1 shows an "onion" representation (a type of abstraction hierarchy) of the different levels of work and process considered in an ecological design approach based on renowned cognitive systems engineer Jens Rasmussen's representations of cognitive work.[16]

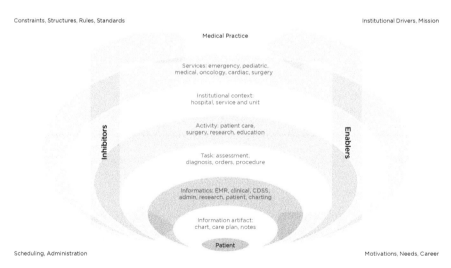

FIGURE 7.1
Cognitive work dimensions in clinical care.

Multiple dimensions of clinical work are performed by a doctor (or nurse or staff person) at any time. At the bottom of the hierarchy is the patient, the purpose of the entire series of functions. The patient is the most concrete "function" in the hierarchy, or the least abstract. Each level represents the next adjacent level of abstraction:

- Information artifacts (capturing patient data in different forms)

- Informatics (that manage this data)

- Clinical tasks (that use informatics)

- Activities (the execution of purposeful work)

Interaction designers usually target the *task* level to optimize discrete tasks in an application. Yet clinicians have multiple purposes and administrative requirements for regulation, oversight, and control. The arrows moving upward (enablers, or drivers) and down (inhibitors, or constraints) indicate the motivating forces in the work ecology that regulate activity.

When determining use cases or task scenarios for system design, the rationale for pushing the abstraction up a level (e.g., from artifact to informatics) may be based on finding motivations that the prospective user will respond to. For example, in the context of disease treatment, tests and procedures may be chosen for a care plan. Physicians must consider the costs and justifications for certain tests (institutional level) to justify the "best procedure" for the situation.

Constraints facilitate behavior in the reverse direction. The limiting factors for choices and actions are "imposed" from the higher levels of abstraction by policies, practice norms, and organizational values. Designers might anticipate these positions and build in checks for institutional policies that a user might not always consider in the rush of decision making.

Clinical Tasks as Cognitive Work

Enterprise EMRs can automate clinical tasks that appear to be manual and inefficient but that have evolved over time as sophisticated practices to enable exchange of tacit knowledge. One such task is patient scheduling in acute care units.

In a design case, Chris Nemeth shows how both clinical and technical work are closely coordinated for the cognitive demands of task coordination.[17] Computer software and artifacts must be designed so that the *technical* work—the background activity of a clinical unit, such as scheduling, organizing resources, setup, managing workload, and patient communication—is maintained efficiently so that *clinical* work can continue unimpeded.

Designing computer information displays for technical work is quite difficult because of the need to maintain distributed cognition in a team environment. Nemeth discovered how clinicians adapt and respond to the information demands in a rapid-paced, fast-changing, team care environment such as an acute care unit (Figure 7.2). Not only is clinical cognitive work highly hazardous and fraught with constant decision risk, the technical work is also highly hazardous. The wrong patient in the operating room at the wrong time, or the wrong team assignment, can mean the loss of vital minutes or even vital organs.

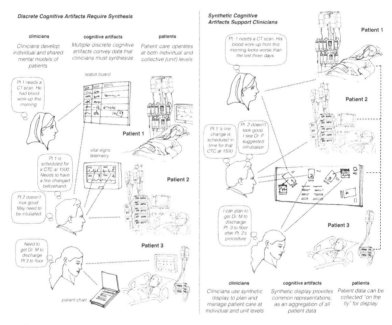

FIGURE 7.2

Discrete and synthetic cognitive artifacts in acute care. (Copyright © 2005 Cognitive Technologies Laboratory. Reprinted with permission.)

Cognitive artifacts assist the technical work of scheduling and managing an anesthesia function in an acute care ward. The master schedule is the primary artifact that a coordinator creates the day before procedures and embeds all of the assignment information that matters in this work setting. It is one of many manual displays created to reduce uncertainty to a minimum, which is essential to effectively manage resource allocation in this variable, ever-changing, contingent, high-risk setting.

The right-hand panel in Figure 7.2 shows the entire unit activity based on history, current activity streams, and anticipated data for each patient. According to Nemeth,

> As data related to each patient changes, the patient's representation changes. . . . Clinicians have the opportunity to probe for more particular data that is related to an individual patient, or to view the unit as a whole. This is not a solution that simply collects vital signs data into one display. Rather, it is an information ecology that is created to assist the way that clinicians work.[18]

Yet there are real cognitive constraints when coordinating technical work with nondigital artifacts such as schedule whiteboards, paper charts, and analog telemetry displays. Using several tangible displays requires *cognitive synthesis* to construct a complete situation awareness, adding to the clinician's already heavy mental workload.

Synthetic information views that integrate data from multiple sources (patient scheduling, clinical staff, room availability) require integration across IT vendors and even internal administrators. Ecological interfaces for team information entails mapping and flexibly integrating data formats, databases, security systems, data feeds, and middleware.

A well-designed synthesis of information could provide all the data necessary for clinical and technical decision making at the time of need in the workflow. Yet these systems still do not exist today. Worse, the institutional lock-in effect of vendor-defined data and formats may actually inhibit the possibility of effective synthesis. Moreover, conversion from paper or "mixed-interactive" artifacts to digital is not a simple translation. These artifacts are difficult to dislodge with new integrated systems that attempt to automate the formerly nondigital information ecology.

Clinical staff are usually not involved in redesigning applications that are assumed (by IT departments) to meet the functional needs of all hospital services. Yet each service area may have significantly different cognitive tasks for administrative processes such as patient scheduling. Disrupting these cognitive routines with a generic application forces every clinician to relearn a "best practice" standard that may be suboptimized (or overkill) for their particular needs.

Integrating Clinical Workflow

Nursing service provides a good case study, being the most hands-on, patient-intensive work in the hospital. In some institutions, nursing is among the last role to finally adopt an EMR because time spent on the system takes away from direct patient care. In US Veterans Health Administration (VHA) hospitals, adoption of the computerized patient records system (CPRS) is universal, yet nursing services continue to employ mixed and alternative practices, such as customized paper forms and binders for local notes and clinical backup, and ward clerks. Different nursing services allocate tasks between CPRS and paper forms, depending on work tempo, support, and local practices.

Figure 7.3 shows the nursing shift change as the start of a day's workflow, when paper forms (usually a shift book) are updated and exchanged between shifts. An IDEO study found that the shift change is a key encounter in which critical timely knowledge is exchanged to maintain continuity of care between shifts and staff.[19] This exchange has been found to greatly benefit patients and care management by raising issues occurring at the front lines that might otherwise be overlooked by a single nurse or clinician.

In IDEO's project with Kaiser Permanente, a high degree of variation was observed in nurse communications and data points during shift changes in the hospital. The researchers correctly identified the shift change as a high-leverage opportunity for improving health communications. They designed the Nurse Knowledge Exchange as a response to the findings, which provides a standard process and visually engaging system for capturing salient patient and clinical information necessary for shift change handoffs.

VHA nurses in acute care meet for roughly half-hour transition periods at shift exchange to share written notes and personal observations about patient conditions. In acute units, patients may experience significant changes in health status during the course of a day or evening, and nurses with different experience and specialization are able to triage problems as they just start to occur. Nurses coming onto shifts can be alerted to possible issues to observe and anticipate, rather than responding to symptoms and signs as they break through to obvious levels.

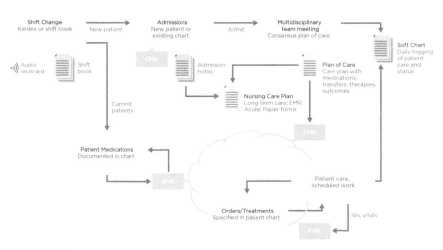

FIGURE 7.3
Nursing documentation workflow.

In the VHA case, the EMR is not used until an event requires its updating, such as a newly admitted patient or a new medication entry. Although complete patient "charting" is supported by the EMR, acute care nurses often use paper forms. Given their constant fast-paced work tempo, they have little time to carefully type into an EMR. Nurses in long-term care units tended to use the CPRS because patient changes are less frequent, and constant updating is rarely needed. They have the time built in to their routines to document patients on the EMR.

Do Nurses Need the EMR?

Just because an event *can* be translated electronically does not mean it *ought* to be. Nurses readily adopt technology when appropriate for their units and environments, but they are not inclined to adopt high-tech as a replacement for high-touch. The shift change is a dedicated time and place for face-to-face communication. An automated tool for shift exchange adds documentation time and trades off interpersonal communication. It could reduce the critical tacit exchange in verbal communication that occurs when nurses describe events and notes inked on paper. In the same way, using electronic communications to exchange information across roles in the care team may introduce the risks of misunderstanding and assumption. Even pharmacists use the phone constantly to discuss medications ordered electronically and remotely.

Nurses, doctors, and therapists in unit activity rely heavily on face-to-face and nonverbal communication to orient each other to possible emerging problems. Oral communication remains the primary knowledge channel for direct patient care, as it supports transfer of verbal and nonverbal tacit knowledge about patient history, current understanding, agreements, and plans of care. Differences in understanding can be immediately repaired in bidirectional speech, unlike in written or electronic communication modes.

Merely recording findings in a sharable location does little to share the embodied understanding learned from direct patient care. Interprofessional communication is exchanged in everyday practice by conversation about patients, relating subtle observations, simple questions and responses, experiences from other patients with similar care regimes, and visual cues and informal reminders. Some acute care units keep a "soft chart" handy for their short-term patients as a visible common paper chart available for any other physician or nurse. In some VHA units, information is entered both on soft charts and in the EMR record and then updated in the CPRS in accord with a local workflow. In future practice, these notes could readily be taken on a tablet interface, but the exchange between clinicians should be seen as essential in acute care.

In many acute and long-term care units at US hospitals, paper records, known as the "Kardex," are maintained as a separate documentation system from the enterprise EMR system. Nurses in particular use these ward-specific artifacts because they enable rapid display and reporting of *only the data that matter* for current or recent patients. The Kardex ensures resiliency—in case of an EMR outage or for any immediate uses, it provides a meaningful data backup available to all clinicians. It displays a tangible common ground reference—the print and written copies are easily and rapidly located, reviewed at a glance, and shared with others.

Is the Kardex an informatics system, even if not automated? Functionally, yes. It enables clinical tasks (at the next level up) perhaps more effectively than the electronic informatics equivalent. Information tools such as the Kardex records are endogenous cognitive artifacts—tools or information displays created by users themselves to navigate an ongoing and consistent information demand. Endogenous artifacts range from simple sticky notes (as reminders or scheduling tips) to complete information "systems" such as the Kardex. These are often maintained even in work environments where IT systems have replaced the supposed obsolete resource.

On the other hand, *exogenous* cognitive artifacts, such as those managed by EMR systems, are designed and created from outside the field of local work. "Exogenous" means they are made and supported by nonpractitioners and require the various practices to adapt to their way of working and thinking.

Paper artifacts, custom forms, and whiteboards are used in nursing and other services to manage a significant proportion of the precise communication required in technical work. Paper artifacts present immediate displays of current and validated information to one or more people. They are reliable, transparent, and traceable. Paper is the original ambient interface; printed artifacts are both highly visible and unobtrusive. They can be left on the desktop or pinned to the wall when needed for an urgent notification. They are created and evolved in use to serve distributed communication and cognition functions in the high-hazard acute care environment.

Nursing is a culture of physical engagement with patient realities, and it has the highest proportion of human interaction of any professional position. The social meaning of nursing culture is found in the necessity to help patients through direct human care and continual healing practices. Even IT design has to acknowledge this reality as the context for use and utility.

Interacting with the EMR

Irrespective of their usability problems, physicians rely on the EMR for comprehensive and updated medical and account status of their patients. Some have taken to improvising with the systems to increase their interactivity. It is becoming more common to include the patient in the data entry, turning the EMR screens toward patients during an interview, or showing data summaries to discuss tests or lab results. In most cases this is not an ideal representation, but the need to both record and share current medical, test, and lifestyle data offers a glimpse into the future. Leading vendors are starting to establish partnerships with specialized technology providers to meet the demand for well-designed interfaces for clinical staff.

The future value of the accumulated health history of all patients in a practice is extremely useful, not only to clinicians but for patient engagement and education. Analytical reporting and assessments based on actual patient historical data will revolutionize clinical advising and prescribing. Clinical informatics are currently designed to evaluate the co-occurrence of risk factors in patient data to identify critical intervention points and to show the effects of treatment or changes in behavior over time. Specialized algorithms can connect diagnostic codes, procedure codes, medications, and vital values over time to present a hard argument for clinical intervention or behavior change. The lagging field of personal health records reminds us (both designers and clinicians) that most people do not yet find it useful to manage their personal health accountancy by entering and tracking health values. Physicians will continue to advise and support health seekers directly.

Health seekers have always had to trust the physician's emphatic advice to make personal dietary, lifestyle, and behavioral changes. Patient education materials such as printed handouts (and now websites) have been used to supplement advice and provide support for healthcare decisions, which are ultimately the health seeker's to make. People have cognitive and habit-based barriers to acting on advice, which shows up as resistance to the demand for "adherence." Seeing one's own health data displayed in a visual context and relating one's lab and blood values and changes in physical response, will make all the difference.

The trend toward tablet and mobile apps for health and personal data management (including *quantified self* applications) are leading candidates for dedicated displays of specialized data types. Massive Health's Eatery app captures and displays dietary data, and can prompt and remind health seekers of their guidelines and limits. This is one of several targeted applications for managing individual health feedback developed by Massive Health. Whether this type of lightweight app could be linked back to the EMR is yet to be shown. It is likely that innovative EMR vendors will spin off healthcare apps for patients once their data is secure and accessible.

Data visualization approaches include the dedicated visual display for disease or condition type. uKare Analytics developed a series of materials for public education on metabolic syndrome, including the print/e-book title *Abdobesity*.[20] Its interactive resources include personal analytics reports and interface design concepts for personal health visualization. The resources are dedicated to specific disease regimes, with the first kit serving as a system for clinicians and healthcare advisors to coach patients in managing cardiometabolic disease and atherosclerosis.

The uKare concept includes the health visualization display and the content platform, including publications and patient education materials. Designed for institutional and mobile devices, uKare provides a natural relationship between the EMR and personal health records (PHRs) for dynamic patient health dashboards. Health education is interactive, based on available personal data directly related to a condition. The concept aims to satisfy "meaningful use stage 3" objectives for patient and family engagement.

The visual display in Figure 7.4 shows a "metabolic grid," a visual map of the individual behavior factors and measures for cardiometabolic health, in color-coded fuzzy logic. The interactive grid provides an overlay display of a patient's current health values and visually illustrates the effects of continued unhealthy activity (smoking, poor diet) in the red areas. Clinicians can demonstrate how behavior change can reverse an unhealthy trajectory and move toward the green areas (from A to B to C) of normal and optimal health.

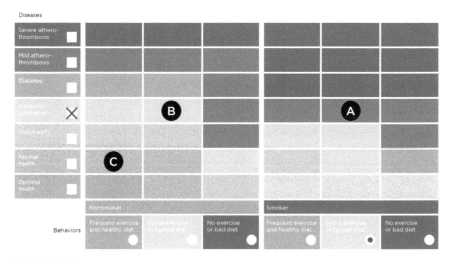

FIGURE 7.4

Patient analytics interface—EMR overlay. (Based on material copyright © 2011 by Anthony Pothoulakis & George Demosthenous. From *Abdobesity: The belly fat that kills*. Dayton, OH: uKare Analytics. All rights reserved)

The authors' variation of the uKare cardiometabolic grid was adapted to further highlight the specific risks of smoking. An active smoker is prevented from an assignment of "optimal" health, but can achieve "normal." The concept of the "fuzzochrome" is indicated by the range of colors, showing relative variations between levels of health.

Clinicians need better tools for representing health data in a meaningful way. Patients cannot easily act on a barrage of numbers reeled off from the printout of lab tests. EMRs will be required to offer health management tools and interfaces to PHR systems, and allow patient-generated data to be imported into the EMR.

DESIGN BEST PRACTICES

- Health IT cannot be designed in isolation from clinical complexity. Observe how practices are performed in the front lines at the points of care and develop solutions for their everyday information practices.

- Though human factors has finally become a standard practice in medicine, user experience is not yet widely supported for health IT. An organization can grow its UX competency through socialization of a core UX practice that creates demand for its skill to improve all IT platforms and Web services.

- Design for EMRs and other health records involves trade-offs between management's IT investment objectives and staff needs for a usable system supporting their clinical workflow. If user experience addresses "staff users" only, management processes may become encoded as infrastructure. Change both together.

- Discover and improve the cognitive artifacts developed by those closest to the front lines of practice. Even paper-based tracking processes and displays (lists and patient data) should be observed carefully for the inherent information needs they reflect. Breakthrough design solutions can be sourced from local tools reframed for use by other services.

- Although UX design can improve task performance, preventing clinical errors is the highest value and return on investment. No EMR field or online display can be treated as safe until it has been locally tested with staff and certified. Remember, your career skills save lives.

- Be very cautious about introducing new IT or Web services into an existing organization. Run pilot tests or full trials and assess the fit of tasks and functions to your staff, patients, and other constituents.

Case Study: VistA—Why It Still Matters

The US government operates one of the largest healthcare systems in the world. Across the VHA, information services are managed by the VistA (Veterans Health Information Systems and Technology Architecture) platform and patient records are managed by CPRS. The VHA is second only to Kaiser Permanente in size, and has a much wider national reach:

- Eight million veterans are enrolled.

- Annually (2006 total), 5.5 million people receive care at 1,400 sites.

- Nearly 60 million visits are made to outpatient clinics, and over 750,000 are treated at inpatient facilities annually.

- The VHA has affiliations with 107 medical schools, 55 dental schools, and more than 1,200 other schools.

- More than 90,000 healthcare professionals train at VHA facilities annually.

- More than half of all US healthcare professionals have received VHA training.

With respect to EMR usability, consider that nearly half of all residents and doctors, and many nursing professionals, have worked in the VHA system and are familiar with CPRS. At the CHI 2011 conference, Ben Shneiderman's panel made the argument that the large-scale VistA project was uniquely successful with respect to human factors appropriate to the healthcare system and clinical needs:

> Transformation of health care at the [VHA] is remarkable. By all objective metrics VHA patients now receive health care better than the average of all U.S. private hospitals. During the same period capacity increased by 60% and cost decreased slightly. The VHA success is attributed to two complementary initiatives: one for continuous quality improvement of care processes, the other for participatory design of an enterprise-wide computerized patient record system, known as VistA.[21]

VistA is the best-known healthcare platform in the United States due both to its longevity and its scale. It includes 99 system modules with 16 infrastructure applications, 28 administrative applications, and 55 clinical applications. VistA applications perform functions in common with other health IT systems, such as managing laboratory, pharmacy, radiology, ADT (admissions/discharge/transfer), and scheduling functions. The core clinical services used by clinicians on an everyday basis include CPRS and the Bar Code Medication Administration (BCMA).

VistA has been in constant development since the mid-1980s, and designers unfamiliar with the health sector might prejudge the platform as aging and running on ancient technology. In January 2010, however, Kaiser Permanente announced plans to interconnect VistA with HealthConnect, the largest civilian health records database, through the new National Health Information Network, a US federal initiative under the HITECH Act established to coordinate the interoperable and secure exchange of health information among institutions through regional health information exchanges.

This level of system interoperability will establish a baseline for connecting systems, data, and services that other vendors may be moved to emulate. *The level of usability expected from such a massive system should not be underestimated.* VistA/CPRS user experience may be much better supported than commercial vendor EMRs, given the VHA's single organizational mandate and longevity of experience in development and support. And because the system was built with tax dollars, the product is noncommercial, with an open version available for free. World VistA, a scaled-down version designed for the case of remote, poorly supported locations worldwide, can be downloaded from the Web.

CPRS: Old Interface, Good Fit?

VistaA's CPRS is a client-server EMR application with a Windows-based, rich-client interface used by all healthcare practitioners in the VHA for managing and using clinical services. CPRS enables physicians and nurses to enter, review, and continuously update patient information. Using a tabbed screen with a patient chart metaphor, it organizes records around a salient problem list. Immediate (one-click) access is available for pharmacy status, physician orders, lab results, progress notes, vital signs, radiology results and images, transcribed and scanned documents, and reports such as echocardiograms. Clinicians can enter and e-sign documents and orders. Nurses can track and update patient information; order and record diets; record adverse reactions to medications; request consults; enter progress notes, diagnoses, and treatments; and submit discharge summaries.

CPRS links clinical decision-making tools and enables review and analysis of summary and individual patient data. Figure 7.5 shows a "cover sheet" for a patient in the default view of the patient record.

From a contemporary information design perspective, the CPRS user interface represents a conventional and outdated presentation layer. Yet the user experience and its fit to practice has been evaluated constantly over the years in many internal reports and in studies as recent as 2008,[22] and it consistently tests better than most leading commercial EMR systems for satisfaction and clinical usability. As recently as CHI 2011, the leaders in interaction design supported VistA/CPRS for its fit to environment of use, and its open, auditable, and adaptable system architecture.

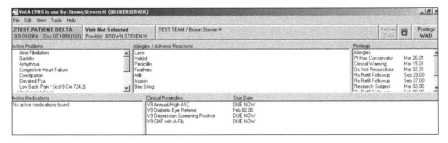

FIGURE 7.5

CPRS cover sheet for sample patient (top of screen), revealing the problem list (left), allergies (center), and reminders (second row). (Courtesy of WorldVistA)

Although digital media designers may think such a claim represents the technology inexperience of large government institutions, direct experience is convincing. The system was specifically designed and customized for the VHA's work practices and organizational routines, which is the primary goal of any enterprise system. Technical usability means little if the system itself is rejected by the organization because it fails to support routines and preferred work styles. VHA clinicians easily navigate the complex network of CPRS screens, and few complaints were documented in my (limited) experience, consistent with published reports. Hundreds of new residents train on the system each year, perpetuating the installed base of trained users and providing sources for continuing innovation ideas.

Integrated Design for Institutional Impact

What opportunities and priorities might designers focus on to best improve EMR systems? From a product design perspective, the most important characteristic of informatics on the front lines is how well *it is integrated with clinical work practice*. According to practice studies and research reviews, current EMRs are found to increase workload and reduce clinical efficiency.[23] However, whereas most commercial EMR systems are designed as generic systems to be customized to fit institutional workflow needs, the CPRS system was designed by the VHA to enable preferred procedures and standards of practice.

Physicians, nurses, and other staff each have specialized EMR information needs. For example, the basic VistA imaging module collects and displays multiple image types (radiology, CT, MRI, ultrasound) in an integrated gallery associated with a single patient's record.

Designers hoping that EMRs contribute to meaningful organizational change may be disappointed—although these systems change *practices*, they may not change operations and will not change the institutional business model. A large-scale EMR aggregates and integrates hundreds of data types in processes much more likely to lock in outdated operational models for the duration of the installation.

The VHA operational model is highly stable and is unlikely to face near-future disruption, even as it expands into community care networks. Where healthcare records and documentation are completely automated, there may be little opportunity to change processes outside of that infrastructure, so new processes tend to be designed and integrated into the standard platform. As standards evolve for EMR systems, open-access interfaces (APIs) or standard software (such as the Columbia Infobuttons standard, OpenEMR, or HL7 specifications) will be more broadly adopted to support integration of add-on vendor tools and homegrown applications within the services.

What Can Future EMRs Learn from VistA?

VistA represents the contributions of deep understanding of full-time internal experts concerned with efficient operations, reliability, and the needs of practice. Because so many clinicians and staff have touched VistA over the years, the CPRS interface has become embedded into routines and practices. Changing system providers would incur needless risks and require extensive transition management and retraining. Replacing the system would require the largest healthcare system in the world to change its effective processes and well-learned behaviors and tacit knowledge. The transition would never recover its true costs, and ultimately be less productive than staying with an aging system that has (by most user and institutional reports) served the VA's clinical practices very well.

There are numerous and notable failed attempts to transform aging information infrastructures used in technical work, such as the roughly 20-year transition to a modernized air traffic control system in the United State. In high-reliability organizations, systems cannot be swapped out or even easily upgraded without risking lives and operations. Navigating VistA to adapt to new standards (ICD-10) and displays (mobile) requires a series of sustaining innovations, supported now by the open innovation model of WorldVistA.

GUI Does Not Equal Usability

Character-based, non-GUI terminal interfaces are extremely efficient once operators are trained and experienced in the codes and shortcuts. These still enjoy wide use in retail, banking, and government, which have in common both high-volume, repetitive transactions and flexible orders and exceptions (which could be tedious on a GUI). Some attempts to change these systems have led to disastrous results in the operational context, especially when the purpose of the upgrade was merely the installation of a GUI.[24]

In high-risk work environments, measures of total system effectiveness become significant. CPRS was designed as a sociotechnical system, and not from a UX or usability context. CPRS functions are integrated into work practices, and tasks are allocated to team roles to optimize overall effectiveness. The VHA has accomplished this by allocating staff and automation to the tasks best performed by each agent.

The VHA medical centers employ ward clerks who organize, translate, and type handwritten orders, test results, and other instructions on behalf of clinical staff. They do not handle all entries, but work as scribes to translate and mediate clinician inputs. It may appear counterproductive to employ people to perform manual tasks to support the information requirements of the enterprise EMR system. However, the "human-in-the-loop" has become a critical resource in the VHA. In such a large system, many physicians are visiting, busy with faculty and other clinical positions, or may lack the time or experience to perform skilled data entry in the CPRS.

In the traditional medical culture, many senior doctors do not enter their own data or orders in an EMR. A good argument can be made for data entry intermediaries serving as clinical team members, freeing up clinicians to focus their attention on patient issues. The human-in-the-loop can be a reliable process to ensure a complementary, human process manages orders and data. Experienced humans can do a much better job of data quality checking than even the most sophisticated rule checking in a database system. By managing the total flow of inputs into a resource management system like an EMR, the human in the middle can often optimize the total throughput of orders and responses from other service areas in the hospital.

With the introduction of complicated EMRs, the role of scribe has started to catch on. Prominent "online physicians" and health issues bloggers, such as Scott Silverstein, have claimed that the human mediation of a scribe is necessary as a workaround for fundamentally defective EMR processes.[25] Author and medical blogger Douglas Perednia claims that scribes add significant overhead costs to practices and may not be as effective as claimed.[26] Both may be right. The increased costs may be a process workaround that enables healthcare organizations to progressively deploy the EMR without interfering with the long-established communications patterns on which care professionals rely.

The fact that scribes are considered effective at all anchors the design axiom: "*Can* does not demand *ought*."[27] *Just because a task can be automated does not mean it should be*. Humans are poor at repetitive data entry tasks and vigilance, as our ability to sustain attention is variable and inconsistent. Yet humans surpass automated systems at tasks such as assessing contexts (Is this order correct for the patient?), verifying the quality and fit of the data

(Does this drug dose look right for a child?), pattern matching (Why is this medication being prescribed when it interacts with these others?), and situation awareness (How does this patient look to you?).

These islands in the stream of automation may add a step and a costly human agent. But people may speed up the overall throughput by saving clinical time, and save lives and liabilities by providing a last-minute check on data validity as it enters the system. People can be employed as centers of agency in an activity design approach. They perform as quality control monitors, task and organizational connectors, and as problem solvers using their adaptive situation awareness.

VistA works well because it was designed by its own organization and represents the contributions of full-time internal experts concerned with efficient operations, reliability, and the needs of practice.

LESSONS LEARNED

- VistA may be among the oldest EMRs, but most of the current market leaders are also based on a MUMPS data architecture.

- VHA hospitals using VistA are among the few that have achieved HIMSS Stage 7 qualification, the highest level of health records integration.

- VistA is a good example of positive lock-in. Because of its history, thousands of clinicians and staff have used some version of VistA over much of their careers and are familiar with its interface and "language."

- The CPRS interface has become so embedded in routines and practices that changing system providers would incur significant transition risks.

- In high-reliability organizations such as inpatient clinics, systems cannot be swapped out or even easily upgraded without risking lives and operations. The best redesign may be a GUI wrapper over the underlying architecture and data model.

- With an open system and information architecture such as VistA, informatics designers can be assured their custom development work will not be obviated by licensing or ownership changes with private EMR vendors.

EMR Design Process

From a care service perspective, the improvement of patient outcomes is the human-centered design goal of every EMR application. Ultimately, patient health (and organizational effectiveness toward maintaining patient health) is the measure of design success. Clinicians are the primary users of the EMR, and strong user-centered design methods are employed in the best institutions today to achieve not just better, more usable applications, but clinical tools that help clinical teams improve care outcomes.

The Center for Biomedical Informatics (CBMi) at the Children's Hospital of Philadelphia has made significant advances in process and EMR design, which they publish and present at their annual Healthcare Informatics Symposium (www.chopcbmi.org). CBMi's human factors designer, Dean Karavite, anchors the interaction design role in their multidisciplinary team of clinicians, researchers, data analysts, and developers.[28]

The CBMi methodology is consistent with modern UX design methods employed in business or commercial software, using an iterative incremental development process (as typical with enterprise applications). Multiple observation and user understanding techniques are employed to learn about clinical users. Although critical, this is rarely enough to understand the complexity of EMR interaction and how that interaction impacts patient outcomes. Therefore, the CBMi team continuously reviews all findings and design work with extensive data analysis, utilizing the EMR itself to not only understand patient care but the behavior of EMR users.

CBMi Design Methodology

1. **Identify the patient population.**

   - Define the patient population, and the outcomes to improve, using literature, research, and clinical guidelines.

   - Analyze EMR data to increase understanding of these outcomes and establish baseline measures (what the design will seek to improve).

2. **Study clinicians and their tasks, and information that impacts outcomes.**

   - Using multiple methods, including contextual inquiry and semi-structured interviews, study clinicians and identify tasks and information relevant to the targeted outcomes.

   - Augment these findings with EMR data analysis applied to the entire (or broader) user population.

3. **Develop use cases.**

   * Develop use cases (or scenarios) that define the most common and/ or important scenarios of patient care.

   * Validate use cases by presenting them back to clinicians, and have them rate in terms of accuracy, importance, and frequency.

4. **Develop the initial design.**

   * Develop low-cost, disposable prototypes that represent the use cases. These prototypes need only convey or simulate interaction and should be in a format that can be developed and modified quickly (Karavite uses the Web-based prototyping tool Balsamiq).

   * Review designs in a use-case format (e.g., sequential, task based, storyboard) with representative clinicians. Adjust designs as required.

   * Iterate, iterate, iterate.

5. **Develop the application.**

   * Build a functioning system.

   * Perform usability testing with representative users to validate the design work to date.

   * Adjust designs as required.

6. **Release the application on the EMR platform.**

   * Release the initial beta version to a small group of users.

   * Identify any remaining issues.

   * Release to entire user population.

7. **Measure the outcomes.**

   * Utilizing EMR data and feedback from end users, analyze the impact of the clinical decision support system or application intervention.

These methods develop the human interaction requirements, which are coordinated with system and functional requirements to provide validated clinical tools. As a design methodology, these activities are led by the human factors team on the EMR project. The steps may not perfectly match the application development process, yet are necessary to ensure that an application serves the highest value tasks for a service. Karavite's organization has developed a sophisticated and consistent process over time with CBMi. An organization just starting its design capacity will of necessity adapt to their local development process and evolve design practices with increasing scope of projects.

Design Methods: Cognitive Engineering

Two of the more basic methods from cognitive engineering are recommended in the context of designing for complex sociotechnical systems such as the EMR in clinical work. Cognitive systems engineering was developed as a research and analytical approach to designing interactive systems with significant human interaction that require cognitive tasks to be shared between human agents and increasingly complex systems.[29] Cognitive engineering has served as the design methodology for complex and high-reliability systems, such as in nuclear energy production and military systems. It has more recently found applications in healthcare with the increasing adoption of health IT.

The abstraction hierarchy is a rapid modeling and reasoning method that follows the canons of cognitive systems engineering. It is useful for mapping out abstract functions for a practice, allowing the design team to understand what essential activities must take place in a healthcare environment or service. The second methodology presented, activity scenarios, may be the most pertinent design approach a team might employ with mixed-discipline teams in a clinical institution. The activity scenario process anchors innovation concepts in concrete examples from real-world experience. The two methodologies cover complementary, nonoverlapping requirements in an EMR design process. Both of these methodologies have widespread application and can be used in other D3.0 and D4.0 contexts, such as management, customer-facing services, and information systems.

Abstraction Hierarchy

The abstraction hierarchy is a powerful aid to analysis and synthesis of essential functions and touchpoints in service design. Employed for means-ends analysis, it maps out the relationships of system elements to each other by both purpose (abstraction hierarchy) and system function level. It has the analytical power to represent large-scale systems by mapping human and system activities across organizational and community or policy levels.

Based on Rasmussen's cognitive engineering and extended by cognitive work analysis,[30] the method offers designers a way to quickly understand the purposes, priorities, and functions in a system. A simpler technique drawn from the methodology (presented here) provides an analytical tool for identifying best options for service design and problem solving.

Creating the Function Matrix

To create an abstraction hierarchy, an analysis is made of a step-by-step identification of functions in a problem space. The levels of *abstraction* (columns) represent the relationship of means to ends, where the ultimate ends of the function are positioned at the top. The *functional decomposition* extends across the row, from the whole system to its parts. This cognitive engineering approach requires (at minimum) two passes of analysis, which can appear like the model in Figure 7.6. A total system view of (idealized) healthcare is simplified (abstracted) in the leftmost column.

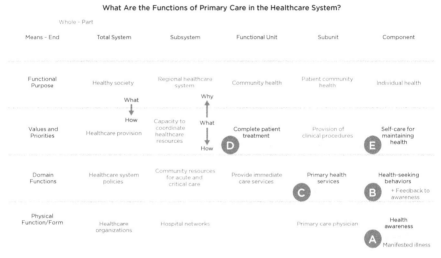

FIGURE 7.6
Abstraction hierarchy for means-ends analysis.

- Within a column, each level shows a *means* relationship, from purpose (top) to physical functions (bottom).

- The means-ends coupling can be tested by determining whether the function at each level is an "end" state for the means function below it. If a healthy society is the function (the "what"), healthcare provision is the "how," or a means to accomplishing that function.

- The upward test is *why* this function is performed in the system. Why do we need local clinics (bottom row)? To provide full care services. Why? To provide complete patient treatment.

Mapping a Pathway

Although the complete matrix is helpful for analysis, service design scenarios are built by defining a subset of activities within the map to establish a system boundary for the service. Figure 7.6 shows a scenario pathway (activities A–E) mapped within the matrix to define a range of typical health-seeking behaviors and patient motivations within the current healthcare system. This set can be labeled as one scenario pathway.

The functions being analyzed are in bold. The activity relationships are shown by indicating a path through the functions, from A to E. A given actor in the social system traverses the functions from health awareness (of a symptom) to health seeking, through a treatment cycle, and then self-care. A feedback loop is shown (not typical of most abstraction hierarchies) to show how completing the activity cycle reinforces health awareness and leads to better self-care.

The pathway defines only functions of interest but helps analysts and designers consider the range of potential activities and options available by increasing scope or narrowing the function. Service touchpoints are defined at the functional level of *values and priorities*—these critical activities can be provided in a service ecology by innovations other than the design plan being mapped.

Activity Scenarios

Activity scenarios are stories or mixed-visual narratives of situations that involve envisioned users (defined as focal personas) in their work activities or life contexts that drive behavior and engagement with services and information. In designing for a service system, scenarios are formulated to test-drive the interactions and touchpoints that various personas will engage in their journey through possible sequences. Activity scenarios provide all organizational team members with a common road map of service functions, presented in examples and terms they understand well.

Scenarios can be defined at macro or micro levels of detail. At different stages in design, different scales become useful. Early design calls for macro scenarios that envision how people (personas) will encounter the service, find it helpful or not, and share information with others. Macro scenarios are formulated to represent observations and actions at the *activity* level.

An "activity" refers to a repeating and ongoing practice that involves multiple discrete tasks typically performed together in support of an objective. "Patient examination" would be an example of an activity composed of multiple tasks that is repeated consistently in principle, and is guided (by rules) by the needs discovered in the situation.

Macro scenarios are best for participatory scenario design because a diversity of perspectives are necessary to reflect what can happen in clinical environments. Furthermore, participation requires facilitating activities that include a wide variety of contributions and expertise.

Activity scenarios developed in workshops can fold into requirements analysis, concept design, and prototyping. For the clinical education context, resident scenarios might include:

- Learning a new procedure in advance of seeing it performed.

- Reviewing a known procedure to evaluate complications (e.g., I've done this before and everything went right, but what could go wrong?)

- Learning how to discriminate between and choose tests when faced with more than two possible diagnoses.

- Finding a guide to a rarely performed procedure.

Micro scenarios are essentially use cases. They focus on discrete actions, or part-tasks, and can require specialized expertise and research observation to formulate with meaningful fidelity. Use cases are developed in middle or later stages, when the product and user requirements are well defined and initial prototypes have been built and tested. Micro scenarios involve the details of interaction given specific interface options that have been realized in design and testing. In early design stages, these details are unproductive to consider because the interface design is usually quite sketchy. Even when redesigning existing systems with well-established patterns of use, focusing on micro scenarios early in conceptual design may prematurely reinforce current interactions and user patterns and prohibit discovery of alternative experience design proposals.

- EMRs reconfigure clinical practice, requiring significant management support and overhead. During implementation, design teams might also advise changes to management practices. A "whole system" of practice involves leadership as much as it does the tasks of practitioners in the service units.

- Management is also a care practice and is subject to design improvement by employing similar design methods advised for care services: activity scenarios, abstraction hierarchy, and sensemaking research.

- Designing for complexity requires agreement on a map of the territory, which the abstraction hierarchy provides. Other system maps (see Chapter 8) are valuable for communication and engagement.

- The abstraction hierarchy can be adapted to any complex design process as a modeling method for systematically decomposing and rethinking the functions in a service or practice. Because it models functions and not specific technologies, designers can substitute different tools or manual activities to enable the abstracted functions required of the system.

- Any method requires multiple diagrams to be constructed and iterated. Every design effort may require slightly different presentations that communicate the possibilities and decisions for that scenario.

- Practice innovation begins with an abstract process first to ensure that common and critical functions are well understood. This can be followed by concrete alternatives that embody or accomplish these abstractions in a process such as activity scenarios.

- Starting with a concrete process leads to "garden path" solutions based on the primary example, essentially paving the cow paths of old practice and making it harder to revise later.

CHAPTER 8

Systemic Design for Healthcare Innovation

Elena's Story: A System Upgrade

Elena returns to the cardiac care center 2 weeks after her scan and diagnostic procedures. She maintained her medication schedule and her rapid heart rate did not return, so now she wonders whether the invasive procedure is really needed. She has second thoughts about agreeing to what feels like an extreme procedure.

Elena arrives at the center at 6:30 a.m. for her appointment with electrophysiologist Audrey Chen. She is greeted by a receptionist, signs insurance and consent forms, and waits briefly. Unlike at the hospital, she is immediately escorted to a prep room by a staff nurse. Elena changes into a flimsy green gown, and the nurse takes vital measurements and discusses the radiofrequency ablation procedure.

Dr. Chen must first initiate diagnostic testing to "map" the arrhythmia. After administering local anesthesia at the catheter entry points, she inserts a needle through Elena's right femoral veins leading up to the right side of the heart. A sheath is run over the needle to guide the catheter's entry, using a fluoroscopic display to guide the ablation needle. Three catheters are introduced to the bundle of His near the aorta, at the right side of the heart. Dr. Chen electrically stimulates several critical points of the heart's circuitry with the catheters in an attempt to reproduce the kind of arrhythmia Elena has spontaneously generated. She looks for the patterns in the real-time ECG to determine when she has reproduced the SVT signals.

Once the arrhythmia is reproduced (a complex process that can take well over an hour), Dr. Chen maps this electrical circuit by locating the nerve signaling positions on the heart. After confirming with the ECG reading, Dr. Chen inserts the ablation catheter through an incision in the groin. She guides it to the heart location using the ultrasound display from a second catheter that monitors the ablation. The ablation catheter is controlled to deliver radiofrequency pulses at selected points in the heart tissue.

Dr. Chen proceeds to "ablate" (electrically cauterize) the absolute minimum that is necessary to stop the arrhythmia. The ablation instruments are powerful and can literally burn a hole in the heart, a potentially catastrophic complication. The entire procedure, from catheter insertion to post-operative recovery, is about 6 hours for Elena's case.

Elena has no way of judging the quality and sustainability of her treatment. As long as the SVT symptoms do not reappear, she has no way of knowing how her body has accommodated the treatment.

There are hundreds or thousands of small errors that could occur in the diagnosis, mapping, and ablation procedure. The fact that the vast majority of ablations are performed without problems during or after attest to the high level of training and the level of trust in the standard of care.

Elena's ablation is an advanced technical procedure that is fully dependent on formal institutional practice. The clinical focus on body systems (e.g., cardiovascular system) translates biomedical research and advances in procedure into innovations for specialized care. The body-system orientation facilitates the development of specialist expertise, but reinforces a tradition of problem-based, not person-centered care.

A successful procedure reinforces the perception that optimal health outcomes have been achieved. It suggests that service delivery is value received, when value is only realized upon improved health as declared by the customer, the health seeker. In many specialist care situations, patients may not realize that other valid therapeutic alternatives may be possible. Between the high-cost standard of care (a business driver) and the customer's knowledge gap, there may be little motive to change the model of care. ■

Disruptive Transformation

Innovation theories celebrate the value of "disruptive" innovation as the most competitive form of innovation. Business authors claim disruptive interventions have the most impact and profit potential, because disruptive entrants displace winners in large economies. Disruption of current practices has become an aim of innovation, if not its very definition. Disruptive or radical innovation promises rapid change with technological interventions—yet healthcare systems are designed as institutions, which are resistant to any type of rapid change.

In healthcare practice, the goals of *transformation* are perhaps more relevant than disruptive innovation. US healthcare and other publicly financed systems face a long-term cost and financing crisis as populations grow, age, and use more healthcare services than are supported by revenues. A large proportion of healthcare services are "delivered" from a centralized care model in which people visit a regional hospital to have emergent or acute problems treated. Yet common chronic illnesses such as acquired diabetes, metabolic syndrome, and asthma are becoming pandemic, and there are no easy design solutions for prevention or intervention at the societal scale.

Innovation in Markets or Services?

Clayton Christensen[1] defines disruptive innovation as the way smaller entrants grab a niche market by offering similar products at much lower cost. Or by providing a single significant feature overlooked by current users, they build a new market that leapfrogs the competition. They eventually overtake established players when their offerings expand to fulfill the larger demand of the market as their value proposition catches on.

We often celebrate innovation for its own sake. But in healthcare, we might be more cautious about the intent of innovation:

- What exactly is being "disrupted"?
- Is a disruptive or radical innovation the right mindset and frame of reference for healthcare innovation?
- Whose values are being optimized when technology is hailed for "disrupting healthcare"?
- Are we learning from the vast history of technology and software failures and unintended consequences in healthcare applications?
- Is new necessarily better, or is any chance to improve good?

Even if many healthcare services are profit-based, should innovation best be envisioned as enabling a *competitive* outcome? It depends on the market being disrupted. In the care market, human lives are at stake, not merely profits. If the market is competing products in the healthcare industry, then disruption or radical innovation may lead to market share dominance. But new products more often incrementally improve well-known care practices than transform them. They maximize care while incurring minimal risk in their adoption.

CT and MRI imaging systems were breakthrough innovations and transformed diagnostics and surgical outcomes by significantly improving diagnostic imaging. Yet even these powerful diagnostic systems—together considered the top medical innovation of the last 50 years—did not reinvent the hospital, streamline inpatient care, or even change clinical workflow. The da Vinci minimally invasive and remote surgical system is one of the newer significant innovations of both technique and workflow. Yet the system does not replace a surgeon's skill as much as it improves options for the patient, with less-invasive procedures and robot-assisted remote operations.

Breakthrough treatments or techniques that transform healthcare services are not disruptive to clinical work in the economic sense of innovation. For example, a new entrant may introduce an innovation into a competitive market, such as the pen-style insulin injection systems for diabetics. The new Timesulin pen cap (Figure 8.1) adapts to pens already in the market and displays the last time of injection. It solves a single problem well.

The Timesulin approach disrupts the competition among insulin devices by providing a better product unavailable from the current providers. Though it does not disrupt clinical *care*, it disrupts the product ecosystem by improving a necessary application by adapting to the most current accepted innovations already in the market.

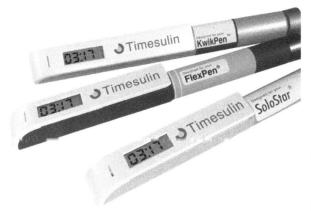

FIGURE 8.1
Timesulin insulin pen
cap. (Courtesy Marcel
Botha, Timesulin)

The healthcare system absorbs new technology and prices it into the existing delivery model. New care services are adopted if they are shown to be effective and are supported by evidence, even if they cost more. New services in *sequential* care modes (such as continuing services for diabetes, allergies, dialysis) have direct patient impact, but may raise costs when first implemented. New services in *iterative* modes (chronic, cancer, cardiac) may not be seen as novel by patients.

Because patients often receive a specific type of treatment only once, they may not be informed or repeating customers. They have little to compare, even if their treatment represents a demand and its fulfillment represents received value. Thus the patient experience of a healthcare innovation may be invisible. The radical improvement is only appreciated by its absence and is perhaps measured by *not noticing*. If a service innovation helps the clinical team maintain awareness, sensitivity, and control over a difficult procedure, the invisible value may also be recognized in the errors or lengthy duration that did *not* occur due to an improved clinical system.

What Is the Target of Innovation?

Reliance on a profit-based business model in healthcare and its supplier industries (pharmaceuticals and IT in particular) has resulted in the expensive, fragmented, and unsustainable US healthcare system. Insurance firms and health maintenance organizations (HMOs) have less incentive to innovate because they have established regional monopolies and have little organic competition. The obvious entry of government as a global underwriter and single payer would disrupt the noncompetitive insurance model.

Although some observers propose that changing market incentives to enable an even freer market of payers could result in fair competition for healthcare business, new entrants are at a serious disadvantage. The entrenched provider-payers enjoy a privileged position; they have influenced policy for decades, have deep pockets to compete with low-cost models, and own proprietary sources of patient data for analyzing risk and underwriting. The insurance model establishes a very high barrier to entry.

The core innovation problem at this level is not the disruption of service models but the transformation of payment systems. There may be no perfect system anywhere, but the US system is uniquely structured to prevent universal care and institutional innovation.

Healthcare policy reveals cases of unwanted, anti-innovative disruption. The insurance industry has by default designed the healthcare delivery system in the United States by mediating payment for care procedures. As policies are instituted to give more oversight of patient services and payments, significant consequences to costs and everyday clinical management will arise, often moving the system in the opposite direction intended by decision makers. The planned implementation of the ICD-10 coding system (with tens of thousands of finer-grained billing categories) will require system-level updates to all US billing and electronic medical record (EMR) systems that track and code medical procedures. Although the standard was intended to enable better cost oversight, ICD-10 will be disruptive, costly, and counterproductive.

The need to account for piecemeal billing has led to fragmented procedures, as clinicians must keep track of every micro-task that could possibly vary for billing and reimbursement. This creates a significant overhead to track, account for, and defend every procedure on a bill. This pressure places perverse incentives on clinicians to identify variants that can be reasonably reimbursed, not to extract from the payer but just to break even with legitimate time spent in clinical consultation. (In US healthcare, there is no way to bill for the procedure known as "conversation." My Canadian family physician spent two hours in conversation with me on our initial intake to the practice. Our appointments have never been rushed for time. Though there are many other contrasts, the ability of Canadian doctors to cultivate a personal understanding is something most US patients may never see.)

There are hundreds of possible targets for innovation, but few have an effect on the system or organization as a whole. A systems view of innovation considers the whole system and its interrelated components. Innovation or disruption is efficient and influential when the least effort has the largest desired effect. Although social systems such as healthcare practices are dynamic and change may not be predictable, there are systems and design methods that enable stakeholders to determine the maximum benefit or influence in innovation or change programs.

The Healthcare Innovator's Challenge

The innovator's challenge is to understand and preserve core values while changing practices for durable social and economic benefit. Although economic value is often a pivotal driver of innovation adoption, cost management is not itself a core value but a sustainability factor to be evaluated in decision making. The related social innovation challenge is perhaps a macro policy problem, not a design issue. A significant social impact from cost savings could be obtained from transferring value from a high-profit sector to facilitate better access to services and improve primary care.

Healthcare is a social and public good that *can* be provided universally, in some form, as in most developed countries. In the United States, this would require a truly disruptive change to public policy and the insurance payer model of the healthcare system. As a recent *New England Journal of Medicine* article declared,

> It is hard to ignore that in 2006, the United States was number 1 in terms of health care spending per capita but ranked 39th for infant mortality, 43rd for adult female mortality, 42nd for adult male mortality, and 36th for life expectancy. These facts have fueled a question now being discussed in academic circles, as well as by government and the public: Why do we spend so much to get so little?[2]

Was there ever a clearer innovation challenge in any sector or business? Healthcare as an industry faces multiple crises that beg for systemic solutions, not piecemeal fixes. System interventions aim for the root issues most closely related to the perpetuation of critical problems. Sustainable solutions are those that economically scale across institutions and regions.

Systemic redesign requires agreement on a shared vision of the future value state. Any project aiming to satisfy multiple stakeholders (not just users or owners) requires a systemic approach, rather than the mere negotiation of service functions. We might reframe the purposes of "disruptive innovation" in institutional healthcare from economic and technical value to that of *co-creating significant service transformations that benefit all stakeholders.*

Systemic Design in Healthcare Service

This book maps to three systems: the individual health seeker, clinical practice, and institutional healthcare. Each is a complex system with different opportunities for system change resulting from services within the system. The design and research methods appropriate to one system context may not transfer well to the others.

Systemic design adapts design practices to sociotechnical complexity. By integrating systems thinking and its methods, systemic design adopts human-centered design to co-create complex, multistakeholder services such as those found in medicine and healthcare.

Any system is an emergent network of deeply interconnected functions that achieves an intended purpose. Every system can be seen as social or human-influenced. Systems researchers report consensus that human intervention has touched all aspects of the planetary ecology. As a result they call our current era the Anthropocene. So we can also say "all systems are social."

Systemic behaviors occur throughout healthcare. Systems (including most medical services) may fail in unpredictable ways if their components are separated from the connected whole. Cases show traditional product development approaches to innovation often fail in a complex system scenario. As planners and designers, we focus on the wrong object for innovation, often expecting an IT application to diffuse into an organization with intended system-wide uses. In complex sociotechnical systems like medicine, the planned adoption becomes fraught with challenges, and the unintended effects outweigh the benefits.

A Systems View of Specialty Medicine

The shortfall of US primary care practitioners is a systemic case. Growing from a primary care *crisis* into a permanent situation, it has evolved into the current specialist-based dominant system. From a systems perspective, specialists create a market of specialist health problems, which satisfy the demands of the "big box healthcare" business model. As the rights to certain procedures are owned by specialists, primary care physicians become busy brokers of referrals to the specialty system.

The specialist body-system model fulfills its intended purposes well—patients with broken hips see orthopedic surgeons, cancer patients see oncologists, cataracts are treated by ophthalmologists. However, the clear societal need in the United States and other national systems is for more accessible primary and preventive care. If primary care were more successful, it would greatly reduce the need for highly profitable specialty services.

The vast majority of all physician encounters are for outpatient treatment, whether specialty or primary care. Medical residencies have prepared trainees for inpatient care at the expense of societal needs. A recent Johns Hopkins study showed that residents trained in community hospitals were better prepared for basic outpatient care than those in the large academic medical centers where most residents are trained.[3] The status and monetary bias toward specialization may prevent many of the best doctors from going into primary care service. This bias is a positive feedback loop that produces more of the same outcomes over time.

Consider Elena's scenario in this chapter. Her patient experience could be enhanced in many ways to reduce anxiety or facilitate quicker restoration.

If her ablation procedure works as intended, is there any payoff for clinics to make incremental improvements in short-term care experience?

Specialist care is necessarily reactive, based on referrals and responding to disease discovery, and is not positioned to proactively prevent health problems. From a preventive care view, specialists are counter-systemic, as their service waits until illnesses erupt into obvious health concerns. Even specialized medical tests are often counter-systemic, as aggressive testing often leads to unnecessary procedures. Specialists (and surgeons) are also not institutionally able to engage patients as whole persons with multiple life and health issues. This may prevent individuals from understanding and tackling the root causes emerging from their lifestyle and behavior. The specialist model has no systemic incentive to deal with underlying root causes, as prevention or mitigation could reduce specialists' income growth. Given the insurance-based payer model, the specialist is incentivized to conduct as many high-paying procedures as possible.

This is not an indictment of specialists. The need for specialty care has also increased with population growth and aging, and with the advancement of technical procedures. Their maximization of profit by procedure type or volume is entirely rational. Proposing radical innovations to their established model will encounter cultural resistance from the current system. Technological innovations (such as the ultrasound-guided cardiac procedure Elena undergoes) do not usually reduce costs but yield clinical goals, easing invasiveness and increasing reliability and sophistication.

Primary care physicians usually have significant patient caseloads and are unable to actively follow referred patients, at least until follow-up. The family doctor is not part of a collaborative care team in the inpatient context, and may only be copied on the clinical report and final ECG after treatment. Continuity represents a major service and IT design challenge for the foreseeable future, even as EMRs become integrated across practices. If a new role of *care coordinator* was introduced across the patient's entire disease cycle—from diagnosis to aftercare consultation—a whole-care experience could be co-created with the patient's health-seeking journey. The patient experience is directly improved by such continuity.

A systemic design considers the entire flow of specialist service. Specialists are not typically trained to engage the whole person or a holistic view of treatment. In fact, in Elena's entire health-seeking journey, no *single* clinician or coordinator attends to all her treatments and medications. Known as *continuity of care*, in multi-condition, multi-specialist situations, a holistic coordination of treatment and medication is, unfortunately, quite rare. It is also a huge opportunity for innovation, as presented in the IDEO case study in Chapter 6.

Chronic disease exposes the systemic weakness of the specialist model. Environment- and lifestyle-induced diseases such as diabetes and cancers increase in the population and complicate any other conditions. Multiple treatments and medications are costly to providers and society. Unraveling these causal impacts is difficult because each is also an effect of other long-term causes, such as environmental degradation and the marketing of unhealthy lifestyles. Unfortunately, the current US market-based system provides no incentive or process for managing multiple combined conditions effectively.

Systemic Innovations in Primary Care

The specialist model will not be changed "by design" because it is profitable and institutionalized. Even minor changes will trigger lobbying in response to policy design. Disruptive change will emerge from innovation on the input side, by reducing the referred patient demand to the specialty practices.

Practice innovation is motivated by business and operational structure more than clinical process. Integrated practices combining primary care and related specialties are growing, as their cost and business models adapt more quickly to changing payers and incentives. Among these new structures are the accountable care organizations (ACO), the manifestation of a major policy innovation emerging in the United States from the 2010 Affordable Care Act. These are decentralized and cooperative clinical practices that promise better cost management and quality care, usually connected to a traditional hospital system or payer network. ACOs are envisioned as evolving toward community-located or distributed health clinics that promote a community-oriented, patient-centered model of care. ACOs are "accountable" in that their risk and reward is based on a defined segment of their population, to which they are responsible for measures of community health and quality goals. Though the ACO is a policy innovation, the result will be a rapid evolution of new clinical business models, allowing innovative practices to experiment with approaches that fit their community needs. The model encourages a coordinated care approach for patients with complex and chronic diseases and for the predominant concerns of a community area.

The ACO model is community-based, not regional, yet it is growing in large urban areas, establishing a cooperative ecosystem with hospitals. According to a 2012 study, 221 ACOs are in operation in 45 US states, primarily in larger urban areas.[4] Most ACOs (67%) are private, single-provider groups comprised of cooperating generalist, primary care, and relevant specialists providers. The growth of ACOs has been largely based on the favorable risk and payment model provided to early adopters.

Another structural innovation is the alternative primary care model, the patient-centered medical home (PCMH). Promoted by the Agency for Healthcare Research and Quality and other foundations and organizations, the "medical home" concept is not home-based care but rather a compact community health center with strong support for localized patient-centered care. The idea has been developing since the 1960s, but has only recently caught on as an alternative practice model. The new PCMH model has a triple aim of quality, improved patient experience, and lower costs while directing the practice toward a personal physician with coordinated and continuous care, a whole-person orientation, and a wider range of communications approaches. The medical home and ACO models have rapidly changed the organizational environment favoring institutional innovation.

To Innovate, Follow the System

Patient-centered service design does not aim for a "user experience" but rather health outcomes. Health outcomes are realized at some indefinite point after care services and self-care, and are both measured and experienced future benefits. Outcomes can be seen as an emergence of many design inputs, most of which are invisible to the patient.

How can innovators move clients beyond the current entrenched system? In commercial healthcare (pharma, HMOs, insurance), we unwittingly maintain the current system when extending a dominant position in a market. Even enhancing *service* (patient-centered or otherwise) within the established business model almost always reinforces the current system and denies system change. Adapting design to improving current service for large, profit-driven organizations may only sustain the injustices of financially driven healthcare. Design thinking, even when "challenging the brief," does not challenge the assumptions of business logic and client economics.

Who is empowered when we design better ideas for clients that benefit from the current system? Our clients will not endorse a scope that aims to disrupt the very system that sustains their revenues and supports their ongoing role and business. Many of these opportunities may be disguised by the rhetoric of "care" and "patient centeredness." The contributions of service design may extend and even lock in regressive practices by making them accessible and easier to use.

Fixing the wrong thing well is a typical system conundrum. Although systems thinking excels in finding ways to navigate complexity, the systems disciplines integrate very few design methods. And design-thinking methods—including fundamentals such as cyclic iterations of prototypes, human-centered design research, and shifting problem-solving contexts— are insufficient by themselves in complex systems.

Systems thinking includes science and design, which both must converge to design social systems. In systems thinking, the *organization* is regarded as a high-leverage target for system change because organizations are functionally coherent and purposeful. Policies and roles can be changed directly. Leverage points for changing behaviors can be defined within the organizational system. Changes to internal medicine practice (as in this chapter's case study) have impact across the clinic and all services that draw from the practice. If a large organization succeeds in a systemic change, the new process has significant leverage across the sector as an exemplar.

Organizations are social systems that stakeholders can directly influence and design (the purpose of Design 3.0). Yet organizations are never *whole* systems as they exist to serve a customer or community, which participate in social (D4.0) and economic ecosystems. The organizational boundary is a powerful frame, so it is typical for innovation teams to ignore the whole system beyond the hospital or the company.

The Four Systems of Healthcare

A "system" can be defined as a purposeful collection of interdependent activities that operate as a single dynamic and complex process, with intentional or automatic regulation over its inputs of resources, energy, and information to produce defined outputs. In any whole system, the parts are inextricably interdependent and the whole has a single identity.

Wharton management professors and systems thinkers Jamshid Gharajedaghi and Russell Ackoff developed an integrated foundation of systems and design thinking spanning several decades. Gharajedaghi articulated five essential qualities of systems that designers can account for:

- Purposefulness
- Emergence
- Openness

- Multi-dimensionality
- Counterintuitive behaviors[5]

Many different system types can be articulated, but for the purposes of system design, we require a reduction of variety to make choices. Ackoff defined a simple four-system model based on whether the whole system or its parts exhibit intentionality, as a way to call out the critical complexity in social systems.[6] For healthcare, the four systems can be viewed within the single context of a large urban clinic as the patient, the EMR system, a hospital, and the city or geographic region it serves (Table 8.1).

TABLE 8.1 ACKOFF'S FOUR SYSTEM MODELS

System model	Parts	Whole	Real system
Deterministic	No choice	No choice	EMR application
Animate	No choice	Choice	Patient
Social	Choice	Choice	Hospital
Ecological	Choice	No choice	City

The connection may be closely drawn from Ackoff's systems to the four design geographies of D1.0–4.0. In general, the design orientation to each system level maps as follows to the four levels of clinical design:

- **CD1.0:** Traditional design for mechanistic IT and communication systems (billing systems, wayfinding)

- **CD2.0:** Products and services design for human systems (medical devices, typical healthcare services)

- **CD3.0:** Organizational design for well-bounded social systems (practices, hospital departments, ACO)

- **CD4.0:** Social transformation design for ecological systems (community, policy, health system level)

The four systems are reviewed briefly for each relationship.

Deterministic Systems

Few systems in reality are purely deterministic (or *mechanical*), especially in healthcare, whose systems are entirely organized around human health. All communications, products, and materials are designed for interaction with a human health context, implying some choice in the use of the system. Generally deterministic systems are defined by their structure and interactions from external functions. Health IT, from Web apps to enterprise EMRs, can be seen as mechanistic in their operation—without human intervention, they exhibit no purposeful choice, and they are determined by their programming. The skills and mindset of mechanistic systems applies to both design and system functions for this level. The highly reliable implanted pacemaker, for example, is a mechanistic medical device designed as a closed system, fully functional once programmed, needing minimal monitoring or control. Although these mechanisms are devices for human systems, they do not function like animate systems.

Animate (Human-Centered) Systems

A human being is a whole *animate* system with choice as a whole, in which components (body systems) have purposes but no choice. Here the human system is an agent interacting with the environment and making choices with respect to physical, objective feedback from the world. Human-centered design often covers both animate and social systems without distinguishing between them. When healthcare service is treated as a traditional body-centered model of the patient, an animate system viewpoint is implicit.

When a human is conceived as acting within a sociotechnical system, as a *person* in other words, his or her role elevates from animate agent to a social actor. The patient-centered care model is an attempt to integrate the patient as a whole person, but it often falls short of the social system ideal. By idealizing a patient's experience, the system is bent to meet the symptomatic, medical, and customer needs as perceived by given human actors. The measure of quality is dependent on an underinformed participant in a complex system (even if patient health is the desired outcome).

Social (Organizational) Systems

Social systems are purposeful, persistent, human-constructed, and highly interconnected networks of processes, activities, rules, and actors. Hospitals are social systems that serve the communities within a geographic region and are constructions of policy, practice, and organizations. Universities, medical schools, clinical practices, and families are all social systems. All services are social systems, whether or not they are defined as such by service designers and client teams. Any organized entity involving multiple stakeholders constitutes a social system, with choice at both part and whole levels of action.

Social systems are designable from both design and systems methodologies. Organizational systems (with the neat boundary of the firm or institution) are researched and redesigned within the frame of D3.0 skills and processes. Open societal systems, nongovernmental organizations (with no defined boundary), and many policy organizations are framed by D4.0, a social transformation approach to change rather than a design-led methodology.

Sociotechnical systems are a type of social system developed in the healthcare research literature. They are defined by dynamic, mutual interdependence among socially organized subsystems (people, their activities, roles, and relationships), technical subsystems (information technologies, practices and techniques, workflow, work settings), and organizational environments. The unit of design and analysis of the sociotechnical system is "the system," although technical activity and workflow are often directly studied to assess and redesign technologies and the underlying social systems.

Ecological Systems (Ecosystems)

Ecological systems are the most complex systems, as they are living systems and subject to interventions of the choiceful systems (animate and social systems). Ecologies respond in a determined causal way (as a whole) to interventions such as animate activity, human outputs, natural forces, and the dynamics of living beings that depend on the ecosystem. Their components are both living systems (humans, animals, plant life) and social systems, and the activities that characterize the ecology as dynamic are largely the choices of these part-subsystems. They are considered extremely complex largely because of their emergent and adaptive behaviors in response to a myriad of inputs, which cannot be predicted by human observers.

The colloquial reference to "ecosystem" as a constellation of interdependent social and technological services should be treated metaphorically. The social ecosystem is just a larger social system, considered as the largest boundary of systemic design action at the D4.0 level.

Encountering a Mess of System Problems

There is no single "whole system" in healthcare identified by a boundary such as "the US healthcare system." Instead, there are many whole systems, most of them overlapping in function, that represent different social systems. Incremental improvements to these service systems may have significant positive impacts on the performance of the whole.

Each system type is identified and innovated differently by design, management, and engineering disciplines, leading to the confusion of distinctions that occur when we discuss design in healthcare. For example, the information systems mindset of health IT orients toward deterministic systems in research, design, and methodology. EMR teams rarely include social scientists or design researchers, and workflow is usually defined as a standard, not a cognitive task. Designers make the mistake of viewing breakdowns and observed frustrations as service design requirements. By elevating the patient "customer" to a sacred construct, systems are designed to produce an optimized experience. However, a service systems approach might sacrifice parameters of patient experience with a life cycle–oriented service strategy that designs for better overall value in realized health outcomes.

Service systems, even if not "designed," function as whole systems. The integration of IT, technical practices, and organizational dynamics becomes shaped into a coordinated, emergent process more powerful than the sum of its parts. The emergent character of these functions operating as a whole creates a resilient, productive system that resists "disruption" as innovation theorists like to imagine. However, small changes to critical functions, so-called high leverage interventions, can result in new practices that become unintentionally innovative.

In real terms, intervention in one system often *excludes* valuable expertise found in the others. The most widely used health records systems are mechanistic—they regulate policies by encoding business rules, billing codes and related forms, and of course, patient records. Social systems within the clinic are largely ignored and are even replaced by "big data." EMRs are not designed for the proactive provision of deep local knowledge of specialized practices, or knowledge of patient and care communities served, or even local practice management.

Consider the obvious "problem" of wait times in care service, such as surpassing target wait times for emergency room patients. Wait times are an effect resulting from a mess of interacting causes. These causes may differ between institutions and even departments—therefore even a hard-won analytical solution to "the problem" may not transfer to other institutions.

When we measure effects as problems, we point to underlying systemic issues. Our problem-solving practices (which include *design*) are often constructed to *produce the right measure*, not to achieve the underlying goal the measure was designed to indicate.

Even with obvious gaps in medical knowledge, designers bring a valuable perspective to clinical and social health problems. Design thinking changes the context for rational problem solving by constantly reframing with stakeholders who may have settled early on "solving the wrong problem." Solving the right problem—or more accurately, finding a better problem—may be design's most important contribution.

Can Systems Care?

We call situations "problems" because they raise shared concerns triggered by values. Problems may not have a common basis in fact or even agreement. They may appear to have existence and their resolution may reduce uncertainty, but all are matters of interpretation.

Many of the problems in healthcare are recognized by their visibility rendered by valuing care (as opposed to efficiency, for example). Values of care are responsive in all "choiceful" system types in which humans are involved—animate, social, and ecological. Only individuals (or beings with choice) can be said to care. Families, communities, and organizations of all kinds are social systems designed for caring for those within the system. The smallest social system, the couple, is also a mutual circle of care. Circles of care are formed as purposeful micro-social systems to facilitate caring and health seeking among a small collective.

Social systems can be designed for providing and reinforcing care, as a preferred or idealized value in the world. Social systems designing requires a design process quite different from products and artifacts. CD4.0 is informed by assembling stakeholders from across organizational and community perspectives to formulate an understanding of values and purposes to develop a strategic frame.

The formative social systems thinkers (e.g., C. West Churchman, Stafford Beer, Alexander Christakis) created system methods that start with understanding stakeholders and their fundamental values and purposes. Social systems design follows laws of systems science. A primary law is cybernetician Ross Ashby's principle of *requisite variety*: the variety of the control system must be equal or greater than the variety of the system being controlled. Social systems design adapted this cybernetics principle by increasing stakeholder diversity (with their domain experience and personal knowledge) in place of controls and feedback loops. Social systems design follows a democratic design philosophy, embracing the diversity of roles, power, practice, values, and risk to design services that all stakeholders in the system can support.

People extend their values as systems of caring into ecologies and for inanimate objects and machines. Individuals and organizations care about their technological choices and the tools and materials associated with practice. We devote care for natural ecologies in our immediate locales and across the planet. The human capacity for empathy can be extended to things as well.

Business Models as Values Systems

Values are enduring preferences that guide personal and organizational behavior, decision making, and managerial action. Values embed tacit knowledge and they perform the same function as knowledge—they are beliefs that enact what we understand to be true and worthwhile. They efficiently move us to act on priorities without the need to pause for deliberation or reflection, as would be expected when values conflict with other organizational demands.

Organizational values are not the inspirational messages printed on wall posters. They are normative rules that encode collective preferences and desired states, and result in hiring decisions, budgets, major investments, internal agreements, and community initiatives. Values systems function *systemically*, as a network of interdependent values that emerge as a whole, often recognized as "the way we do things here."

Real values are built in to business models and routine processes, each of which have values systems. A hospital's emergency department operates from different values than the IT or clinical research departments.

A hospital's *business model* acts as a process guideline and arbitrates values conflicts when they occur. Hospital business models generally reflect values in use, which are typically grounded in efficiency and safety. If we intend to innovate the *institution*, the business model is the place to start. The dominant logic of the clinical enterprise is a centrally managed collection of independent service lines. If the hospital was organized as a service system with a distributed logic, enabling cooperative services, staff, and payment across business lines, a whole-system approach could develop. New business models follow the development of new service lines.

Business models are artifacts, whether formalized or not, that are designed by management as road maps of intra- and interorganizational relationships and their commitments to people, resources, and economic logic. Business models serve as maps of the decision territory for organizational stakeholders to identify relationships between contributing resources, customers, and revenues. Ultimately, business models are planning tools for effective design of an enterprise social system.

The business models of care organizations can be reenvisioned to formalize agreement on the partnerships and operational processes that ensure the well-being of patients, providers, and the served community. However, business models rarely consider the strategic value of the *ecosystem* (natural capital, water access, air quality) or the health value of a region's environmental management. In fact, most hospital business models overlook the necessity of accounting for social sustainability, providing resources for improving health access, and equity. Urban medical centers embrace social welfare in their outreach and community partnerships, and are becoming responsive to social needs for home care, community awareness and education, transportation, and health hazards. Yet even these core social functions are not yet strategic services in the organizational business model.

Leading healthcare centers in the near future (within 5 years in progressive cities) will begin exploring sustainable business models beyond the current "triple aim" strategy of care, health, and cost.[7] (They will have to develop new business models because the big box healthcare facility will be seen as a relic in roughly 5 to 7 years.) A new triple aim of *strongly sustainable* business models will encourage organizational design and accounting for financial, social, and environmental well-being, beyond individual care satisfaction. The new community-based clinics are well positioned to design and champion novel business models to lead the sector. They have a historical opportunity to lead health and other service sectors in a moral and social transformation of healthcare service systems as sustainable community-led enterprises.

We know that poorly planned neighborhoods, mediocre education, inadequate public transportation, and unregulated food and water sources all contribute to poor health outcomes in the near and long term. The public centers of health and research have the position and influence to promote community-level health, and can sponsor the alignment toward new value systems for ecological and social capital.

Patient-Centric Design Values

The patient-centered care movement started as a way to relocate the appreciation of the patient from a "case" in the clinic to the central meaning of care. Though perhaps nursing has always been patient-centered, the slow change to patient-centricity across medicine has emerged from strong advocacy, education, and most critically, designing care services in ways that respect the needs of the whole person.

Patient-centered care was succinctly defined by Don Berwick of the Institute for Healthcare Improvement as "the experience (to the extent the informed, individual patient desires it) of transparency, individualization, recognition, respect, dignity, and choice in all matters, without exception, related to one's person, circumstances, and relationships in health care."[8]

How might service designers act on these values? As care services continue to align toward these guidelines as moral anchoring points, we will observe situations in which values conflicts emerge and we may also have to make choices. "Choice in all matters" as a principle affects every touchpoint.

Patient-centered medicine has developed into a meaningful and desirable value system in the 10 years since the publication of the Institute of Medicine's *Crossing the Quality Chasm.*[9] But it is not yet truly mainstream because cultural change is slow, as evidenced by the equivocating commitment to patient-centered care in actual practice. Patient-centered care represents just such a systemic change requiring redesign of processes and socialization of values across nearly every function of institutional care. It involves:

- Inclusion of the cultural traditions of health seekers (patients).

- Personal values and preferences.

- Understanding and accommodating family situations.

- Recognition of personal lifestyles.

- Integration of health seekers and their families, close supporters, and caregivers with healthcare providers in making clinical decisions as an extended care team.

- Respectful, coordinated, efficient transitions between providers, departments, and healthcare settings.

User-centered design improves human interaction with technology, but does not challenge the logic of practice.

No clinician works from "anti-patient values." But values conflicts show up in practice not as fundamental disagreements but as differences in method—in how things get done. Differences between clinicians and administration, doctors and nurses, and one unit and another are a source of conflict when each group has different preferences and priorities. Consistency and routine are maintained for coordination and safety purposes, and values differences are rarely examined. These stakeholders may not share a common values base, even if they serve the same explicit goals.

What are the unique values and roles served by design in co-creating care?

- How could human factors, UX, and service designers develop resources that connect to the culture and values of care and caregiving?

- Can we better contribute to healthcare transformation if design collaboration is treated as a care practice?

- Will design research be respected and included in decisions involving care delivery, based on a shared ethic and accountable contributions?

- Should informatics courses include a service and design track taught by design professors?

- How might we learn to create and design better clinical services as "attending" design professors?

There are *many* ways to express a caring design ethic, yet each discipline views their meaning of care differently. We can create a design practice of care—such a change in values is supportable and authentic. In design, several disciplines contribute to human and social care: inclusive or universal design, human factors design, empathic design, and human-centered design.

These fields share a common technical language of design and evaluation, methodologies, user behavior, and focus on the human use of and interaction with technology and systems. We are missing the recognition of care professionals, a shared language between professionals acknowledging the primacy of human care, and our own realization of a tacit values system now shared by physicians, nurses, and all clinical staff. These are not small gaps.

Care Design and Institutional Change

Organizational change programs, such as movement to patient-centered care, offer an opening for rethinking and redesigning other systems interacting with business processes. Yet when that opening arrives, the methods and experience bases of most designers/researchers may be unprepared for the complexity. Collaborating with domain experts and recruiting cross-functional teams are only starting points. Innovation projects engage larger, diverse groups of possibly disagreeing stakeholders to get to breakthroughs in understanding any complex situation.

Large-Scale Healthcare Innovation

The healthcare system is technically a "mess," the pithy term used by Russell Ackoff to describe entangled, interconnected, wicked problems.[10] Ackoff leveled the term *mess* at healthcare at a conference in 2004:

> Study after study has shown that much of the need for the care that is provided is created by the care that is given; excess surgery, incorrect diagnoses, wrong drugs prescribed or administered, unnecessary tests. The fact is that the so-called health care system can survive only as long as there are people who are sick or disabled. Therefore, whatever the intent of its servers, the system can only assure its survival by creating and preserving illness and disability. We have a self-maintaining sickness- and disability-care system, not a health care system.[11]

The United States and other developed nations face a near-future crisis driven by the following well-known shared concerns:

- *Demographics*: Baby boomers are aging and living longer than any cohort in history.

- *Health needs*: Healthcare service demand is shifting from acute care to chronic and long-term care; at the same time, there is pressure to reduce costs across the system.

- *Economics*: The lack of common payer or universal coverage is forcing more people to use emergency and outpatient services.

- *Industry*: Competition is driving institutions to grow, absorb rivals, and differentiate by investing in new and expensive equipment.

- *Organization*: Healthcare staff face growing stress and work demand, and staff-to-patient ratios are declining.

- *Medicine*: Awareness and interest in patient-centered and family-centered care is increasing, while the number of primary care or family doctors is steadily decreasing.

In a "mess," any isolated issue is connected to many others, all of which are symptoms of deeper causes, which themselves have evolved into new symptoms. Attempts to intervene in one problem (e.g., improving cancer diagnostics) may result in consequences that reinforce the mess (e.g., increasing and expensive false positives). Changing any process (e.g., to improve wait times for patients) without planning for a larger scale may create an exception for that problem that healthcare staff must work around. If clinical and communications processes are not redesigned to lead (not lag) IT deployment, the risk is high that IT vendor solutions—and their process values—will by default design the de facto clinical process.

Designing Inside the System

We are on the cusp of a major trend in systemic design in healthcare, based on the cost and management drivers for system-level change of organizations and practices. In lieu or in spite of national policy innovation, organizations will be forced into fundamental change of business and practice models that many are ill prepared to accomplish. Few consulting design firms and fewer institutions have the experience and method skills to accomplish the sociotechnical analysis, multidisciplinary design, and cross-organizational facilitation for these complex CD3.0 and CD4.0 projects.

A Case for Service Systems Design

Two schools of services design and management have developed recently: the design-led *service design* school and the scientific, whole-system approach of *service systems*.

Service systems science has become a leading methodology for systemic design in large-scale, high-complexity, high-risk service environments. Service systems are "dynamic value co-creation configurations of resources" connected through the fulfillment of value propositions with customers.[12] Service systems fulfill consumer demands and provider requirements, coordinating people, organizations, shared information, and technology in a service-oriented business model. Services are designed as social systems.

Consider a complex service system example. The regional clinic has evolved into a "big box care" business model that is no longer sustainable. It reveals itself in the inflexible (nonreconfigurable) routines imposed by both administration and service areas. It is revealed in the siloed organizational structure that separates services by specialist profit center. In Chapter 6, one root cause of the primary care crisis (too few family physicians for societal demand) was found in an institutional business model that rewarded specialist care and not generalist medicine. In the meantime, increased patient loads in primary care were not mitigated by increasing equitable payments for the volume, leading to inevitable system-level inequities and bottlenecks in basic service. These service problems are consistent with the operating business model of hospitals.

Other cost factors contribute to the whole system. High-technology investments (new scanners, surgical suites, cancer treatment facilities) keep hospitals competitive by promoting their advantages in regional markets. Large medical centers consider such technology investments a preferred pathway to service innovation and a means of building market share. These investments shift costs and development to procedures and medical technology, creating the necessity to gain returns on investment for extremely expensive high-tech purchases.

Taking a systems view, this approach to "buying innovation" reveals a possible values conflict. Capital investments dominate budgeting and squeeze total funding, effectively limiting the capacity to support community-level care.

Systemic root causes are not yet business drivers in the health marketplace. Consider the impact of several causal trends on healthcare delivery: aging demographics, dramatically poorer health of families in poverty, increasing proportion of multiple chronic diseases, increasing population of large urban centers. All institutions are poorly prepared in general for these readily identified trends that will soon be root-cause drivers of future health crises.

A more effective innovation stance in healthcare services recognizes the need for top-down systemic redesign of institutional processes, practice and delivery, and business models. Bottom-up co-creation approaches (and what we normally call design thinking) does not intervene at the institutional scale, but co-creation methods are employed in the design of artifacts. Service redesign requires intentional organizational willpower to surmount the established mindset. Management sponsors and their protection during the research and design stages are essential for the project to survive the exploratory stages and inevitable criticism.

Iterative prototyping is not enough when the risks involve millions of dollars and human lives. Research on defined alternatives is required to build an evidence case for system-level change. To effect system change, a systems approach to research and design is needed. Solutions applicable to entire healthcare systems at the sectoral level can be envisioned by service systems design teams and assessed in iterative research processes (developmental evaluation[13]) or democratic stakeholder methods (dialogic design[14]).

Understanding Problems as Systems

Design and design thinking create artifacts and services that bring a preferred state into being. Designers proactively discover deficiencies and promote creative opportunities in hope of maximizing overall betterment. We are educated and rewarded to solve problems and help people resolve difficulties. But because of this, designers share a single bad habit—the compulsion to solve problems. We resolve those gaps between the way things are and the way things should be. High complexity requires the suspension of this cognitive style and helpful reflex. The combinatorial complexity of interacting social and clinical factors, unforeseen consequences, and emergent outcomes of healthcare require a systems thinking approach.

Every sector of the healthcare industry is riddled with problem systems with interconnected and insoluble situations. Because most designers do not have professional training in health sciences, we risk introducing unforeseeable errors and unexpected outcomes when pursuing conventional problem solving in highly complex interactions. Yet we are discouraged by institutional culture from using unconventional means of inquiry, design research, or generative design. Our clinical clients and users are educated in analytical methods and may have limited patience for discovery and collaborative design. We risk the appearance of "not knowing" in an environment where confident knowing is all important.

A Better Way to Problematize

Problems are "preframed" by members of organizations as they collectively attend to similar gaps and deficiencies. We can assume these problems often represent the *effects* of an unknown cause (e.g., an increase in medication errors) or data reflective of past history (e.g., clinic wait times). When we attempt to solve these "thin problems" as given, we underconceptualize their complexity and set ourselves up to, effectively, fix the symptom. By attempting to rapidly understand and simplify a situation, we are forced to ignore the complexity of systemic causes that may have interacted to produce these effects.

In a complex social system, analysis of its effects (e.g., acting on measures) is a path to slow failure, not resolution. If a problem is wicked, then traditional problem solving just wastes valuable time.

Traditional organizational and project management processes are poorly suited for complexity or innovation. Whenever we organize to fit the established steps of (1) problem definition, (2) analysis, (3) solution (or design), and (4) execution, an analytical deductive process is employed. In clinical situations, the problem definition is often based on a measured deficiency (e.g., emergency wait times) or a high-profile recognized need (e.g., EMRs). These are well-known shared processes for organizational action.

Systems thinking addresses the rationalizing bias as the central cause of problematic outcomes we attempt to address. In some sense, the ultimate root causes of individual, service, and organizational problems in healthcare are our own thinking processes and an unreflective reliance on scientific method.

A problem in clinical and scientific research is the reliance on a single epistemology, when multiple modes may be necessary to understand perspectives, dynamics, and consequences. Systems scientist West Churchman advanced a general theory of systems inquiry, being the process by which human knowledge is produced (e.g., research and design).[15] Churchman mapped five eras of epistemology, or ways of knowing, and identified their modes of inquiry. Each frame has a signature philosophy and method, and each is legitimized—"guaranteed"—by a different type of evidence (Table 8.2).

TABLE 8.2 CHURCHMAN'S SYSTEMS INQUIRY

System of inquiry	Guaranteed by	Healthcare examples
Empirical, inductive	Consensus	Social proof (e.g., checklist practices)
Rational, analytic-deductive	Logical consistency	Evidence-based medicine
Idealism, multiple realities	Range of perspectives	Patient-centered care
Dialectic	Conflict	Policy making
Pragmatic, systems inquiry	Progress	Service design, iterative practice

Conventionally, these modes are in conflict, as different people in different settings disagree on what counts as legitimate evidence. A systems context considers them complementary methods for reasoning and research. Design thinking has no similar concept, but the Churchman modes might serve to integrate systems and design. For example, ethnographic research is based on inductive empirical observation, and its evidence and methods are misunderstood by those who require "hard" or quantitative evidence from experimental traditions or deductive hypotheses. In law, multiple realities are contested by the adversarial dialectic used to force a jury to a single claim on reality. Design research iterates over multiple observations and makes abductive connections between each sweep of the data.

The methods for "progress" require creative reasoning and mixed-methods research. In social sciences, methods are "triangulated" (combined) with complementary research to develop a stronger set of findings than produced by a single method. In a systems inquiry, methods are iterated progressively, allowing observers to learn from each session and review questions, methods, and participants as necessary. A progressive systems inquiry enables a research or design team to identify multiple, possibly conflicting causes and relationships in a problem, ensuring that the right problem and the best level of its complexity are pursued by the team's limited resources.

Mapping Complexity in a Problem System

We can identify many sources of complexity in services and systems design. The most complex service problems are not those with inherently difficult *content*. Difficult clinical problems may have constraints that only allow certain approaches, and they can be treated as puzzles with a known best answer based on current evidence. Problems turn wicked when they live in the social realm. Stakeholders have varying goals and perspectives, incomplete knowledge, and insufficient collective understanding of the problem space.

Achieving consensus on socially complex problems requires we reach an understanding before attempting to design solutions. For multi-organizational and multistakeholder situations, that understanding should be *co-constructed*. Stakeholder management is a design problem, not an expert issue.

In such a case, we can choose generative design approaches and deliberative, structured design approaches. In high-reliability sociotechnical systems, using a generative design (co-creation) approach can significantly underconceptualize the problem, thereby coming up with interesting but essentially unworkable design concepts. The aesthetics of co-creative design workshops may not be congruent with the seriousness of the given problem in a medical environment. A range of appropriate design methods may be needed.

Strategic and structured dialogues provide a deliberative social design approach for complex services in serious domains such as medical procedure, practice organization, and service reconfiguration. Methods known as dialogic design provide a rigorous and engaging approach to elicit collective wisdom and collaborate on strategic solutions. In dialogic design, stakeholders are facilitated in group work to dive deeply into a shared inquiry, identify factors and systemic relationships, and then choose priorities and the best leverage among priorities.

Dialogic design produces a collaborative map of the problem system, or *problematique*, a systems model that reveals interdependent relationships in a diversity of perspectives. All of the viewpoints and priorities expressed in an inquiry can be considered and consensus reached.

The methodology has a deep history going back nearly 50 years. Wharton's systems scientist Hasan Özbekhan developed the problematique as a framework for assessing relationships between overlapping and co-evolving problems. Özbekhan criticized conventional problem-solving approaches as antisystemic and ignorant of the cognitive basis of complexity: "We proceed from the belief that problems have 'solutions'—although we may not necessarily discover these in the case of every problem we encounter. This peculiarity of our perception causes us to view difficulties as things that are clearly defined and discrete in themselves."[16]

A problem system is mapped to reveal challenges and potentially high-leverage solution pathways in a map of problems structured by their mutual influence relationships. A published case study from the Chronic Kidney Disease Initiative sponsored by the American Society of Nephrology illustrates their problematique for the complex set of factors involved in chronic disease management (Figure 8.2).[17] A workshop of 48 stakeholders representing 38 organizations engaged in structured dialogue to reach consensus on the problematique, using the Structured Dialogic Design (SDD) method (see the Methods section on page 288).

The SDD workshop facilitated consensus across a range of issues facing the 38 constituencies (of which only the consensus is shown in the problematique). The influence map is employed in strategic planning and group decision making, as it shows the agreement on foundational issues (at the bottom of the map) that influence all other issues (following the influence indicated by the arrows).

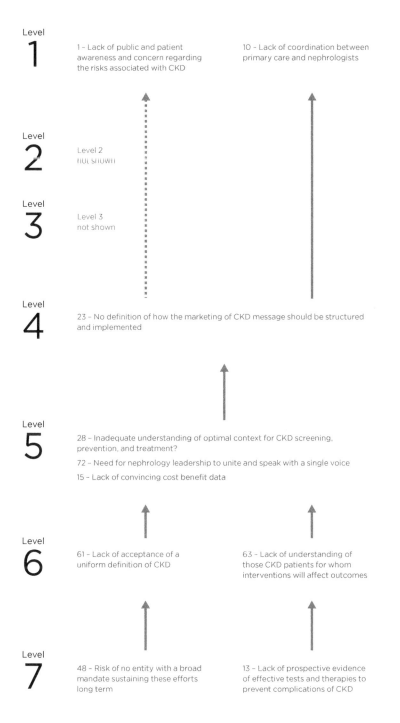

Level 1

1 – Lack of public and patient awareness and concern regarding the risks associated with CKD

10 – Lack of coordination between primary care and nephrologists

Level 2

Level 2 not shown

Level 3

Level 3 not shown

Level 4

23 – No definition of how the marketing of CKD message should be structured and implemented

Level 5

28 – Inadequate understanding of optimal context for CKD screening, prevention, and treatment?

72 – Need for nephrology leadership to unite and speak with a single voice

15 – Lack of convincing cost benefit data

Level 6

61 – Lack of acceptance of a uniform definition of CKD

63 – Lack of understanding of those CKD patients for whom interventions will affect outcomes

Level 7

48 – Risk of no entity with a broad mandate sustaining these efforts long term

13 – Lack of prospective evidence of effective tests and therapies to prevent complications of CKD

FIGURE 8.2

Partial problematique for the Chronic Kidney Disease Initiative.

As an action research and planning approach, SDD leads to organizational commitments to highly influential "root cause" actions. The map supports the resolution of issues with the most reach or leverage across the system. The goals of the Chronic Kidney Disease Initiative are common across healthcare:

- To understand the anticipated barriers that stakeholders will face in improving patient outcomes

- To build commitment to an action agenda to address these barriers systemically

- To forge a chain of partnerships that embrace the variety of stakeholders in implementing the agenda for improving patient outcomes

Stakeholders in the nephrology community generated the map in Figure 8.2 as one of several representations of dialogue constructed throughout the session. Participants engaged in a moderated workshop process that elicited individual responses to a framing question about barriers to action (problems). These "barriers" were transformed in several group language processes, using software (CogniScope II) to vote between issues to co-create this influence map. In this structuring of dialogue, root-level issues emerge in a consensus process and are recognized as those with the highest leverage to produce change in the system.

Issues at the top (level 1) represent the "most influenced" problems and are the visible effects. Barriers shown at the bottom (level 7) are the most causative or influential. The bottom two levels (6 and 7) tell us that (a) no group had a mandate to sustain efforts to improve patient outcomes, and groups acting independently would be unable to make progress; thus *a systematic solution was necessary*; and (b) *physicians had no consensus on evidence* for the relative effectiveness of therapies.

Some of the original factors were removed to better enhance the readability of the map. In the original, a single *unconnected* level I issue indicated the pervasive "worsening shortage of health care providers" as a major problematic effect. This is the same system-level issue known as the "primary care crisis." It was disconnected because it was an independent outcome, and was not reinforced or influenced by any other problem in the map. It becomes a deep driver for the action plan, regardless of the chosen strategy.

The strategic planning outcomes were reported in a society journal to generate commitment across the specialty toward the initiative. Solutions were formulated in a second SDD workshop that mapped strategic design options—solutions to the "barriers" identified in the problematique.

System-Level Innovation

The chronic kidney disease case suggests the difficulty of effecting change at an institutional scale across organizations. In this model, clinicians (or any stakeholders) associated with organizations, regions, and subspecialties organize to accomplish agendas they have developed and socialized within their networks. Significant planning and a common determination are required to bring players to such a design and planning context. Yet when the system boundary is expanded beyond the organization, domain, or discipline—to achieve higher variety and broader impact—the difficulty of coordinating action increases.

Complexity increases when considering other chronic diseases that co-occur with kidney disease. If Type 2 diabetes and cardiovascular disease were included in the problem system (as occurs in the health seeker's contexts), the root cause and barriers would expand beyond the specialist scenario.

The formation of mass opinion for a defined position has been necessary to motivate institutional change in the United States and Canada for the entire history of state-supported healthcare. Consensus building among competing stakeholders is a vital process necessary for changing business models and decision making at the systems level.

Today the enormous health sector has more in common with government and policy innovation than with business innovation. Simply implementing business-led innovation practices will not create a collaborative or innovative culture and has failed in institutional settings. The institutional values (of care) conflict with business (financial value) at a fundamental level. Design-led practices lend both cultures effective skills and means—D3.0 adapts well to organization and business contexts, and D4.0 methods to institutional and community contexts.

Changing System Behaviors

Systems thinking historically divides roughly into two major schools of thought: soft systems and hard systems methodologies. Soft systems includes social systems and dialogic design, and stakeholder-led processes. Soft systems have evolved from interpretive approaches, viewing social behaviors and purposive systems as outcomes of human agreement. Social systems may reflect actual organizations, but the systems are viewed as sociotechnical, cognitive, or languaging constructions.

Alternatively, hard systems are presented as engineering processes, with inputs, conditions, and feedback loops. Hard systems include system dynamics and cybernetics, including modeling and simulation—methods based on natural sciences and observable measures employed in information systems and living and ecological systems. Most hard systems methods define a clear system boundary and consider a system to be a real thing, an observable set of co-occurring behaviors "out there" in the world.

Both schools position the designer as leading "interventions" within a system as defined. For any type of system, an intervention is an action that disrupts system functions to enable a preferred shift of performance and behavior. The design role is to identify the range of options and choose the type of action, precise point of application, and timing of action or policy that creates a sustainable effect.

Systemic design as *intervention* is well accepted in the systems sciences. Perhaps the best formulation of leverage concepts is found in "Leverage Points: Places to Intervene in a System" by the late systems thinker Donella Meadows.[18] Her "12 ways to change a system" still stands as an actionable and testable proposal for systems thinking approaches (Table 8.3). Their leverage is high because, if applied at the right point (and time) of force, the power of a single idea could reform an entire global system. However, these are the very ideas filtered and ignored by those maintaining the paradigm.

For example, John Thackara, a systemic designer who is not a physician, suggested that healthcare practice could become more like the system in Cuba, where 95% of the population is treated initially by family physicians located within neighborhoods.[19] Care in Cuba and the United States is very different, as are socioeconomic conditions and resulting lifestyle diseases. Yet a distributed, low-intensity family care model has promise for rural and remote communities as well as large cities with dense neighborhoods. Today's healthcare planning might screen out such proposals as infeasible or alien; yet such proposals may apply as well in developed countries.

Remarkably, Meadows' formulation harmonizes across systems methods and removes some causes for disagreement. Hard systems modelers are able to identify leverage in their models and changing values, delays, flow rates, and so on. Social systems designers tend to focus on leverages 1–5, but have a meaningful checklist to map stakeholder ideas to their potential impact. This is a general, more functional approach to leverage than the barriers shown in the influence map (see Figure 8.2). The deepest barriers to patient outcomes in kidney disease were fundamental definitions and agreements that had leverage on everything else in the system. When determining solutions to those same barriers in the design stage, the understanding of leverage points would be very helpful indeed.

TABLE 8.3 LEVERAGE POINTS IN A SYSTEM

1.	The power to transcend paradigms (e.g., patient-centered or evidence-based medicine)
2.	The mindset or paradigm out of which the system—its goals, structure, rules, delays—arises
3.	The goals of the system (e.g., efficient medical care or healthy communities)
4.	The power to add, change, evolve, or self-organize system structure (e.g., healthcare design roles)
5.	The rules of the system (e.g., incentives, constraints)
6.	The structure of information flows (who does and does not have access to information)
7.	The gain around driving positive feedback loops (e.g., reinforcing hand-washing practices)
8.	The strength of negative feedback loops, relative to the impacts they are trying to correct against
9.	The length of delays, relative to the rate of system change
10.	The structure of material stocks and flows (e.g., transport networks, population, age)
11.	Constants, parameters, numbers (e.g., taxes, subsidies, standards)
12.	Sizes of buffers and other stabilizing stocks relative to their flows (critical to concepts such as wait times for procedures or stocks of hospital beds)

System Dynamics as Design Thinking

System dynamics encompasses a robust quantitative methodology for measuring the functions of a complex system and modeling their throughput and interactions. It is a popular approach in systems engineering, but not in design practice. However, key ideas in system dynamics can support design thinking and visual understanding of complex system behaviors In healthcare services, care management, and policy outcomes, it helps to understand and illustrate patterns following the well-known language of system dynamics.

MIT's Jay Forrester developed the system dynamics modeling approach as a way to formulate better decisions through prospective evidence for large-scale industrial and policy planning.[20] Adapting the comprehensive WORLD model, Forrester identified ranges and assumptions to model behaviors of global population, industrial growth, energy consumption, food supply, and other trends. The simulation resulted in scenarios of unsustainable growth and resource collapse that were published in the best seller *The Limits to Growth*.[21] When those scenarios failed to appear within a few short years, the exercise was debunked by business and growth advocates. Rejecting the move toward global stewardship, this sparked the unforeseen and unintended consequence of a generational culture shift toward consumption and away from precaution with respect to energy, environment, and global industrialization.

System dynamics has contributed prominently to healthcare research and to process design in hospital process and wait time studies. However, it remains unclear where systems thinking contributes to service or interaction design problems. For surprisingly complex design problems—for example, achieving adoption of hand-washing routines to reduce iatrogenic infections—we can plot expected behaviors against observed current states to elicit patterns to be mitigated.

Systems have a purpose. Systemic behaviors repeat their operational functions on inputs to produce defined outputs. In so doing, they seek *homeostasis* (called "equilibrium" in mechanical systems). In social systems such as healthcare, homeostasis regulates a process to ensure that the human purposes of the system are met.

Human purposes have explicit goals (to provide health services) and implicit or tacit goals (to maximize profit from the payment system). The hidden goals are often the most powerful in systemic design problems because they are the source of the deficiencies we are trying to correct. They are especially powerful because we often cannot identify or discuss them directly.

First, consider the critical behaviors selected from a defined problem of interest. The functions are primarily based on *stocks* (measured supply of a material or state) and *flows* (inputs, outputs, exchange, and behavior). Often a simple stock-and-flow diagram is sketched to identify the basic mechanics of system operation. System dynamics excels at representing the forces of positive and negative feedback on system constituents.

Figure 8.3 shows a causal loop diagram, the signature visual representation of a system dynamics analysis. It is a sketch of the relationships between system components and their patterns of feedback. Causal loop sketches are portrayed by identifying commonly recurring problem patterns among the selected components to illustrate the dynamics of a complex situation.

A positive, or reinforcing, feedback loop is drawn as a curved line with a plus sign (+). It amplifies the flow associated with the arrow, or increases the gain in the component. It is not always an increasing (or "positive") direction, as positive feedback loops can equally increase a destructive effect.

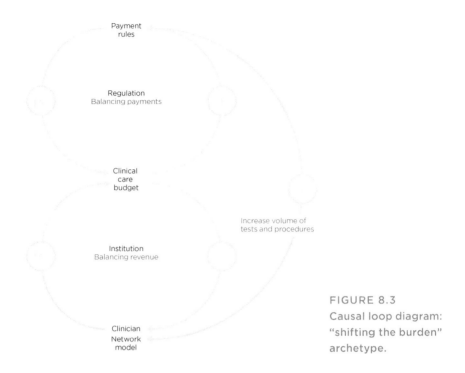

Payment
rules

Regulation
Balancing payments

Clinical
care
budget

Increase volume of
tests and procedures

Institution
Balancing revenue

Clinician
Network
model

FIGURE 8.3
Causal loop diagram:
"shifting the burden"
archetype.

Negative feedback is shown as a balancing (B) loop and regulates the rela-tionship between two things. A car's cruise control is a classic negative feedback loop—it uses a continuous balancing loop to regulate power to maintain the desired speed setting.

The diagram represents a common system *archetype* called "shifting the bur-den." Archetypes are recurring systemic patterns, the knowledge of which enables systems designers to quickly recognize dysfunctional patterns in a system. This pattern illustrates how physicians bypass the regulatory intent of managed procedure costs by increasing the number of related procedures as a workaround that maintains the expected income. Also called "over-treatment," this function can be seen to have a systemic cause that has more to do with practice management than ethics.

Two balancing loops (associated with "regulation" and "institution") each have a positive and negative loop, joined at "clinical care budget" (where the symptom appears). A third reinforcing (+) loop bypasses the *symptomatic solution* (payment rules) to shift the *fundamental solution* (managing physi-cian revenue). This reveals the unintended consequence of regulation aimed at reducing healthcare costs across the system.

The "shifting the burden" archetype illustrates the problem with setting rational incentives as policy targets and expecting outcomes to match. *Incentives* have been identified as a recurring problem dynamic at the institutional level of healthcare, and like other "rules of the system," are potent interventions. The trap of "perverse incentives" occurs when the unintended consequences of a defined incentive results in behavior precisely contrary to the intent of the incentive.

Another archetype called "success to the successful" is evident in the imbalance between primary and specialty care at the healthcare system level. A differential allocation of resources is positively reinforced for the "winner" and continues to draw from the "loser" (primary care). The United States spends roughly 5 times on physicians as its peers, such as Japan and the United Kingdom, which show equally good clinical outcomes and life expectancy. One analysis shows that the most significant driver is the much higher costs of specialists.[22] Higher fees in the United States are driven largely by higher rates paid per procedure, and a larger proportion of higher-paying private (insurance) payers.

This is another design problem. The "success to successful" archetype is reinforced by the supply of residents in specialty medicine. The existing imbalance of specialists in US healthcare leads to poorly designed policy and distorted incentives. Society needs more primary care doctors, but there are no financial incentives to draw medical students toward this choice. Because subspecialists can outearn primary care providers on an immediate and lifelong basis, even idealistic medical students will choose the higher-paying career paths. Design at the level of policy could certainly help, by creating financial offsets for primary care, for example, or subsidizing school loans if residents choose to go into primary care. But the most difficult function in design is seeing execution through to making those decisions.

Reframing Design and Systems Methods

How does systems thinking help the designer in everyday practice? How can systems thinking be integrated with design thinking for improving health-care services? Design and systems thinking are not integrated disciplines, despite many mashup attempts. They approach problem definition and problem solving in almost incompatible ways.

Systems thinking was developed over half a century of research, from systems theory, and applies scientific principles to social practices (healthcare services) and engineering problems (medical device design). The systems perspective is both holistic and analytical—by discovering whole-system behaviors and outcomes, human-centered design can be targeted to the sources of those effects.

This process is easier said than done—systemic design requires time *up front* to conduct the research, to unearth discoveries, or to organize stakeholders in the design process. Design projects are usually launched to target critical business cases, which may not even have an allocated research budget. Designers have to make the case for an integrated systems/design/research approach. Clinicians and clients need to be convinced on each case's basis.

Designers have their own barriers to the process. We do not pitch or perform methods we do not understand. Systems methods may appear too structured to be considered "creative" practices and may even appear to inhibit the possibilities for design ideation. Improvisational design practices (design thinking techniques such as brainstorming or affinity mapping) are preferred by designers to structured systemic processes because of their agility—their ability to produce rapid results that are sufficient to the problem (as framed). The learning and planning costs are much higher for systems methods, and if their execution does not yield outstanding results, second chances may be harder to win.

Design thinking changes the game board when the rules of play cannot be touched. We can skip over the necessity to fully analyze problem structure and behavior by envisioning a different frame and outcome than the situation as given. In classical terms, this is called "reframing the brief." Design researchers Bec Paton and Kees Dorst have shown how designers modify and negotiate the framing of design briefs.[23] They describe an abductive reasoning process to identify new metaphors and a "better problem" to resolve than the issue as given. Although this process risks possible avoidance of the complex set of problems a healthcare client may present, the systemic inquiry process (which they term a "journey") reduces the risk of expending resources solving symptoms and bringing superficial relief.

The reframing process is driven by three steps:

1. *Use of metaphor and analogy*: reframing by adopting visual abstractions to rethink a situation

2. *Contextual engagement*: inquiry with problem owners to deeply appreciate the context

3. *Conjecture*: co-creating new ideas as "what if" scenarios

And reframing is inhibited by three barriers:

1. *Cognitive fixation*: following the "garden path" of predetermined projects and ideas

2. *A problem-solving mental model of design*: attempting to fix a deficiency as stated

3. *Resistance to the journey*: unwillingness to explore variations over time

A team's initial understanding of a concern or a "fuzzy situation" is always insufficient and is often biased by precedents, groupthink, or prior work. Design and health cultures are biased toward action and outcomes, and dialogue (inquiry) is discouraged when schedules are compressed and stakeholders hold an expectation of professionalism. We need good techniques to deftly slow the rush to action and sustain an inquiry.

The Third Thinking

Healthcare problems are known to be complex. They demand a combination of systemic and human-centered design methods. Yet in health practice (and in consumer sectors) wearing two thinking hats is not enough—we need a third hat of domain knowledge. A care service orientation requires thinking like a care professional, one with a holistic view of patients and their communities, healthcare practices, technology, and policy.

The designer role, while still a creative activity, leads by facilitation and co-creation with stakeholders in designing care service. They convene and lead circles of stakeholders, designers, care providers, and patients to collectively gain and visualize a deep understanding of complex issues.

The structure, organizational collaboration, and evidence are precisely why these methods are effective in healthcare. Organizational project management is not the best approach for wicked problems. We often have a single chance to plan or propose a new project, and winning proposals have to account for a complex range of decision holders. Internal stakeholders may include clinical services, administrators, business and finance, and marketing. External stakeholders can involve community advocacy groups, policy makers, regulators, corporate partners, and other community members and organizations. Not to mention the patients!

This level of complexity becomes unworkable with innovation practices that rely on the creative emergence of ideation. These stakeholders represent significant positions and histories in their communities, and they do not share common goals or outcomes. Collaborative governance and decision processes are not facilitated by creative brainstorming. Social systems design methods discussed in this chapter (such as SDD), and the Positive Deviance and Simplexity methods described in Chapter 6, have been integrated with design practices and rest on formidable bases of evidence. For high-risk, multistakeholder complexity, these industrial-strength methods can be engaged, at least within a spectrum of practices.

- Systemic design integrates services and IT systems to the entire organization and its ecosystem. Systemic design achieves design goals through D3.0 practices (within the organization) and across institutions and health ecosystems or within communities (D4.0).

- A primary goal of systemic design is to gain collective understanding about a problem system and to discover effective interventions based on shared wisdom. Design methods are used to create artifacts that bring scenarios, options, and leverage points to life within abstract system and behavioral models.

- Systemic design requires multiple sketches or views be made of the whole system. Methods of system mapping and life-cycle workflows visualize the processes, boundaries, and systemic relationships among actors and other systems.

- Experience and systemic design are complementary to each other. Systemic design maps services and IT interactions for a given area. Experience design maps the individual health-seeker life cycle to services and systems.

- A clinical service system is concerned with fulfilling care, the outcome of service. The design of processes and procedures are reconfigured to achieve human system goals.

- An organization's business model reflects its values and operational principles. The business model is a top-down process model that can be redesigned for new collective goals. A sustainable business model can be designed to produce value in the clinic and the community as an integrated service system.

- Service systems touch a large number of stakeholders and require multiple socially oriented design methods such as moderated group processes and design workshops. These methods may be novel to stakeholders, and organizations should engage skilled design support when first learning and using these methods.

- Systems and design thinking methods are enhanced by consciously framing and reframing the problem as given or stated. Reframing is itself a design process and is improved by collaboration, sketching, and critiquing ideas.

Case Study: Mayo Mom
Community Health Service

The following case was a proposal illustrating the direction of integrated service design. It offers a model for service innovation based on a deep appreciation of long-term business goals, health values, and community needs, and the systemic drivers that link these.

A team from OCAD University's Strategic Foresight and Innovation program won the 2011 Rotman Design Challenge with a unique service design proposal to facilitate children's health.[24] Sponsored by the Mayo Clinic's Center for Innovation, the concept employs an online social network to connect new and experienced mothers in both live and online communities.

The Mayo Mom concept leverages the understanding of deep drivers in a social system and enables motivators for learning and behavior change. Mayo Mom is designed to facilitate breastfeeding, one of the earliest life determinants of future health, and therefore a powerful preventive health practice. The US Surgeon General's 2011 Call to Action to Support Breast-feeding provided framing and impetus.[25] Breastfeeding is correlated with fewer infections and diseases, such as pneumonia, asthma, diabetes, and obesity. The United States has one of the lowest rates of breastfeeding of any country in the developed world (only 13% of children are exclusively breast-fed for the first 6 months). If 90% of US babies were breastfed for their first 6 months, more than $13 billion per year could be saved in healthcare costs.

Mayo Mom helps new mothers adapt to the experience of breastfeeding as a pathway to preventive health for mother and child. It demonstrates how simple design methods, even in prototype form, can inspire the development of critical social system changes that improve health. By taking a systems view of the breastfeeding experience, it was possible to look outside the traditional boundaries of the healthcare system to design an intervention that could improve a first-time mother's experience when it matters most. Helping to shift the perceived problem around breastfeeding from one of education and access to one of social and cultural breakdown, the design team ultimately reframed the role of the targeted service provider, the Mayo Clinic, to a facili-tator of community health, rather than just a provider of care.

Preventive Health as a Service System

Preventive health is a classic wicked problem, as the right actions must be taken and ineffective actions not only waste time but allow a health problem to evolve further without a response. Preventing a disease from occurring later is "counterfactual" and impossible to measure within a person when it does not occur. (Prevention is measured across population samples.) Community-level prevention programs usually focus on social determinants (such as housing and education) and root causes (such as early childhood diet in obesity), while advising at-risk individuals when they show up in primary care. The results of investment in root causes may not register for years, and programs must maintain a consistent campaign for years to collect longitudinal data.

What unique contributions can service innovation make to the prevention of multiple diseases across a population? How does a healthcare design team decide the best level of investment for the fuzzy return?

The immediate and long-term benefits of breastfeeding are well documented, and the opportunity for Mayo was identified to help new mothers by establishing a distributed community of care. The design team started from a set of design principles to effectively design for prevention:

1. Be human-centered.

2. Intervene in key moments of wellness.

3. Be focused, simple, and decentralized.

4. Create personalized knowledge, not information.

5. Start early (really early).

The service design team followed a design research strategy portrayed in Figure 8.4, adopting an exploratory approach (diverge) to formulate the right problem framing, and then using focusing methods (converge) to design for the best alternative solution. They engaged mothers and childcare experts in interviews on the experience of breastfeeding, exploring the root causes and sociocultural constraints that inhibit mothers from reaching that 6-month mark. Critical to the design process was the search for a "key moment of

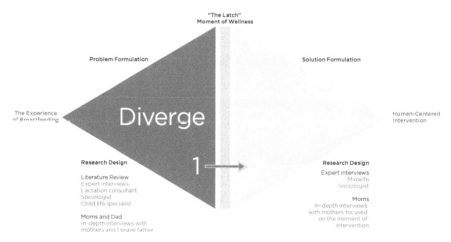

FIGURE 8.4

Service design research plan for Mayo Mom.

wellness." Without finding a specific moment grounded in time, space, and deep emotional need, a systems intervention can remain too abstract, losing critical focus and sensitivity to its context.

The initial "divergent" phase of the research process concluded in the identification of a specific moment called "the latch"—the critical period during a new mother's breastfeeding experience in which she tries to establish her first connection with her baby. Success in this moment had a significant effect on a mother's relationship with breastfeeding. This discovery gave designers clarity about where to "converge" and focus efforts to design a service system capable of improving her chances of success.

The research uncovered that US society's aversion to the topic of breastfeeding creates a climate in which the deep physical and emotional challenges of achieving a good latch are not openly discussed, even among family and friends. Instead, a myth is perpetuated whereby new mothers are led to believe that a good latch will "come naturally." Without disbanding this myth, the almost inevitable struggle of achieving a good latch can cause an otherwise confident and stable mother to doubt her own body, and even her ability to care for her child. Although not the only cause, this emotional turmoil creates enough personal doubt and feelings of failure to play a prominent role in a mother's decision to turn to formula prematurely. This emotional experience remains pervasive among first-time mothers, despite the current healthcare support systems and educational programs in place, suggesting that because it is primarily a social problem, its resolution is beyond the scope of the existing healthcare system.

Designing a Sensitive System

Mayo Mom was designed to complement existing breastfeeding services by leveraging one of the most abundant resources across local communities: the wisdom of experienced mothers. The Mayo Mom concept is based on an accessible online network that connects experienced Mayo-certified mothers in the network with first-time mothers who hear of the program during their prenatal care. The network facilitates personalized and emotionally supportive one-to-one relationships during the stressful time leading up to and during breastfeeding, focusing mainly on the month before and the month after birth.

Mothers who volunteer for the program complete a simple online certification module before they are entered into the service's database and matched with a new mother in the online network. An essential component of the service system design, the certification enables new mothers to trust their Mayo Mom and builds a community of practice between Mayo Clinic and the certified advisors.

Before birth, the Mayo Mom relationship helps prepare new mothers for the emotional and physical challenges of breastfeeding. After birth, the experienced mother is there to offer socially unconstrained (potentially anonymous) emotional support and positive reinforcement as the new mother seeks to create a good latch. Mayo Mom reframes the Mayo Clinic's role from that of a primary provider of care to a key facilitator of the network and a beacon of credibility for the service. Mayo Mom shows the possibility of care services that extend the clinic into the community. After all, most illness and wellness experiences occur outside the walls of the traditional healthcare system, and this is where many solutions are to be found.

LESSONS LEARNED

- Health value is realized in the ability of people to participate in their work and communities. New sources of value for clinical institutions will be found in the regional community of health seekers and their caregivers.

- Most everyday health needs are localized in people's homes and communities. For clinical service lines to expand their reach into the community, they will need to coordinate both social networks and place-based human networks.

- Creative approaches to new health services will be discovered in response to both declared needs and small-scale prototyping. First Lady Michelle Obama's concern for breastfeeding brought social attention to an overlooked issue, creating an opportunity for a new service that might otherwise falter. On the other hand, such a novel service would require the safety net of multiple iterations of design and testing before its public announcement.

- Unhealthy circumstances reinforce disease processes that might originate from a person's network. Healthy communities support restoration of individual health. Design for communities considers home conditions, friends and family circles, autonomy and mobility, neighborhood safety, and food supply.

Design Methods for Systems Innovation

Most healthcare service design projects embrace common goals—to improve the delivery of healthcare, sustainably maximize the value of available resources, and enhance the health-seeking experience for people. At the system level, different measures of effectiveness are needed beyond usability and patient experience satisfaction. The customer defines the quality of a user-centered approach. Stakeholder satisfaction in a complex service system accounts for quality, staff performance, process, and of course, health outcomes.

Services are designed to fulfill customer value over a cycle from request to fulfillment, a series defined in a service journey. A service journey involves a series of products or communications delivered at each touchpoint or engagement. Incremental products are delivered over time to customers or subscribers, with a user-centered design focus on touchpoints. The atrial fibrillation (AF) case in Chapter 5 contrasts the design for service level (AF communications) and system level (practice redesign for chronic AF patients).

Both service design and service systems methods bring real value to healthcare design, but they have different purposes and outcomes. Selection criteria for the right methods are not yet well defined. For service design practices, the practical research and design methods are based on experience from fields with a well-defined customer and setting (as in retail). There is a need for relevant service theory that indicates when and how to select methods from one context to apply in another.

As the health sector has become heavily invested in during the last decade, a highly competitive environment has resulted. Therefore we have insufficient sharing of project experience for effective comparison of methods, as many providers prohibit sharing of their work and practices.

The D1.0–4.0 geographies are one set of criteria for method selection based on complexity and scale. The association of design methods with *research goals* is another. Design and system research methods can be mapped to their purposes in a simple framework (originally proposed for selecting information research methods[26]). Figure 8.5 maps the types of design research methods for service and social design based on four primary (non-overlapping) purposes or research goals.

When planning service systems, several phases of research and design are typical. Each phase may have a different purpose, initially to *understand* activity and the environment (phase 1), to *design* and prototype options (phase 2), and then later to design for system *change* (phase 3).

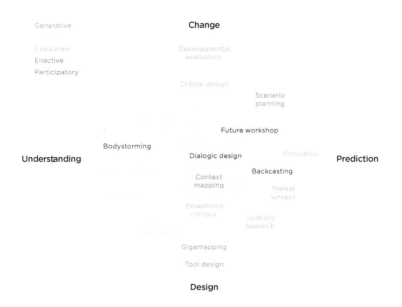

FIGURE 8.5
Design research methods by purpose.

Research methods are rarely conducted once just for a single phase—they are repeated to build a deeper base of knowledge applicable to each purpose. In UX projects, research does not always progress from understanding to change. Pure *understanding* methods such as sensemaking and empathic design research are often employed early in a project to construct a shared model of human social behavior.

Ethnography is a primary method for understanding, yet is relevant for all research purposes in a service systems context. Ethnographic field research provides some predictive capacity for cultural trends, often with a further intention to create change (design or social action) based on understanding. On the *prediction* side, market surveys as well as expert analyses (task analysis and usability research) and foresight enable analytical assessment and some degree of prediction based on qualitative or mixed data.

Change research purposes are system-level. Dialogic design and social participatory methods connect a bridge of action from understanding to change. Research for service systems requires both system and user understanding, and connecting those insights to design and organizational change. *Design*-oriented methods specialize in defining artifacts or services, not primarily the goals of change.

Service design at the system level requires a holistic understanding of organizational goals, management and caregiving capacities, and patient/community touchpoints. Nearly all new services in healthcare are necessary for managing the increasing complexity of (mixed morbidity) patient conditions, changing demographics, and institutional pressures for cost reduction and IT and service integration. UX-only methods, such as ethnography, surveys, and prototyping, are too user-focused. Design of complex services should be guided from the beginning with multistakeholder change planning and process/service design.

Dialogue as Participatory Design

Participatory methods are foundation methods for complex social systems. Designers have limited medical expertise, and most services cut across organizational lines, so a cooperative design approach draws from across service lines and management levels. We cannot work alone—even small efficient study teams can generate idealized models that can ignore or hide reality. We need participatory cycles built in to the process.

Design practitioners have adapted participatory workshops into the entire spectrum of design projects, from ideation through design to delivery. We must meet to make meaning together. Participatory design requires deep transdisciplinary communication, written and pictorial expression, and argumentation.

Workshop methods focus group attention on co-creation for a defined shared outcome, requiring planned facilitation. This trend has inspired facilitated design based on convening nondirective ideation (Open Space, World Café) and more structured facilitated methods such as Appreciative Inquiry. Organizations are increasingly adopting participatory and co-creative practices in their innovation life cycles, involving stakeholders directly in the design of their services. Methodologies for co-creation for complex systems are necessary, beyond the capabilities of open generative approaches.

Figure 8.6 shows dialogic methods across the range of systemic design applications, by structure and scale. These range from open and generative (brainstorming and its variations) to structured and democratic.

Appropriate methods are selected by identifying required outcomes and the appropriate stage of engagement and style for the stakeholders and context. Different design outputs are created with each of these methods, and though they can be joined in sequences, the relationship of one method's outputs to the inputs of another is largely understood by practitioner experience. Several of these methods are commonly adapted together to accomplish stakeholder design.

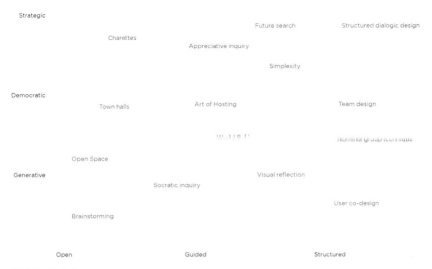

FIGURE 8.6
Mapping dialogic practices in design.

Each method in the map follows a different process, but a common design language can be drawn from their process logic. The design language of divergence > emergence > convergence (see Figure 6.7) expresses a fundamental sequence of social design process found in Appreciative Inquiry, SDD, and Simplexity.

Generative methods (e.g., brainstorming, visual reflection) tend to be wholly divergent. Simple dot voting helps groups "rapidly converge," but group voting elicits well-known errors and biases that result in suboptimal decision making. The first bias is thinking that generative divergence is sufficient to develop the field of options for selection; a related error is insufficient understanding of the options for selection; finally, simple multivoting leads to people selecting desired outcomes as their priorities, which always result or emerge from deeper systemic causes. Reaching agreement on outcomes (such as cost reduction) is antisystemic. System solutions are located in the highly leveraged actions that relate intended actions to each other to yield those outcomes. Those ideas are usually not big vote-getters (a principle known as the erroneous priorities effect).

Dialogic Design

Dialogic design deals with the problem of sociotechnical complexity increasing beyond the capacity of experts and management. Rapid progress can be made when stakeholders can visualize their understanding of the relationships among shared concerns and solutions.

Dialogic design was structurally formed to require the democratic inclusion of the requisite variety of diverse stakeholders for both ethical and design reasons. It is a true dialogue process. Dialogue is viewed as a multistakeholder inquiry by systems thinkers, a method of group research inquiry or designing.

Unlike common facilitated methods such as Open Space (as used in "bar camp" and unconferences), World Café, or idea brainstorming, dialogic design directly enables the following:

- Large-group democratic decision making
- Policy design and decision conferences
- Complex (wicked) problem solving
- Complex business service design and business planning
- Strategic and long-horizon collaborative planning
- Portfolio allocation and business strategy
- Problem identification and root cause analysis

We can never achieve complete understanding of a complex domain. We can use democratic, well-structured dialogue to maximize the wisdom of individual observations toward a more complete understanding.

Structured Dialogic Design

Dialogic design was formulated to enable stakeholder groups to resolve communication and decision issues common in organizational and innovation management. Its primary method, SDD, is a collaborative design methodology composed of multiple techniques that are "structured" following defined language patterns to facilitate effective group planning, design, and decision making. SDD is usually coordinated as a workshop with associated group decision software (for mapping and voting), but its essential methods can be facilitated as entirely manual processes.

Dialogic design evolved from Interactive Management, developed by systems scientists Alexander Christakis[27] and John Warfield[28] as a scientifically grounded method for social systems design. The method is validated by 50 years of planning and operations research, 40 years of scientific research, and 30 years in practice. As defined by Christakis, dialogue is "the participation of observers engaged in creating meaning, wisdom, and action through communication and collaborative interaction."[29]

SDD employs design principles for a facilitated method of dialogue for decision making for wicked problem assessment and solution and scenario creation. SDD is based on reaching strong consensus across stakeholders.

All collaborative processes require sufficient facilitator capacity. Although SDD requires a level of training to accomplish well, a collaborative design process can be considered as effective as its facilitation, a paradox of collaborative design that is rarely acknowledged.

In a typical workshop, a distinct series of questions and prompts are presented to participants, based on the underlying logic of the language patterns shown in Figure 8.7. To facilitate process usability, SDD's complexity is kept intentionally hidden. It is consistent with ensuring clarity of each step and the sense of true dialogue created in the live session by these methods.

1. **Define the problematic situation:** A problematic situation is articulated and framed by a core team.

2. **Focus and frame a triggering question:** A focus question is carefully defined as both invitation and inquiry, capturing the essence of the situation shared by all envisioned participants.

3. **Articulate observations:** Stakeholders generate responses to the triggering question. Ideas are refined into statements; labels are posted.

4. **Clarify meaning:** Facilitated group dialogue ensures all responses are clarified to the satisfaction of the idea owner (stakeholder). A catalogue of the responses and clarifications is circulated for real-time review.

5. **Inductively cluster:** After clarification, stakeholders vote on the ideas they believe should receive deeper consideration in the system design. These ideas are clustered based on exploration of similarities.

6. **Create shared language:** The group reflects on the formation of their first consensus structure pattern. Dialogue is captured as verbatim text associated with each statement.

7. **Assignation:** A group vote identifies the responses that will be included in structuring.

8. **Abductively structure:** With software support (employing the interpretive structural modeling algorithm), stakeholders vote on all ideas selected. Voting establishes the influence network among selected ideas, showing the collective assessment of influence relationships.

9. **Interpret learning:** The influence map is discussed in reflection for group learning and meaning creation.

10. **Evaluate cross-impact:** When both the challenges (problematique) and the solutions are mapped, the relationships of solutions to specific items in the problematique are constructed.

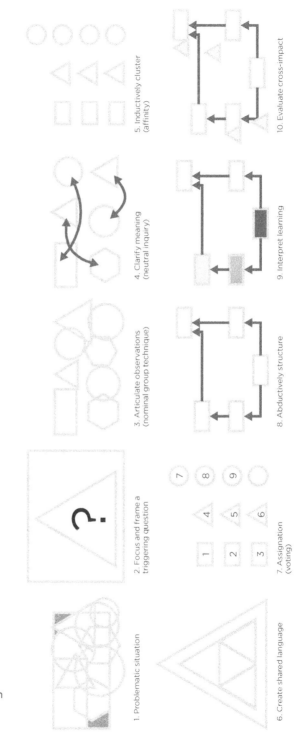

FIGURE 8.7
Language patterns in
Structured Dialogic
Design.

1. Problematic situation

2. Focus and frame a triggering question

3. Articulate observations (nominal group technique)

4. Clarify meaning (neutral inquiry)

5. Inductively cluster (affinity)

6. Create shared language

7. Assignation (voting)

8. Abductively structure

9. Interpret learning

10. Evaluate cross-impact

Each phase of SDD involves a separate, documented step, but there is significant flexibility and control in tuning the design for a planned application. These are basic language patterns, and experienced design planners can choose different techniques applied to accomplish the purpose of each step.

SDD is convened as a highly engaging, disciplined dialogue involving every stakeholder's voice and input. Figure 8.8 shows how printed and handwritten statements for language patterning are organized visually for tangible group presentation.

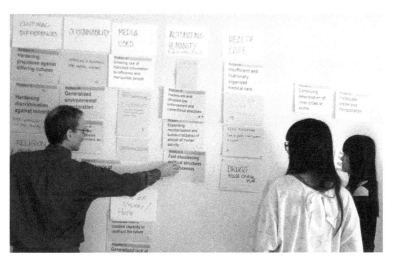

FIGURE 8.8
Group clustering and labeling. (Photo by Linda Blaasvær)

- Dialogic and participatory design methods share a common perspective on the necessity for democratic participation of all relevant stakeholders.

- Participant recruiting for good requisite variety (multifactorial diversity) is one of the most critical factors in successful systemic design.

- Mixed-method approaches are typical in systemic design and supporting research. Compatible methods are selected for the targeted purposes of each stage (understanding, design, change). However, dialogic and participatory methods might be employed productively to some extent in every stage for complex design projects.

- Generative participatory design workshops are not inherently good techniques for systemic design problems. Generative workshops (ideation, open process, prototyping) have no system methodology for reaching a collective understanding or identifying system patterns.

- Dialogic design is uniquely powerful for systemic design in complex problems. But unlike open methods such as Open Space or World Café, SDD requires a significant level of facilitator experience to do well.

CHAPTER 9

Designing Healthcare Futures

Elena's Story: A Change of Heart

Elena's ablation procedure is clinically successful. The most difficult part of the procedure was lying flat on her back for 6 hours in postoperative recovery, a necessary precaution. Elena's chest area feels sore and bruised for about 2 weeks, and she is instructed to avoid heavy work.

While resting at home, Elena finds herself back on some of the online forums she encountered in her earlier research. She visits MedHelp.com and finds dozens of responses to questions about SVT. She sees similar discussions at HealthBoards and eHealthForum. Several discussions have thousands of views and hundreds of threaded posts. Having time and a renewed interest in the problems, Elena is compelled to participate and post.

Elena had set up a profile on the site PatientsLikeMe during her earlier research and had posted a few times before the ablation. She was fascinated by the respectful discussions, the compassionate level of response to experiences, and the sense of caring. Returning to the community site after the treatment, she considers it worthwhile to post about her feelings and her personal impressions, and to browse the journals of people with similar disease profiles and treatments. A feature called InstantMe allows her to post a daily feeling, color coded from "very good" to "very bad" and tagged with a brief phrase. She clicks "good" for the day, but then adds "Sore and healing from ablation." She updates entries for Quality of Life, and enters a few notes to describe Treatments (her prescription for bisoprolol).

Elena begins to see how the world of healthcare is changing at the level of patient engagement and peer interaction. She would never substitute the expertise of medical advice and clinical experience for the collected posts of other health seekers she does not even know. But there is a sense of community, mutual respect, and genuine caring among people suffering from the same physical misfortunes and emotional concerns. Elena may yet have to wait weeks or months to find out whether the clinically advanced procedure restored her heart and her well-being. But she finds the online circles of care a possible new mission for her future as a health seeker—helping others on their journeys to care and health. ◾

In the Adjacent Future

Healthcare is an enormous industrial, research, and practice sector with increasing job growth and increasing economic impact, as measured in national surveys. According to the US Bureau of Labor Statistics, the occupation with the highest job growth is nursing, with a projected increase of nurses from 2.75 million today to 3.5 million by 2020. According to the American Medical Association, there are 815,000 licensed US physicians. Including pharmacists, allied health practitioners (in nearly 60 professions), dentists, and administrators and staff, the US healthcare sector is the largest private employer. In many countries with public healthcare, it is the largest employer, with the United Kingdom's National Health Service notably the largest public employer in Europe.

Hospital jobs were one of the few bright spots in employment during the recent recession: while more than 47 million jobs were lost, hospitals added nearly half a million new jobs. Although the big box healthcare model of large centralized medical centers has been faulted for sustainability, impersonal care, and wasteful expense, healthcare is often the largest economic and employment system in any region. Policy changes to the organizational and process structures of healthcare facilities could affect the jobs of many thousands. Policy innovation means cutbacks will happen somewhere in the sector, and every profession has a defensive strategy to prevent economic disruption, if not process change.

In 2011, futurist David Houle predicted that one-third of all US hospitals in operation would not survive to see 2020.[1] The driving trends are considered significant enough to tip the sector into a phase of creative destruction. In this scenario, economic forces will force the hand of decision makers and policies will change by necessity. These trends include the following:

- Employer healthcare costs as a proportion of wages are extremely high ($12,000 annually) and increasing 10% a year. This rate is unsustainable.

- The performance of traditional hospitals has historically been poor if measured by the Hippocratic Oath standard of "first do no harm." Estimates vary, but the *Journal of the American Medical Association* has reported 100,000 inpatient deaths annually, 80,000 of which originated from preventable hospital-acquired infections. The public is expected to wise up and avoid bad hospitals.

- Due to long wait times and poor customer service, hospitals will improve or die.

- Open data and connected services will provide the public with honest information about performance and value.

These are bold predictions, and their radical prescription predicts decentralized market-driven solutions. This transition is suggested as "inevitable," but an experienced view of foresight suggests that the inevitable never happens the way we think it will. There is a high likelihood of healthcare costs destructively transforming the US institutional system as we know it. Many hospitals balance on the edge of sustainability at close to a 1% operating margin.

The business models of healthcare organizations will change to navigate these trends, perhaps not by ending operations but by creatively reconfiguring practices, organizational structure, and shared overhead. These challenges assume that large clinics may not have learned from their mistakes and that market alternatives may earn the public's trust. Hospitals are already starting to decentralize, more due to the implications of Accountable Care Act policy than to market pressures. In fact, many hospital brands will strengthen. Large care organizations move slowly, require time to build consensus, and usually reinvent their own solutions to known issues.

Large-scale system innovation can be greatly accelerated when funding and values shift. In the case of big box healthcare, both have happened. The emergence of new community-based practice models has converged at the same time that many clinical leaders have called for values change. The patient-centered paradigm is rapidly becoming the new norm at many large institutions. At the same time, many traditional facilities are leading the way toward distributed, community-centered care centers.

In response to Houle's claim, we might ask: "What will we call a hospital in 5 or 10 years?" If the big box model is already distributing into regional centers, we could see it becoming a constellation of storefronts with a big-brand, central, acute-care hospital.

Near-Term Design Challenges

What are the most critical service or system design issues we all face in healthcare? What problems should we focus on now? At least five "grand challenge" social design problems recur across the sectors (the whole system), none of which are healthcare IT or digital design.

- **Redesigning care services:** How can healthcare be reimagined and reinstitutionalized as a caring service? If the customers are a "market of sick people," is it ethical to encourage this market's further growth by creating new ways to help people identify themselves as being sick? Can health seekers and communities form durable circles of care to recover the meaning of care?

- **Reenvisioning professional relationships:** Have health professions created a self-serving system of professional services that converts people into patients? How can new service approaches enable patients to recover a sense of autonomy and choice in their health seeking?

- **Working with multiple payers:** US healthcare will be burdened with multiple market entities for the foreseeable future, and the trend continues toward market, not single-payer, systems. Here the treatment of disease and injury has been packaged for insurance, which hurts those who need it most. How might a systemic approach to service design reframe these offerings so that the consumer has the ultimate power of choice, not the provider?

- **Health awareness and healthy societies:** A healthy society emerges from individual health awareness. How can care service design educate people about the discrete and cumulative effects of choices and lifestyle results?

- **Future position of healthcare:** What if, over the next generation, the right to care was treated as a human right? How would personal and public health change to afford universal and inclusive care?

Design education and academic conferences are currently exploring these emerging topics (as well as conventional technology scenarios). A recent CHI conference workshop engaged current issues and shared common whole-system problems.[2] Responses from more than 70 participants (consultants, academics, and representatives from private firms) identified critical themes and emerging issues at the whole-system level of healthcare. Responses for each question were clustered in four problem areas: management and policy, systems and services, design, and research (see sidebar on page 302).

Designers report struggling with the pragmatic issues of validating their contribution to the clinical workplace and appropriate technology design. One of the biggest conflicts is the acceptance of design thinking and practice in the evidence-based clinical and institutional setting. Professionals in differing sectors report issues with recognition of their value to the organization, difficulty in project collaboration, and limited access to clinical practice and patients for service and informatics design-oriented research. These organizational issues are perhaps barriers to collaborative innovation, but are not the primary systemic problems. A summary of trends and themes reveals:

- Management and policy issues are the most significant barriers to whole-system design.

- A strong focus on IT is often the focus for system-level design. This may not be the most effective means for design intervention in clinical practice. How can a service-oriented approach drive appropriate IT design and selection?

- A clear call is made for establishing systemic and integrated practices—interdisciplinary projects, design bridging groups, professional integration, multistakeholder engagement.

- Designers are seeking better ways to model, map, and framework the multiple systems, services, and data they deal with to help teams and organizations better plan and integrate multiple resources.

The workshop discovered that priorities and barriers involved both *structural* (policy, roles, and work practice) and *organizational* (process routines and management) issues. Organizational redesign is a primary aim of systemic design and organizational change, but not UX or services design.

What are the highest priority design or research issues in healthcare today?

MANAGEMENT/POLICY

- [Designers] achieving credibility within organizations
- Getting design practice into healthcare planning
- Risk management when making decisions
- Educating management and clinicians about systemic risks and lock-in
- Educating leadership in design, healthcare, IT systems
- Leverage social groups and support of patients to relieve burden from professionals

SYSTEMS/SERVICES

- Integrating multiple systems, dealing with huge amounts of data
- Systems-level road map—model of whole clinical services
- Finding agreement on frameworks for service-level systems
- EMRs [electronic medical records] do not support true clinical workflow. How to redesign for scaffolding support?
- Quality of EMR design and task flow
- Secure accessibility and sharing of electronic patient records
- Common users and different needs for same device
- CPS (cyber-physical systems) for healthcare (system of systems)

DESIGN/PRACTICES

- Matching effective design practices to systemic contexts in healthcare
- Co-design with patients and practitioners
- Identifying design issues as a cause rather than human error

RESEARCH

- Need for interdisciplinary design research
- Research support to promote interoperability of EMRs and shared databases
- The role of emotional wellness in general healthcare
- Not understanding priorities/mental models of different roles in the hospitals

What are the most significant *barriers* to complex health services design today?

MANAGEMENT/POLICY

- Most design decisions are financially driven. How do we counter this?
- How does IT design fit into wider intervention?

- [How might systemic design] change current practice procedure?
- What cultural change is necessary from the medical side? How can designers meet them halfway?
- Without EMR mandate by 2014, compliance is probably (significantly) lower
- Lack of coordination among disparate, well-intended activities
- Barriers from HIPAA or other healthcare laws
- Convincing clinicians of the importance of design
- Poor responsiveness from health IT vendors

SYSTEMS/SERVICES

- Lack of standardization; lack of interoperability, even in the same systems and settings
- Lack of motivation; users are (not) motivated to contribute to system
- Integration across different healthcare providers (hospitals vs. PCPs [primary care providers])
- Enabling designers to collaborate with clinicians (How do they?)
- Dramatically lower system costs/availability
- Integrating PHRs [personal health records] and EHRs [electronic health records]

DESIGN/PRACTICES

- Focus on clinicians, overlooking support and administration as resources for system understanding
- Paper artifacts still play a crucial role in clinicians' workflow. How can we bridge with the digital system?
- Balancing user/practice personalization with a standardized EMR system
- Clinically relevant content needed at the ready
- Streamline clinical and support workflows
- Lightweight applications with high privacy/security
- Getting clinicians and designers to speak to each other, share goals and similar language
- Countering the ~50% decrease in doctor/patient interaction due to EMR implementation
- Sharing case study–style success and failures of various approaches

RESEARCH

- How to bring researchers in different disciplines working toward healthcare together?
- Inter/transdisciplinary and clinical and diagnostic research
- Funding and academic focus require researchers to position in narrow and often inconsequential research areas for publication and continuity

Considering the precarious position of design teams reported within the current organizational culture, design-led approaches are not yet recommended (but may be practical after several years of practice development). In hospitals, multidisciplinary collaborations led by senior clinical staff with senior design partners would be the best route toward integrated organizational change. New leadership roles for designers and researchers will be effective in interdisciplinary practice research, IT project design and development, and service design applied to clinical offerings in the institution.

Mid-Future: Resolution of Critical Healthcare Problems

Canada faces serious headwinds as costs rise, as do all health systems. Although the single-payer systems of the United Kingdom and Scandinavian countries are held as examples of cost-effective healthcare, the burdens on funders are unsustainable. In the most recent Quebec budget, 45% of all provincial spending went to healthcare, up from 31% in 1980. The opportunities for business and policy innovation are compelling and necessary.

Canada's federal government sponsored several healthcare commissions toward system-level reform and sustainability of their universal access Medicare system. In 2001, the Commission on the Future of Health Care in Canada recommended policies and measures to improve the system and its long-term sustainability. The subsequent Romanow report surveyed thousands of citizens and churned through statistics to produce an analysis and a set of 47 recommendations.[3] Even though these recommendations were generated a decade ago, they remain current issues in policy and are considered long-term trends. They are well suited as mid-term to long-term trends for assessment in foresight.

Graduate students from the OCAD University Strategic Foresight and Innovation program constructed an influence map analyzed from the Romanow report, showing the continuous challenges in Canadian healthcare.[4] The diagram represents policy agreement on the significant drivers affecting costs and quality, most of which are applicable to the systems in the United States and other nations. Figure 9.1 shows the connectedness between the most critical problems as determined by their influence (revised by the author).

The graduate design research team produced the map using a dialogic design method (as defined in Chapter 8). The purpose of the mapping was to identify the highest-leverage problems that, once resolved, would propagate and resolve much of the connected system of problems.

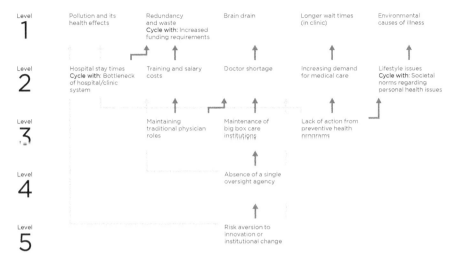

Level 1 — Pollution and its health effects | Redundancy and waste **Cycle with:** Increased funding requirements | Brain drain | Longer wait times (in clinic) | Environmental causes of illness

Level 2 — Hospital stay times **Cycle with:** Bottleneck of hospital/clinic system | Training and salary costs | Doctor shortage | Increasing demand for medical care | Lifestyle issues **Cycle with:** Societal norms regarding personal health issues

Level 3 — Maintaining traditional physician roles | Maintenance of big box care institutions | Lack of action from preventive health programs

Level 4 — Absence of a single oversight agency

Level 5 — Risk aversion to innovation or institutional change

FIGURE 9.1

Influence map of Canadian healthcare system issues.

Notice in Figure 9.1 that some of the traditional points of intervention to improve patient experience (based on an open source survey and experience) include "longer wait times in clinic" and "doctor shortage." These points are convenient targets of action as they are observable and tangible, and resolution appears feasible. These also indicate the effects of deeper causes. Efforts expended toward these goals may not even touch the deeper problems. Because these appear at the top of the diagram, they are highly influenced, not influential. The pattern analysis reveals these are the resulting outcomes of multiple influencing causes, some of which appear in the lower levels of the diagram.

Working on the wrong problem perpetuates the cause and tends to shift the burden to another symptom. Many of the most common complaints in healthcare service, such as the shortage of family doctors, long wait times for certain specialists and procedures, and the ever-increasing costs of care, are the highly visible symptoms of overlooked (or delayed) systemic causes.

The influence map helps stakeholders visualize the complexity of the relationships among various issues in order to evaluate the problem system and make better decisions on actions that have the best "reach."

With even a cursory evaluation of the deep drivers in the problem system we see a different story. The two deepest issues are "risk aversion to innovation and change" and "absence of a single oversight agency." These drive up the costs of maintaining expensive existing institutions without regard to their actual efficacy in providing care.

At level 3, two other root cause drivers influence *all* of the level 1 and 2 problems, and thereby the rest of the map. "Maintaining traditional physician roles" and "lack of action from preventive health programs" are perfect systemic design issues that future practice scenarios could address.

We particularly examined how the blind maintenance of existing healthcare institutions might limit the possibilities for systemic redesign. Do the traditional professional roles of medicine (e.g., doctor, nurse, specialist) represent optimal functions in the system, or were they only reflecting a continuation of past institutional structures? What if the conventional one-on-one relationship of patient to family doctor was revisited? Would the system work better if it were organized around *teams of practitioners* with different skill sets? An expanded role for the community in maintaining public health was envisioned, a movement that is now gathering momentum.

Whole Care Triage Funnel

Ultimately, the analysis from dialogic design converged on three potential areas of intervention that required further consideration:

1. The existing institutional norms that dictate the distribution of medical expertise among currently defined professional roles

2. Individual versus team-based practice

3. The role of the community in health

Powerful insights and future scenarios for system-level change emerged from these three proposals. A new paradigm for the organization of healthcare practices was envisioned for stakeholders using this method. The traditional role boundaries of the doctor as the single (and ultimate) bearer of responsibility for medical diagnosis should relax to enable shared roles in team constructs. Health services will increasingly be delivered outside the hospital system and into community or decentralized practices. Hospital visits will be minimized by increasing the opportunity points for health conversations initiated with immediate caregivers (and the community), instead of the often already critical and rushed centralized care facility.

Today the physician is usually the single point in the system through which all patient data and decisions must flow. A team system was envisioned to extend the triage principle through a "funnel" of increasingly specific diagnosis and responsibility. In traditional triage, patients are assessed as they enter the system, and they are given priority according to the urgency of their condition. In the proposed system, this initial assessment would merely be the beginning of a progressive triage focusing on multiple patient health needs treated as a whole.

In Canadian emergency rooms, a staged triage manages variable and high-volume workloads, where an incoming patient starts with a triage nurse, an emergency room or specialist nurse, or a resident, and is then treated by a senior resident or attending physician. The proposed "whole care triage" engages a physician's assistant or nurse practitioner with diagnostic responsibility and the ability to call in supporting assessment and treatment.

The triage funnel works in two directions: broad community engagement and advocacy at the top, and increasingly specialized expertise at the point. Physician assistants mediate and filter out the appropriate cases before they enter the emergency room. Those that require specialized attention or assessment are passed down to the next level of the funnel.

The funnel introduces a process for organizational resiliency by distributing labor and expertise to the point of need, and optimizes the time cost of medical labor and workload. Other professionals and community advocates are given explicit locations in the process for participation. A wider range of caregivers are equipped to triage, assist, or advocate, enabling the time and capacity to translate patient needs and health requirements. As a result of this systemic process, patients with multiple chronic diseases are given progressive treatment respecting their total health, fewer specialists are utilized for emergency situations, and perceived emergency wait times are greatly reduced.

Similar processes have been put in place for large-scale emergencies (known as continuous integrated triage). However, these are based on efforts to manage resources, not to optimally treat patients with complex care needs. This triage funnel is similar to the proposal for iterative clinical care in the Innovate Afib case study in Chapter 5. By changing the purpose of the service system from internal resource management to patient-centered care, the triage process is repositioned as multidisciplinary guidance for complex care.

Longer-Term Healthcare Foresight

Designing for even longer-range complex design problems—10 or 20 years or more—requires practices from strategic foresight to account for the uncertainty and variation of possible trajectories of social trends and technology. Strategic foresight is not forecasting or future prediction, or as commonly thought, a design process of generating "future alternatives." It is an art and research discipline of constructing possible formulations of future outcomes that enable better long-term planning and reasoning about risks in the present. It identifies trends and drivers from present culture that can be found to significantly influence possible future social and technological outcomes.

Strategic foresight consists of numerous practices for envisioning, reasoning about, planning, shaping, and designing future possibilities (Figure 9.2). It requires understanding current trends, ranges of choices, and anticipating change for strategic design and planning. Strategic foresight identifies emerging trends from technology and scientific research, emerging sociocultural and political trends, and global and economic policies for making sense of possible outcomes. Strategic foresight also attempts to translate trends in innovation (products, services, experiences, and systems) to align or lead the human needs and institutional changes among stakeholders.

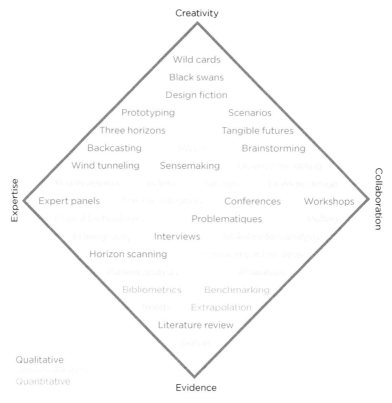

FIGURE 9.2
Strategic foresight methods. (Adapted from R. Popper, 2008)

Foresight research fellow Rafael Popper organized methods from contemporary foresight practice to help practitioners select an appropriate balance of techniques.[5] These are mapped by four dimensions and their evidence type— qualitative, quantitative, and what he calls semi-quantitative. The four points of the diamond indicate whether the method is a creative generative exercise or more evidence-based; or horizontally, whether an expert-based method or a collaborative practice. The diamond applies to clinical culture as a guide to both research and foresight methods, as it is currently heavily weighted toward evidence-based and expert methods. Integrating appropriate methods from the generative and collaborative positions into projects provides opportunities for collaborative teams to explore creative methods complementary to established evidence-based approaches.

Specific foresight methods are not detailed here, although many should be familiar from earlier chapters. Several social systems and emerging future methods have been incorporated into a revised model based on Popper's diamond model (here replacing an equal number of methods).

Given the high social stakes and predicted costs of healthcare services in just the near future, the value of strategic foresight in healthcare should be apparent. Numerous "Future of Healthcare" projects are conducted every year by well-known groups such as the Institute for the Future and the Global Business Network, as well as design firms such as IDEO and PFSK. Not all future studies involve strategic foresight. Many future studies are conducted as "What if?" exercises in the possibilities of technological advancement or as speculation for design thinking.

One axiom of practice is that foresight research requires the investment of participants in the outcome of the future scenarios. The meaning of future possibilities and scenarios must matter to the design team. Professional futurist Joseph Coates lists three principles that underlie foresight thinking:

1. We can see the future to the extent that it is useful in planning.

2. We can influence the future to make the good and the desirable more likely and the undesirable less likely.

3. The ability to anticipate and to influence creates the moral obligation to study the future.[6]

Ethical concerns arise in the "ownership" or personal commitment to healthcare futures, as human lives are at stake in the policy decisions and strategies chosen from these scenarios. It is an ethical requirement to consider all relevant stakeholder perspectives in future scenarios that have a wide social impact. Technological opportunities and breakthroughs do not determine the future of healthcare. The choices of leadership and engaged stakeholders determine the design of healthcare service systems.

One of Hasan Özbekhan's early foresight axioms recognized that people allow technology to determine future outcomes, in that "Can Implies Ought."[7] He argued that just because we *can* develop a technology, the capability implied by that technology should not be implemented unwittingly. Innovation does not obviate the ethical demand to envision the possible future consequences and to fit the technology into appropriate service.

This necessity is an ethical requirement for designers, as well as managers, policy leaders, and citizens. This principle is crucial to ethical social foresight.

Two foresight design methods are explored in the cases that follow: three horizons and gigamapping.

Case 1: Three Horizons of Future Specialty Healthcare

Systems thinker and foresighter Anthony Hodgson's *three horizons* is a method by which three overlapping time curves, or horizons, give rise to group thinking about the emergence of change over time.[8] Three horizons can integrate multiple foresight and design scenarios within the context of sequential timelines, showing when and how trends and technologies might be integrated or fully developed. The method allows practitioners to relate drivers and trends to emerging issues, and links futures studies to organizational and social change.

A current case adopting three horizons was conducted by a team of foresight researchers working with the Mayo Clinic's Center for Innovation. The study, titled "The Future of Specialized Health Care Providers," defined a complete strategic foresight model for the evolution of specialty care.[9]

Following a STEEPV (social, technological, economic, environmental, political, and values) trend and environmental scan, a trend map was developed and key drivers analyzed. Integrating other methods (cone of plausibility, wind tunneling, scenarios, backcasting), the study mapped trends, drivers, and barriers to the three horizons in near-, mid-, and long-term scenarios. Three robust strategies were identified for specialty care:

- Build a smart electronic health system.

- Integrate service delivery.

- Improve the patient experience.

These strategies were developed into their own three horizons timeline maps. The timelines indicate narratives for managing change to a preferred future state, represented by horizon 3 (H3), a patient-centric care system.

Figure 9.3 illustrates the major trend and shift from current practices in H1 to the "preferred future" practices in roughly 20 years (H3). The curves between H1 and H3 indicate the overlapping timelines and the change processes toward which stakeholders must attend in H2.

The study shows the dominant specialty care system declining over the next 10 years, during a transition state, as centralized (big box) healthcare systems reorganize a higher proportion of care in community and distributed practices. Figure 9.4 describes the tensions and concerns faced during the transition, yet there are "pockets of the future" throughout H1 in the next 5 years.

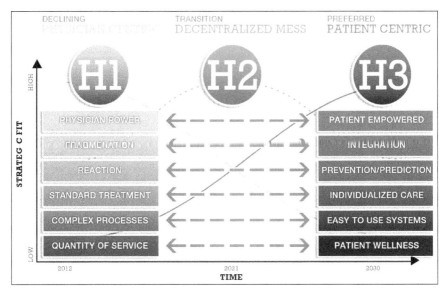

FIGURE 9.3

Three horizons of specialized medicine. (Courtesy of P. Sihavong, U. Maharaj, and J. Vink, OCAD University)

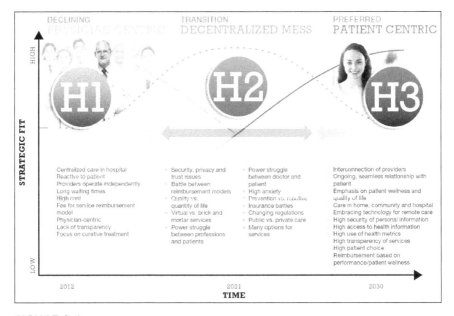

FIGURE 9.4

Challenges in horizon transition. (Courtesy of P. Sihavong, U. Maharaj, and J. Vink, OCAD University)

Weak signals recognized as indicators of new practice include the changes in patient empowerment as active health seekers, changes in payment, and the huge potential for integrated systems and services not being realized in current systems. Rapid changes in access to health information and online e-patients are prevalent indicators of the present that presage everyday future practices. Tensions between standard treatment approaches and the future potential of personalized medicine will be encountered and resolved during the H2 timeframe. The fragmented healthcare services and information systems will be forced to integrate over this period. These signal behaviors are not yet predominant values, but the potential for their trend to become driving values in new institutions becomes apparent.

For the purposes of the case, one of the three strategies is shown as integrated service delivery (Figure 9.5). Over the three horizons model, three scenarios play out between 2012 and 2030. H1 finds the healthcare system maintaining "business as usual" with incremental enhancements to service. As clinics across North America face a significant increase in baby boomer patients in the next few years, it makes sense to manage the demographic onslaught with predictable, known practices that minimize the risks of transition. Over the next 10 years, H2 practices (already in evidence) become widely implemented. Care teams, chronic care coordination, and whole-patient triage become common practices during the decentralization phase. These organizational changes are precursors to the establishment of integrated services delivery between 2020 and 2030.

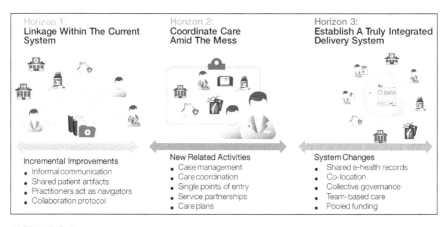

FIGURE 9.5

Integrated service delivery across three horizons. (Courtesy of P. Sihavong, U. Maharaj, and J. Vink, OCAD University)

The emerging practices in H1—collaboration protocols, sharing information with patients, new roles for clinicians—are necessary improvements. But they are seen to evolve in H2 with more established processes for personalized patient case management and care coordination across multiple professionals, similar to that described in the whole-care triage funnel. Both of these horizons consist of incomplete innovations that enable specialized care providers and care teams to better coordinate complex patient care and collaborate on decision and planning.

Care planning is already a consistent practice in most acute and long-term care facilities. In many cases, care planning is recognized as the best opportunity for interprofessional dialogue on care strategies before significant treatment decisions are made. In the horizon mapping, care planning offers a platform for initiating collaborative healthcare, leading the institution toward integrated delivery. The future service system envisioned in 20 years consists of integrated EMR and information resources and fully transparent shared health records with patients. Clinical services will be collocated in communities, consistent with scenarios foreseen under the accountable care organization movement. Clinical networks will be organized under new management models of collective governance, giving all practitioners and patient/community health representatives a voice in healthcare investment and care practices.

The three horizons model provides a pathway for strategic planning based on foresight, enabling designers and decision makers to make sense of possible future outcomes. Although the service examples in this case are not radical changes, they are entirely plausible and will require years of learning and reorganization to be fully implemented. The strategic foresight methodology enables planning teams to envision these pathways and decision points, and provides a road map with which all stakeholders can engage.

Case 2: Intervening in Childhood Obesity

Systemic design based on systems thinking, evidence analysis, and visualization is a powerful approach for strategic foresight as it clarifies relationships in a system that occur over long periods. Future scenarios can be envisioned as with any foresight method, and interventions can be targeted to critical system functions that occur over a longer horizon. Gigamapping, developed at the Oslo School of Architecture and Design by professor Birger Sevaldson, offers such a visual thinking process and social systems design.[10]

Gigamapping is a visual representation that integrates classical systems diagrams (e.g., influence maps, causal loop diagrams, system maps) and visual thinking templates (e.g., timelines, infographics, rich pictures) into a pictorial narrative. The gigamap frames and describes both the problems and proposed interventions in a complex situation. A design team formulates the map over the course of research as its ever-present canvas, layering their evolving concepts and representations to show a narrative of the system story and its possibilities for design intervention. It analyzes the thick complexity discovered in research and presents a visual map of the salient, systemic drivers and solutions.

A design research team developed the system gigamap in Figure 9.6 as part of an investigation into systemic causes and interventions for childhood obesity.[11] Childhood obesity, and individual and social health issues in general, is considered to be complex because the symptoms (effects) mask deeper causes, some of which may progress over long periods.

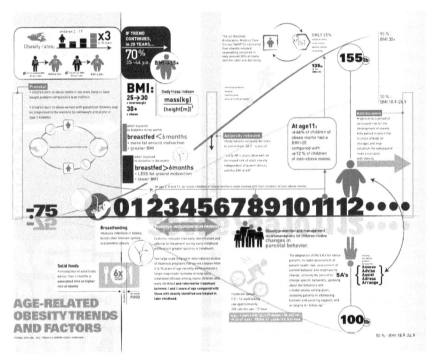

FIGURE 9.6
System map for childhood obesity intervention. (Courtesy of George Shewchuk)

The problem of obesity, a true epidemic syndrome affecting one-third of all adults in the United States and up to one-sixth of children, is a major systemic health problem of our time. Most efforts to address the wicked problem of obesity focus on dealing with behaviors to mitigate the effects—changing eating habits, inspiring regular exercise, and improving lifestyle behaviors overall. The gigamap simplifies the facts and data from evidence and presents systemic behaviors on a timeline.

The case considers the system of childhood obesity within the boundary of North American youth to the age of 16. The prenatal period was discovered as an extremely important window for determining or preventing obesity. The timeline also shows the relative increase in obesity (inclining curve toward higher weight) or decrease (declining curve) depending on factors illustrated at the different critical periods (shaded for emphasis).

A number of different system representations were necessary to organize a complete description of the system. Several map types were integrated here: a mind map, stakeholder analysis, causal loops, and an influence diagram. The history of the research process itself was also captured in the diagram.

The mind map helped identify the stakeholders and influencing factors, based on the literature. Stakeholder interviews and analysis clarified three points during a child's life during which positive intervention could occur: the prenatal period, a spike in body mass index (BMI) at age 2, and then another period during ages 5 to 7. This information was presented in an influence map to identify the points in time at which different stakeholders play a role in the childhood narrative. For example, the mother and clinicians are most influential during the prenatal period, and school and media become influential only after age 5. Therefore, the level of influence and importance of each stakeholder in the system can be understood in relation to the time lag that dominates the system.

The effects of obesity ripple throughout society and the economy for generations; therefore, it is critical to evaluate the influences of stakeholders. Primary stakeholders are the child and his or her family, who constitute a first-order social system. The second-order stakeholders are educators, healthcare providers, government, and food providers. Third-order (indirect) stakeholders include community centers, special interest groups (e.g., ballet programs or sports leagues), and public programs such as parks.

A widely held view is that the best solution to the obesity epidemic is to focus on prevention and education to encourage healthy lifestyle changes. However, the social determinants of obesity are multifactored and affect all age groups and social strata. Interventions tackling individual determinants or narrowly targeted to one group of individuals will have a limited impact on a large scale and will not significantly reduce the magnitude of the problem.

Because of significant time delays within the total system, interventions targeting younger age groups are unlikely to have significant positive effects at the population level for many years. The cost-effectiveness profiles of such interventions may be favorable in the long term, but may be hard to justify during the contentious planning stages when programs and interventions are selected and budgeted.

According to some research, the influence of parents and the home environment is the primary determinant to setting the stage for healthy habits in children. Babies breastfed for less than 4 months have a much higher risk of obesity than other children. An intervention in mother-baby nurturing requires a change in behavior and a shift in priorities. The socioeconomic status of a family may determine the priority given to weight gain. Better nutrition takes more time and attention, and is less affordable than prepackaged and junk foods. Issues are compounded by an early lack of physical activity. This may be a result of a number of barriers that a family confronts, including the lack of financial resources to pay for participation and/or transportation to sporting events.

Although the most efficient interventions are found outside the health sector, healthcare can impact obesity and related chronic conditions by focusing on higher-risk individuals at stages when early obesity is identified. This factor suggests possible design interventions in the clinical setting to help new mothers identify the early symptoms of obesity and to introduce education and support for healthy diets and breastfeeding.

The visual description of the system of childhood obesity "system" helps stakeholders identify the best leverage points for interventions available to their resources. There are many other factors not illustrated here, but the selection of salient targets identified through research provides a basis for stakeholder dialogue and foresight over the 10-year horizon of the incubation of serious obesity.

Future Roles for Healthcare Design Leadership

This book presents three healthcare sectors found across the world: the consumer, medical practice, and institutional sectors. These three nested levels (which include education and community) comprise the primary touchpoints with systems of care. Several major sectors with significant design import were not included—IT, pharmaceuticals, insurance, and architecture. Although any of these sectors may today employ more design professionals than all clinical institutions combined, they are largely commercial entities and have employed designers in product and service roles for years. According to discussions with designers, there seems to be surprisingly little crossover of practice between the consumer and clinical sectors.

Achieving design leadership across these sectors will require a long-term engagement of design roles, not just the increased placement of design skills within IT, Web, and clinical service organizations. Leading roles are currently interaction (IT and UX) designer, service designer, design researcher/ ethnographer, and communication (graphic) designer. Emerging placements include practice and management roles in innovation management, patient-centered research, experience design, and service integration.

Healthcare designer roles and tasks are not clear cut. Designers, ethnographers, and design researchers face a challenge in positioning their new roles in healthcare to make the most difference in health outcomes *and* business outcomes. New roles within established cultures will take time—a year or more—to fully socialize across departments and service lines. Design disciplines and skills may compete with or confront established norms in clinical culture. For organizations (hospitals and firms), discovering the best allocation of design talent will require trial and error, and experimentation across projects. Though some designers may be domain experts in a clinical field or in healthcare organizational strategy, most are not. The new value and values of design leadership will be co-created.

Consumer Health Sector

Throughout this book the roles of patient and consumer that we take for granted were critiqued and the person as health seeker was presented as a centering for design. For the sake of clarity, "consumer" is here, in closing, returned to the sector where it belongs. The consumer health sector is defined by its market and end-user products and services. These include IT (Web services, technology firms, start-ups), consumer products (personal health and consumable products), and health management services (wellness, employer health services, health insurance). The sector is defined by business-to-consumer offerings and is largely independent of the medical sector (clinicians as users) and the institutional (patients and stakeholders).

The majority of healthcare design roles are currently found in consumer health. With mandates to innovate and product revenue streams, commercial firms offer the promise of creative projects and bringing products to commercial markets, serving the health seeker as the primary customer.

The consumer sector carries the highest risks of product failure. With extensive competition and thin margins, consumer firms drive innovation by continuous product development. By some counts, there are up to 35,000 health apps in a widely distributed, fragmented marketplace. Given the interest in healthcare among start-up incubators, there seems to be consensus that consumer demand will follow. Yet the sheer number of single-purpose apps cannot be sustained. Within 3 years, the health app marketplace will consolidate, not expand. This cycle occurs with every technology surge and should be expected. Apps may be less expensive to produce than software or Web services, but they are expensive to maintain, update, and market over multiple platforms. Moreover, they are difficult to monetize.

Consumer-driven online business models may not be sustainable in the long term. Products, not services, rule the consumer health market. Web users do not pay for health applications; they have learned from Web 2.0 that free resources are supported by aftermarkets in user data. Consumer users will not readily pay for health apps when there are dozens of similar free services. (The same goes for physicians as users, who can afford subscriptions but will use free services plus their judgment to qualify the resource.) Advertising is a sustainable source for only the proven, popular sites and resources.

Among Web services, design quality is not yet a differentiator, indicating the field is still in early stages of adoption. None of the popular health sites were design leaders (although WebMD was recently redesigned and may have somewhat better usability). When consolidation reduces the number of viable services, design quality and usability will drive success among the preferred sites. Findability and content will continue to make more of a difference because health-seeking users tend to be intermittent, locating sites from searches and not assessing their relative quality from known sites.

The quantified self segment has emerged as one of the most vital developments in consumer health. The essential value of quantified self applications is converting biophysical measures of everyday behavior and physical activity into responsive feedback for enhanced performance in preferred activities. The availability of inexpensive data-acquisition sensors and durable activity monitors has reduced the barrier to entry for personal monitoring. As with classical disruptive innovations, the first products are directed toward a niche segment, in this case primarily amateur and professional athletes interested in measuring physiological performance improvements in physical activity.

The Nike FuelBand and the start-up Fitbit product use accelerometers to measure movement and track patterns, adapted to quantify energy exertion from walking and running, sleep patterns, and even caloric intake and output. Providing Web and mobile data exchange, the wearable devices gather data on an ongoing basis to track longitudinal patterns or training intensity for runners. Simple smartphone apps, such as the RunKeeper app that tracks running and cycling miles and times, encourage performance monitoring for defined self-health goals.

Portable personal feedback systems have been available for a decade or more in different forms and have been made significantly easier to use with ubiquitous mobile devices and Internet platforms. As a health trend, the quantified self will not necessarily be adopted by large numbers of followers; as a "movement" it is currently driven more by technology innovation than the need for health management. Yet the shift to wider consumer health might occur when small tracking devices can be prescribed by physicians and used for brief periods for health tracking and clinical feedback. As ultra-small sensors are packed into tiny wearable devices, massive amounts of personal data—from everyday activities and movement, to diet and blood sugar, to cardiopulmonary measures—can be tracked and synthesized into patterned displays for clinical decision making. Tracking feedback, responses to treatment and medication, and measuring adherence will make a huge difference in assessing the effectiveness of prescribed drugs and calibrating personalized therapies.

The consumer market for health services is so widely diffused that the consumer healthcare sector may be seen as many small sectors with their own followings and interests, with little crossover. Based on trends, the current and future consumer markets cluster into the following categories:

- Healthcare management and advising

- Personal health management

- General health, wellness, and lifestyle

- Medical diagnosis, treatment, and disease information

- Patient communities by disease or interest

- Medical devices, products, and information

- Health and beauty products and personal services

- Pharmaceutical products and their evaluation

- Nutritional supplements

- Health insurance and financing

- Employer-based wellness and health planning

- Clinician and hospital information

From a service design perspective, it is helpful to understand conventional market sectors as possible adjacent service lines. Yet from the health seekers' perspective, the boundaries between services may be meaningless. If a nutritional supplement or meditation practice can ease a sleep disorder, the conventional categories of health "care" will not matter. Boundaries between consumer services are merging categories wherever the opportunity arises.

Clinical Practice Sector

Designers will find emerging opportunities for service design in healthcare practice and education, where complexity is high and the effect on improving patient outcomes is apparent.

Healthcare practices and therapies are constantly reviewed and researched for effectiveness, and their coordination for patient experience and cost management is receiving close attention from the business and policy decision makers. Design and systems research offer better ways to redesign care at the front lines in full partnership with clinical staff. Clinical design partnership works with interprofessional teams and provides access to real care situations for designing for clinical needs and directly improving patient experience.

Service design for improving patient experiences will become a mainstream trend, and the modes of design research and clinical research will converge as program effectiveness projects are enabled by design leadership. Patient-led service improvements and new healthcare organizational forms (such as the accountable care organization) will change our approaches to service design. Much of the design for patient experience is currently focused on big box healthcare and the enhancement of admission to discharge journeys, wait times, and the experience of care treatments. Even without a standard measure for patient experience, hospitals are rapidly adopting patient satisfaction surveys and incorporating patient-experience measures into their service quality reporting. Specialized clinics and group practices can be even more responsive, and managers and clinical staff are enhancing the direct experience of service provided to their patients. Design-led improvements are performed in very few cases, but the opportunities for design engagement are rapidly opening. In the course of the research of this book, the acceleration of new cases in the last 6 months outstrips the total examples identified over 3 years. There are many new stories of radically improved patient experience and clinical service.

Much of the push for better experience has been promoted by patients themselves, and by their advocates, nurses, and business services staff in hospitals. Though certainly stakeholders, those closest to the patients are not the decision drivers in the organization. Making the return-on-investment case for better patient experience is difficult because it is intangible and without standard accepted measures of merit.

Remember that patients have an unusual customer position in medical care, unlike any other service situation they will encounter. They have very incomplete knowledge of treatments, tests, and hospital procedures. The best "experience" might be the least experience. Large medical centers present risks that far outweigh a clumsy service experience. Doing no harm (or as sociologist Ross Koppel suggests, merely *less harm*[12]) should be the absolute baseline standard of care. This is not yet perfected by any means. Yet such a quantifiable assurance should be the patient's primary concern.

Improving the patient experience is a primary focus for human-centered service design. Yet the end experience of clinical care is an effect of many causes. Focusing on the effects of care is not the most effective way to redesign the cause. Many factors that show up as better patient experience are end results like those in the influence map in this chapter (see Figure 9.1). Most of these are immediate and short-term touchpoints:

- Shorter wait times
- Easier hospital navigation
- Better room accommodations
- Attentive clinical and direct nursing care
- Simpler and easier payment processes
- Better physician communication
- Knowledge of all available choices, not just those prescribed

The systemic factors must be identified that result in consistently better care for health seekers undergoing a hospital service. These are nearly all longer-term management and education issues:

- Better procedure and process design
- Wayfinding that helps the infrequent visitor/patient
- Better housewide bed-management systems
- Clinical education that trains for empathic communication
- Education and practice modes for care teams
- Revamped insurance and Medicare policies

These are all interconnected design issues. Designing directly for better patient experience is indeed a care design problem, but it is not independent of these other factors. It is an outcome of care practices and can be used as a measure of improvement of these causes.

The solution for complicated problems of bed management or education may take much longer than direct redesign of symptoms, but this leads to repeatable and system-wide results. As practice research on hand-washing has shown, the everyday problems in practice are not resolved by verbal instruction or direct habit change. A fundamental change in the system is needed before the results of the change show up visibly.

Institutional Sector

Healthcare is the largest sector and business in North America, with 1 of every 8 Americans employed in the industry. And it is growing, both in dollar volume and population served. The institutional sector includes the clinical organizations, their business and policy ecosystem, practices of all sizes, universities, and medical schools. Think of this level as the employers, decision makers, and management for clinical practice and all the suppliers, IT support, and government organizations.

We have only a few short years to evolve a unique and developing role in the field before organizational routines may fold design roles into well-established, reliable, and repeatable design practices. Processes change slowly in large, rule-bound, risk-averse institutions. Before significant cultural change will be evident, designers will have to adapt to current practices while promoting innovation. Patience and a commitment to learning will be required.

At the institutional level, a service systems design approach is called for, given the complexity of operations, impacts to practice, and the integration with IT. There are several "grand challenges," including:

- Formulating "triple aim" sustainable business models (financial, social, and environmental sustainability).

- Designing the transition to distributed community care.

- Designing the transition to ICD-10 procedure billing integrated with patient service.

- Information integration across technology providers and change management.

- Facilitating patient access to EMR records and health data.

- Managing transition to new practice models for chronic care.

- Leading and selecting appropriate innovation.

As the healthcare applications map in Figure 4.4 illustrates, clinicians have access to and use at least 10 *classes* of information tools for patient and house records, research and reference, clinical decision making, and practice. Most of these are complex applications requiring a user's focused attention on information search and results for the purposes of analysis and decision. These applications are instruments of knowledge and policy that encode clinical practice and organizational routines.

Clinical services may be the primary end users of IT and information services, yet the information function is institutional and centrally managed.

Public-facing Web services, patient portals, EMRs, billing and coding, and patient satisfaction services are organizationally intensive central functions. These systems require the investment in user research and design for ensuring ease of access and use, productivity, safety, and business and community relationships. In practice, these are frequently developed and evaluated without significant insight (deep usability testing) from frontline clinicians or other constituents. Experienced design researchers in the clinical organization might start their tenure with interactive usability research as a way to make significant improvements rapidly and to expose the organization to evidence-based design research in health IT.

As more design-led innovators engage the challenges of this changing sector, a new challenge emerges to increase the cooperation and knowledge sharing across design and research fields. Currently, knowledge sharing is impaired by institutional secrecy, misplaced privacy concerns, and the scholarly approach to knowledge translation. Innovations are often reported in clinical journals and conferences, which require months of secrecy and peer review before being communicated. If both innovations and actual research findings are treated with the same internal protection and inability to circulate, it does not help institutions and practices learn from one another.

The current approaches to knowledge sharing are driven by evidence-based culture and the fact that clinicians are rewarded for publishing in peer-reviewed channels. This adherence to tradition is reinforced by the necessity to publish and teach; therefore, every successful project, even if highly practical, becomes a new research paper. With nearly 700,000 biomedical journal articles published each year, the medical corpus is vast beyond effective searching.[13] Mere publication is not effective communication, as new articles become lost in the noise.

Community Context

A whole-system view helps us extend innovation beyond market segments (defined as customers) and reach people where their health concerns actually originate. All three sectors overlap a fourth context not considered a business sector: the local community where people live and participate. The community (a cultural region or neighborhood) is the primary context for public health, a domain currently characterized by health research, public engagement, and large-scale health interventions.

In the community context, health seekers are not isolated consumers with physical health issues (patients). People occupy dwellings and live in places that are more or less health enabling and are situated in communities that enable or discourage different social and lifestyle behaviors. Neighborhoods can be reasonably safe and socially engaging, or regions of uncertainty, social disharmony, and hazard. The social and lived experience a person lives within each and every day may be the most powerful determinant of health and risk.

Adopted social behaviors, such as smoking or poorly considered diets, may be among the most determining factors for health outcomes. Nicholas Christakis and James Fowler's work on social contagion reveals the statistically significant health impact of close connections among people in geographically proximate networks.[14] Their theory strongly suggests that people sharing similar locations and attitudes will adopt similar lifestyle behaviors that influence better health (happiness) or unhealthy habits (smoking, obesity, even depression). The theory and its support in public health projects show that systemic design (communication and program interventions) can influence the socially prominent influencers in networks and break unhealthy habits where they emerge and spread.

How might service and experience design treat the community as an object for social design? The most common examples are the community care services co-produced by residents as human services, which are not in the least consumer oriented. Circles of care are a well-known community care practice, providing support services such as transportation, errand running, and companionship for elders with regular health needs. Local food co-ops are a kind of caring practice, providing healthy food alternatives to local community members who share in volunteering. Soup kitchens and shut-in visitation are traditional forms of community care. Although these are grassroots community services, they are valued because they are authentic expressions of care that serve real human needs in the local community. Community participatory care can be considered the antidote to the consumer mindset and identity. People find meaning and connection in their communities, a source of relationship, and a source of healing or recovery from personal and family care concerns.

Several case studies in this book present community-level design concepts for reaching health seekers and caregivers within the community context. The Health Design Lab's video documentary series of unscripted cancer stories described in Chapter 4 was developed as a public health communication artifact, sponsored by Cancer Care Ontario as a regional system intervention. The Innovate Afib clinical system redesign (Chapter 5) was conceived as a scalable (province-wide) system, but one that reached cardiac-risk patients within their local community's points of access to the healthcare system. The Mayo Mom concept was specifically designed as a trusted local network sponsored by Mayo Clinic but delivered as an interpersonal service among mothers in their local regions.

The influence of the community on a health seeker's experience and health cannot be overstated. Healthy communities can be considered the ultimate goal of public health and even medicine in general. The D4.0 approaches for societal transformation have only recently been articulated, and similar methods of social system intervention are rapidly being taken up around the world. The opportunities for the impact of social and systemic design thinking are limitless in the richly connected world of the community.

Innovation's Adjacent Possible

The successful innovation—whether a product or institutional change—stands upon an installed base of applications and prior decisions and policies. It reaches a new boundary state compatible with the installed base of stakeholders and infrastructures. The next alternative, the near-future system state, is fully dependent on a preceding context—the social context and technologies that made the current state possible. Systems biologist Stuart Kauffman[15] named "the adjacent possible" to describe the range of possible biochemical changes that any living system—a cellular state, an organism, its social states, and the biosphere—could reach without destroying its internal organization (or homeostasis). The adjacent possible applies to the nearest future opportunities for growth or innovation connected to present development.

Each sector remains coupled to its history and infrastructure, and each has differing adjacent possible states. Next-generation EMRs are not going to replace the installed base without first accommodating their data models *and* the base of expensively trained professionals. Medical education changes within a long period of institutional trials with pedagogy and technologies. Institutions change when they must. The changes triggered by service innovations may remain bounded within their sector and context.

Foresight views are not the same as innovation or direct design applications on real, current problems. Rather, building models of the long view helps designers and stakeholders make sense of possible configurations of the trends we all see and hear about. Design leadership has been nearly absent to date in the rational, modernist approach to care, IT, and organization prevalent in healthcare culture. Design-led innovation in the new multidisciplinary practice provides a circle of imagination and human-centered knowledge that can advance care in novel ways. Design is the adjacent possible for healthcare innovation.

Conclusion

We have explored the possible territory for designers as members of integrated care teams, and for a new base of design skills and applications for clinical care, healthcare institutions, and deeply informed consumer healthcare. Designers are not considered professional caregivers—yet. Increasingly, designers in healthcare are situated and working beyond the known domains of IT, interaction design, and communications to bring human-centered design to clinical practice, service planning, and system-level prototyping. The necessity for highly qualified design in the healthcare enterprise is growing, certainly in major applications such as EMR interaction design, public websites and intranets, patient portals, and patient service experiences. As organizational managers recognize the value and return on compelling design and system usability throughout their organizations, interest will arise in adopting design processes for all types of complex problems.

Regardless of other organizational imperatives that may entail design skills, designing and improving technology for technical functions and everyday use serves a primary role that cannot be substituted by other skills.

However, the design disciplines are not a *critical* clinical function, and so they will not expand and succeed solely by way of executive advocacy. Design does not diffuse well by implementing top-down strategies, such as by hiring chief design officers or by executives evangelizing design to the clinical practices. The direct approach may be seen as competing with the highly contested terrain of IT, with skilled practice work routines, as well as with all strained budgets competing for other improvements. Also, in the healthcare world, outcomes are ultimately measured by the health seeker's quality of life. We cannot always quantify design's contribution.

We diffuse through organizations and projects much more effectively as creative developers of service concepts and products working on the front lines, while working toward the highest aspirations of the enterprise. Design as caring serves the discoverable opportunities for transforming work, organizations, and care experiences with radically better approaches to information, communications, and service delivery.

References

Introduction

1. Mayeroff, M. (1971). *On caring* (p. 50). New York: HarperPerennial.

Chapter 1

1. Kanter, R. M. (2011, February 22). Why innovation is so hard in health care—and how to do it anyway. *Harvard Business Review*. Blog series on innovations in health care.
2. McCallister, M. B. (2009, February). Keynote speech at the Wharton Healthcare Business Conference, Philadelphia.
3. Jadad, A. R., & Enkin, M. W. (1997). Computers: Transcending our limits? *British Medical Journal, 334*, s8.
4. Norman, D. A., & Verganti, R. (2012). Incremental and radical innovation: Design research versus technology and meaning change. Retrieved from www.jnd.org/dn.mss/ incremental_and_radi.htm.
5. Rittel, H. W. J., & Weber, M. M. (1973). Dilemmas in a general theory of planning. *Policy Sciences, 4*, 155–169.
6. Buchanan, R. (1992). Wicked problems in design thinking. *Design Issues, 8*, 5–21.
7. Jones, P. H., & VanPatter, G. K. (2009). *Design 1.0, 2.0, 3.0, 4.0: The rise of visual sensemaking*. New York: NextDesign Leadership Institute.
8. Berg, M., Aarts, J., & Van Der Lei, J. (2003). ICT in health care: Sociotechnical approaches. *Methods of Information in Medicine, 42*(4), 297–301.
9. Ulrich, W. (1987). Critical heuristics of social systems design. *European Journal of Operational Research, 31*, 276–283.
10. Patten, S., Mitton, C., & Donaldson, C. (2006). Using participatory action research to build a priority setting process in a Canadian Regional Health Authority. *Social Science & Medicine, 63*(5), 1121–1134.

Chapter 2

1. Mayeroff, M. (1971). *On caring*. New York: HarperPerennial.
2. Ormandy, P. (2010). Defining information need in health—assimilating complex theories derived from information science. *Health Expectations, 14*(1), 92–104.
3. Pennefather, P. (2008). Health information intermediary skills needed by primary health care providers for supporting decision making by current and potential disease survivors. Unpublished report. Toronto: University of Toronto.
4. Taylor, R. (1962). The process of asking questions. *American Documentation, 13*(4), 391–396.
5. Coulter, A., Entwistle, V., & Gilbert, D. (1999). Sharing decisions with patients: Is the information good enough? *British Medical Journal, 318*, 318–322.
6. Jones, P. H. (2005). Information practices and cognitive artifacts in scientific research. *Cognition, Technology, and Work, 7*, 88–100.
7. Ulrich, W. (1987). Critical heuristics of social systems design. *European Journal of Operational Research, 31*, 276–283.
8. Nielsen, J., & Molich, R. (1990). Heuristic evaluation of user interfaces. In *Proceedings of the SIGCHI Conference on Human Factors in Computing Systems* (pp. 249–256). New York: ACM.
9. Ulrich, W. (2003). A brief introduction to critical systems thinking for professionals & citizens. www.wulrich.com/cst_brief.html.

Chapter 3

1. Klein, G. (1999). *Sources of power: How people make decisions*. Cambridge, MA: MIT Press.
2. Simon, H. (1957). A behavioral model of rational choice. In *Models of man, social and rational: Mathematical essays on rational human behavior in a social setting*. New York: Wiley.
3. Goetz, T. (2009). *The decision tree: Taking control of your health in the new era of personalized medicine*. New York: Rodale Books.
4. Klein, G. (2009). *Streetlights and shadows: Searching for the keys to adaptive decision making*. Cambridge, MA: MIT Press.
5. Jones, P. H. (2010, April). Why do senior clinicians ignore CDSS? A case for clinical sensemaking. Paper presented at the Advances in Healthcare Informatics Conference, Waterloo, Ontario.

6. Young, I. (2008). *Mental models: aligning design strategy with human behavior.* Brooklyn, NY: Rosenfeld Media.

7. Reed, R., & Cabinaw, J. Personal interview, August 2, 2010.

8. Ibid.

9. Ibid.

10. Ibid.

11. Ibid.

12. Leonard, D. A., & Rayport, J. (1997). Spark innovation through empathic design. *Harvard Business Review 75*(6), 102–113. (HBS Working Paper No. 97-606.)

13. Kouprie, M., & Sleeswijk Visser, F. (2009). A framework for empathy in design: Stepping into and out of the user's life. *Journal of Engineering Design, 20*(5), 437–448.

14. Ibid.

15. Portigal, S. (2008). Persona non grata. *Interactions, 15*, 72–73.

16. Maslow, A. H. (1954). *Motivation and personality.* New York: Harper & Row.

Chapter 4

1. Fox, S. (2009). *Pew Internet and American Life Project.* Washington, DC: Pew Family Trust.

2. Andreasson, H. K., Bujnowska-Fedak, M. M., Chronaki, C. E., Dumitru, R. C., Pudule, I., Santana, S., Voss, H., & Wynn, R. (2007). European citizens' use of E-health services: A study of seven countries. *BMC Public Health, 7*, 53.

3. Fox, S. (2009). *Pew Internet and American Life Project.* Washington, DC: Pew Family Trust.

4. Simon, H. (1957). A behavioral model of rational choice. In *Models of man, social and rational: Mathematical essays on rational human behavior in a social setting.* New York: Wiley.

5. Joint Information Systems Committee. (2102). Digital Public Library of America: The biggest library the world has ever seen? *Inform, 33*, 2.

6. Dubberly, H., Mehta, R., Evenson, S., & Pangaro, P. (2010). Reframing health to embrace design of our own well-being. *Interactions, 17*, 56–63.

7. Deming, W. E. (1986). *Out of the crisis.* Cambridge, MA: MIT Press.

8. Boyd, J. (1986). *Patterns of conflict.* Unpublished study.

9. Maqubela, K. (2012, March 11). The reason Silicon Valley hasn't built a good health app. *The Atlantic.* Retrieved from www.theatlantic.com/technology/archive/2012/03/the-reason-silicon-valley-hasnt-built-a-good-health-app/254229/

10. Ibid.

11. Shreeve, S. (2007). *The canonical Health 2.0 representation.* HealthNex blog. Retrieved from http://healthnex.typepad.com/web_log/2008/02/scott-shreeve-m.html

12. Eysenbach, G. (2008). Medicine 2.0: Social networking, collaboration, participation, apomediation, and openness. *Journal of Medical Internet Research, 10*, e22.

13. Van De Belt, T. H., Engelen, L., Berben, S., & Schoonhoven, L. (2010). Definition of Health 2.0 and Medicine 2.0: A systematic review. *Journal of Medical Internet Research, 12*, e18.

14. Eysenbach, G. (2008). Medicine 2.0: Social networking, collaboration, participation, apomediation, and openness. *Journal of Medical Internet Research, 10*, e22.

15. Evans, M. Personal interview, July 15, 2010.

16. Ibid.

17. McGaw, H. Personal interview, September 2, 2011.

18. Evans, M. Personal interview, July 15, 2010.

19. Ibid.

20. Ibid.

21. Ibid.

22. Illich, I. (1973). *Tools for conviviality.* New York: Harper & Row.

23. Goodson, L., & Vassar, M. (2011). An overview of ethnography in healthcare and medical education research. *Journal of Educational Evaluation for Health Professions, 8*(4). doi:10.3352/jeehp.2011.8.4

24. Neuwirth, E. B., Bellows, J., Jackson, A. H., & Price, P. M. How Kaiser Permanente uses video ethnography of patients for quality improvement, such as in shaping better care transitions. *Health Affairs, 31*(6), 1244–1250.

25. LeCompte, M. D., & Schensul, J. J. (2010). *Designing and conducting ethnographic research: An introduction* (2nd ed.). Lanham, MD: AltaMira Press.

26. Wasson, C. (2000). Ethnography in the field of design. *Human Organization, 59*(4), 377–388.

27. Millen, D. R. (2000). Rapid ethnography: Time deepening strategies for HCI field research. In *Proceedings of the 3rd Conference on Designing Interactive Systems* (pp. 280–286). New York: ACM; Kumar, V., & Whitney, P. (2007). Daily life, not markets: Customer-centered design. *Journal of Business Strategy, 28*(4), 46–58.

28. Ylirisku, S., & Buur, J. (2007). *Designing with video: focusing the user-centred design process.* London: Springer.

29. Moore, J. (2007). Video sensemaking. In S. Ylirisku & J. Buur (Eds.), *Designing with video: focusing the user-centred design process* (pp. 111–116). London: Springer.

30. Blais, E. (2011). Design documentaries. Research pattern project. Toronto: OCAD University.

31. Raijmakers, B., Gaver, W. W., & Bishay, J. (2006). Design documentaries: Inspiring design research through documentary film. In *Proceedings of the 6th Conference on Designing Interactive Systems* (p. 229). New York: ACM.

32. Dervin, B. (2003). Human studies and user studies: A call for methodological inter-disciplinarity. *Information Research, 9*(1). Retrieved from http://informationr.net/ir/9-1/paper166.html

33. Dervin, B. (1999). On studying information seeking methodologically: The implications of connecting metatheory to method. *Information Processing and Management, 35*, 727–750.

34. Dervin, B., & Dewdney, P. (1986). Neutral questioning: A new approach to the reference interview. *Research Quarterly, 25*(4), 506–513.

Chapter 5

1. Kahneman, D., & Tversky, A. (1979). Prospect theory: An analysis of decision under risk. *Econometrica, 47*(2), 263–291.

2. Fox, W. (1995). Sociotechnical system principles and guidelines: Past and present. *Journal of Applied Behavioral Sciences, 31*, 91–105.

3. Bohmer, R. M. J. (2009). *Designing care: Aligning the nature and management of health care.* Boston, MA: Harvard Business Press.

4. Ulrich, R. S. (1984). View through a window may influence recovery from surgery. *Science, 224*, 420–421.

5. Ulrich, R. S. (1991). Effects of health facility interior design on wellness: Theory and scientific research. *Journal of Health Care Design, 3,* 97–109.

6. Schumacher, R. M., & Lowry, S. Z. (2010). *NIST guide to the processes approach for improving the usability of electronic health records.* NISTIR 7741. Washington, DC: National Institute of Standards and Technology.

7. Evenson, S., & Dubberly, H. (2010). Designing for service: Creating an experience advantage. In G. Salvendy & W. Karwowski (Eds.), *Introduction to service engineering* (ch. 19). Hoboken, NJ: Wiley.

8. Mager, B. (2007). Service design. In M. Erlhoff & T. Marshalle (Eds.), *Design dictionary: Perspectives on design terminology.* Basel, Switzerland: Birkhäuser.

9. Evenson, S., & Dubberly, H. (2010). Designing for service: Creating an experience advantage. In G. Salvendy & W. Karwowski (Eds.), *Introduction to service engineering* (ch. 19). Hoboken, NJ: Wiley.

10. Ibid.

11. Maglio, P. P., & Spohrer, J. (2008). Fundamentals of service science. *Journal of the Academy of Marketing Science,36*, 18–20.

12. Morra, D. Personal interview, December 18, 2010.

13. Ibid.

14. Ibid.

15. Morra, D., Bhatia, S., Leblanc, K., Meshkat, N., Plaza, C., Beard, L., & Wodchis, W. (2010). *Reconnecting the pieces to optimize care in atrial fibrillation: A white paper on the management of AF patients in Ontario.* Toronto: University of Toronto.

16. Morra, D. Personal interview, December 18, 2010.

17. Oulasvirta, A., Kurvinen, E., & Kanjaunen, T. (2003). Understanding contexts by being there: Case studies in bodystorming. *Personal Ubiquitous Computing, 7,* 125–134.

18. Schleicher, D., Jones, P. H., & Kachur, O. (2010). Bodystorming as embodied designing. *Interactions, 17*, 47–51.

19. Cooper, A. (1999). *The inmates are running the asylum*. New York: Macmillan.

Chapter 6

1. Simon, H. (1969). *The sciences of the artificial*. Cambridge, MA: MIT Press.

2. Ackoff, R. L. (1989). From data to wisdom. *Journal of Applied Systems Analysis, 15*, 3–9.

3. Irby, D. M., Cooke, M., Lowenstein, D., & Richards, B. (2004). The Academy movement: A structural approach to reinvigorating the educational mission. *Academic Medicine, 79*(8), 729.

4. Harrison, M. I., Koppel, R., & Bar-Lev, S. (2007). Unintended consequences of information technologies in health care—an interactive sociotechnical analysis. *Journal of the American Medical Informatics Association, 14*, 542–549.

5. Cooke, M., Irby, D. M., Sullivan, W., & Ludmerer, K. M. (2006). American medical education 100 years after the Flexner Report. *New England Journal of Medicine, 355*, 1339–1344.

6. Jones, P. H. (2010, April). Why do senior clinicians ignore CDSS? A case for clinical sensemaking. Paper presented at the Advances in Healthcare Informatics Conference, Waterloo, Ontario.

7. Gawande, A. (2009). *The checklist manifesto: How to get things right*. New York: Metropolitan Books.

8. Provonost, P. (2006). An intervention to reduce catheter-related bloodstream infections in the ICU. *New England Journal of Medicine, 355*, 2725–2732.

9. Rees, J. (2005). The problem with academic medicine: Engineering our way into and out of the mess. *PLOS Medicine, 2*(4), e111.

10. Christensen, C. M., Grossman, J. H., & Hwang, J. (2008). *The innovator's prescription: A disruptive solution for health care*. New York: McGraw-Hill.

11. Bakken, S., Currie, L., Lee, N., Roberts, W., Collins, S. A., & Cimino, J. J. (2008). Integrating evidence into clinical information systems for nursing decision support. *International Journal of Medical Informatics, 77*(6), 413–420.

12. Dreiseitl, S., & Binder, M. (2005). Do physicians value decision support? A look at the effect of decision support systems on physician opinion. *Artificial Intelligence in Medicine, 33*(1), 25–30; Kawamoto, K., Houlihan, C., Balas, E. A., & Lobach, D. F. Improving clinical practice using clinical decision support systems: A systematic review of trials. *British Medical Journal, 330*(7494), 765.

13. Jones, P. H. (2010, April). Why do senior clinicians ignore CDSS? A case for clinical sensemaking. Paper presented at the Advances in Healthcare Informatics Conference, Waterloo, Ontario.

14. Klein, G. (1999). *Sources of power: How people make decisions*. Cambridge, MA: MIT Press.

15. Klein, G., Moon, B., & Hoffman, R. R. Making sense of sensemaking 1: Alternative perspectives. *IEEE Intelligent Systems, 21*(4), 70–73.

16. Mamede, S., Schmidt, H. G., Rikers, R., Custers, E., Splinter, T., & van Saase, J. (2010). Conscious thought beats deliberation without attention in diagnostic decision-making: At least when you are an expert. *Psychological Research, 74*, 586–592. doi:10.1007/s00426-010-0281-8

17. Frankel, A. S., & Leonard, M. (2011). Practical experience with collaborative models in the health professions. In L. Olsen, R. S. Saunders, & J. M. McGinnis (Eds.), *Patients charting the course: Citizen engagement and the learning health system*. Washington, DC: National Academies Press.

18. Jones, P. H., & Nemeth, C. P. (2005). Cognitive artifacts in complex work. *Lecture Notes in Computer Science, 3345*, 152–183.

19. Patel, V., Zhang, J., Yoskowitz, N. A., Green, R., & Sayan, O. R. (2008). Translational cognition for decision support in critical care environments: A review. *Journal of Biomedical Informatics, 41*, 413–431.

20. Basadur, M. S. (2004). Leading others to think innovatively together: Creative leadership. *Leadership Quarterly, 15*, 103–121.

21. Zeitlin, M. (1991). Nutritional resilience in a hostile environment: positive deviance in child nutrition. *Nutrition Reviews, 49*(9), 259–268.

22. Gardam, M., Reason, P., & Rykert, L. (2010). Healthcare culture and the challenge of preventing healthcare-associated infections. *Healthcare Quarterly, 13*(Special Issue), 116–120.

Chapter 7

1. HIMMS EHR Usability Task Force. (2009). *Defining and testing EMR usability: Principles and proposed methods of EMR usability evaluation and rating.* Chicago: Healthcare Information and Management Systems Society.

2. Armijo, D., McDonnell, C., & Werner, K. (2009). *Electronic health record usability: evaluation and use case framework.* Rockville, MD: Agency for Healthcare Research and Quality.

3. Greenhalgh, T., Potts, H. W. W., Wong, G., Bark, P., & Swinglehurst, D. (2009). Tensions and paradoxes in electronic patient record research: A systematic literature review using the meta-narrative method. *Milbank Quarterly, 87*(4), 729–788.

4. Shneiderman, B. (2011). Tragic errors: Usability and electronic health records. *Interactions, 18*(6), 60–63.

5. Calman, N. (2007). *HIMSS Davies public health award of excellence.* New York: Institute for Family Health.

6. Halamka, J. (2012, October 10). Why meaningful use stage 2 is so important. Life as a Healthcare CIO blog. Retrieved from http://geekdoctor.blogspot.com/2012/10/why-meaningful-use-stage-2-is-so.html

7. Wu, R. C., Morra, D., Quan, S., Lai, S., Zanjani, S., Abrams, H., & Rossos, P. G. (2010). The use of smartphones for clinical communication on internal medicine wards. *Journal of Hospital Medicine, 5*(9), 553–559.

8. Romano, M. J., & Stafford, B. A. (2011). Electronic health records and clinical decision support systems. *Archives of Internal Medicine, 171*(10), 897–903.

9. Koppel, R., Metlay, J. P., Cohen, A., Abaluck, B., Localio A. R., Kimmel, S. E., & Strom, B. L. (2005). Role of computerized physician order entry systems in facilitating medication errors. *Journal of the American Medical Association, 293*(10), 1197–1203.

10. Himmelstein, D. U., Wright, A., & Woolhandler, S. (2010). Hospital computing and the costs and quality of care: A national study. *American Journal of Medicine, 123*(1), 40–46.

11. Ledue, C. (2009, November 23). Health IT savings estimates are "wishful thinking," say Harvard researchers. *Healthcare IT News.*

12. Mostrous, A. (2009, October 25). Electronic medical records draw frequent criticisms. *Washington Post.*

13. Jones, P. H. (2008). *We tried to warn you: Organizational innovations for the learning organization.* Ann Arbor, MI: Nimble Books.

14. Koppel, R., & Kreda, D. (2009). Health care information technology vendors' "hold harmless" clause: Implications for patients and clinicians. *Journal of the American Medical Association, 301*(12), 1276–1278. doi:10.1001/jama.2009.398

15. Jones, P. H., & Nemeth, C. P. (2005). Cognitive artifacts in complex work. *Lecture Notes in Computer Science, 3345,* 152–183.

16. Rasmussen, J. (1985). The role of hierarchical knowledge representation in decisionmaking and system management. *IEEE Transactions on Systems, Man, & Cybernetics, 15*(2), 234–243.

17. Nemeth, C. L., O'Connor, M., Cook, R., & Klock, P. A. (2005). Mapping cognitive work: The way out of healthcare IT system failures. *AMIA Annual Symposium Proceedings, 2005,* 560–564.

18. Ibid., 562.

19. Brown, T. (2009). *Change by design.* New York: Harper Business.

20. Pothoulakis, A., & Demosthenous, G. (2011). *Abdobesity: The belly fat that kills.* Dayton, OH: uKare Analytics.

21. Butler, K. A., Brennan, P., Payne, T., Shneiderman, B., & Zhang, J. (2011). Re-engineering health care with information technology: The role of computer-human interaction. In *Proceedings of the CHI '11 Conference on Human Factors in Computing Systems* (pp. 451–454). New York: ACM.

22. Cam, K. M., Efthimiadis, E. N., Hammond, K. W. (2008). An investigation on the use of computerized patient care documentation: Preliminary results. In *Proceedings of the 41st Annual Hawaii International Conference on System Sciences* (pp. 235–245).

23. Park, S. Y., Lee, S. Y., & Chen, Y. (2012). The effects of EMR deployment on doctors' work practices: A qualitative study in the emergency department of a teaching hospital. *International Journal of Medical Informatics, 81,* 204–217.

24. Jones, P. H. (2008). *We tried to warn you: Organizational innovations for the learning organization*. Ann Arbor, MI: Nimble Books.

25. Silverstein, S. (2010, September 6). The ultimate workaround to mission hostile health IT: Humans. *Health Care Renewal*. Retrieved from http://hcrenewal.blogspot.com/2010/09/ultimate-workaround-to-mission-hostile.html

26. Perednia, D. (2010). Scribes lead to unintended consequences from electronic medical records. KevinMD blog. Retrieved from www.kevinmd.com/blog/2010/11/scribes-lead-unintended-consequences-electronic-medical-records.html

27. Özbekhan, H. (1967). The triumph of technology: "Can implies ought." Los Angeles: King Resources.

28. Koprivica, D. (2011, October 20). The scribe of the double house of life. Informatics 360. Retrieved from http://chopcbmi.org/2011/10/20/the-scribe-of-the-double-house-of-life/

29. Rasmussen, J., Pejtersen, A. M., & Goodstein, L. P. (1994). *Cognitive systems engineering*. New York: Wiley.

30. Vicente, K. (1999). *Cognitive work analysis: Towards safe, productive, and healthy computer-based work*. Mahwah, NJ: Lawrence Erlbaum Associates.

Chapter 8

1. Christensen, C. M. (1997). *The innovator's dilemma*. Boston: Harvard Business School Press.

2. Murray, C. J. L., & Frenk, J. (2010). Ranking 37th—measuring the performance of the U.S. health care system. *New England Journal of Medicine, 362*, 98–99.

3. Sisson S. D., & Dalal, D. (2011). Internal medicine residency training on topics in ambulatory care: A status report. *American Journal of Medicine, 124*(1), 86–90.

4. Muhlestein, D., Croshaw, A., Merrill, T., & Peña, C. (2012). *Growth and dispersion of accountable care organizations: June 2012 update*. Leavitt Partners.

5. Gharajedaghi, J. (2011). *Systems thinking: Managing chaos and complexity*. Burlington, MA: Morgan Kaufman.

6. Ackoff, R., & Gharajedaghi, J. (1996). Reflections on systems and their models. *Systems Research, 13*(1), 13–23.

7. Berwick, D. M., Nolan, T. W., & Whittington, J. (2008). The triple aim: Care, health, and cost. *Health Affairs, 27*(3), 759–769.

8. Berwick, D. (2009). What patient-centered should mean: Confessions of an extremist. *Health Affairs, 28*(4), 555–565.

9. Institute of Medicine. (2001). *Crossing the quality chasm: A new health system for the 21st century*. Washington, DC: National Academies Press.

10. Ackoff, R. (1974). *Redesigning the future*. New York: Wiley.

11. Ackoff, R. (2004, May). Transforming the systems movement. Keynote speech at the Third International Conference on Systems Thinking in Management, Philadelphia.

12. Spohrer, J., Anderson, L., Pass, N., Ager, T., & Gruhl, D. (2007). Service science. *Journal of Grid Computing, Special Issue on Grid Economics and Business Models*.

13. Patton, M. Q. (2009). *Developmental evaluation: Applying complexity concepts to enhance innovation and use*. New York: Guilford Press.

14. Christakis, A. N., & Bausch, K. (2006). *How people harness their collective wisdom and power to construct the future in co-laboratories of democracy*. Charlotte, NC: Information Age Publishing.

15. Churchman, C. W. (1971). *The design of inquiring systems*. New York: Basic Books.

16. Özbekhan, H. (1970). *The predicament of mankind: A quest for structured responses to growing world-wide complexities and uncertainties*. Club of Rome proposal. Institute for 21st Century Agoras. Retrieved from www.globalagoras.org/publications

17. Parker, T. F., Blantz, R., Hostetter, T., Himmelfarb, J., Kliger, A., Lazarus, M., Nissenson, A. R., Pereira, B., & Weiss, J. (2004). The Chronic Kidney Disease Initiative. *Journal of the American Society of Nephrology, 15*, 708–716.

18. Meadows, D. (1999). *Leverage points: Places to intervene in a system*. Hartland, VT: Sustainability Institute.

19. Thackara, J. (2011, September). Community interventions. Mayo Clinic Center for Innovation 2011 Transform Symposium, Rochester, MN.

20. Forrester J. W. (1994). System dynamics, systems thinking, and soft OR. *System Dynamics Review, 10*, 2–3.

21. Meadows, D. N., Meadows, D. L., Randers, J., & Behrens, W. W. (1972). The limits to growth: A report for the Club of Rome's project on the predicament of mankind. New York: Universe Books.

22. Laugesen, M. J., & Glied, S. A. (2011). Higher fees paid to US physicians drive higher spending for physician services compared to other countries. *Health Affairs, 30*(9), 1647–1656.

23. Paton, B., & Dorst, K. (2011). Briefing and reframing: A situated practice. *Design Studies, 32*(6), 573–587.

24. Ryan, M., Mills, J., Vink, J., Sihavong, P., & Chow, J. (2011). Mayo Mom: Case study in healthcare social systems design. Rotman Business Design Challenge, April 27, 2011. Toronto: University of Toronto.

25. US Department of Health and Human Services. (2011). *The surgeon general's call to action to support breastfeeding*. Washington, DC: Office of the Surgeon General.

26. Braa, K., & Vidgen, R. (1999). Interpretation, intervention, & reduction in the organizational laboratory: A framework for in-context information system research. *Accounting, Management & Information Technology, 9*, 25–47.

27. Christakis, A. N., & Bausch, K. (2006). *How people harness their collective wisdom and power to construct the future in co-laboratories of democracy*. Charlotte, NC: Information Age Publishing.

28. Warfield, J. (1990). *A science of generic design: Managing complexity through systems design*. Salinas, CA: Intersystems Publications.

29. Christakis, A. N., & Bausch, K. (2006). *How people harness their collective wisdom and power to construct the future in co-laboratories of democracy*. Charlotte, NC: Information Age Publishing.

Chapter 9

1. Houle, D., & Fleece, J. (2011). *The new health age: The future of health care in America*. Naperville, IL: Sourcebooks.

2. Jones, P., Cronin, D., Karavite, D., Koppel, R., Dalrymple, P., Zheng, K., Rogers, M., & Schumacher, R. (2011). Designing for whole systems and services in healthcare. In *Proceedings of the CHI '11 Conference on Human Factors in Computing Systems* (pp. 359–362). New York: ACM.

3. Romanow, R. (2002). *Building on values: The future of health care in Canada*. Ottawa, Ontario: Commission on the Future of Health Care in Canada.

4. Kachur, O., Resnick, J., & Schroeder, K. (2010). *Healthy healthcare*. Toronto: OCAD University.

5. Popper, R. (2008). How are foresight methods selected? *Foresight, 10*(6), 62–89.

6. Coates, J. F. (2010). The future of foresight—a US perspective. *Technological Forecasting & Social Change, 77*, 1428–1437.

7. Özbekhan, H. (1967). *The triumph of technology: "Can implies ought."* Los Angeles: King Resources.

8. Curry, A., & Hodgson, A. (2008). Seeing in multiple horizons: Connecting futures to strategy. *Journal of Futures Studies, 13*(1), 1–20.

9. Sihavong, P., Maharaj, U., & Vink, J. (2012). *The future of specialized health care providers*. Project whitepaper. Toronto: OCAD University.

10. Sevaldson, B. (2011). *Gigamapping: Visualization for complexity and systems thinking in design*. Helsinki: Nordic Design Research Conference.

11. Shewchuk, G. (2012). Childhood obesity Gigamap. In M. Komori, L. Read, & G. Shewchuk, *Age related obesity trends and factors for children*. Toronto: OCAD University.

12. Koppel. R., & Gordon, S. (2012). *First, do less harm: Confronting the inconvenient problems of patient safety*. Ithaca, NY: ILR Press.

13. US National Library of Medicine. (2012). *MEDLINE® Fact Sheet*. Retrieved from www.nlm.nih.gov/pubs/factsheets/medline.html

14. Christakis, N. A., & Fowler, J. H. (2013). Social contagion theory: Examining dynamic social networks and human behavior. *Statistics in Medicine, 32*(4), 556–577. doi:10.1002/sim.5408

15. Kauffman, S. A. (2008). *Reinventing the sacred: A new view of science, reason, and religion*. New York: Basic Books.

Index

A

open knowledge
  moral argument for value of, 92
Open Space, 290, 292
operational studies, outcome measures
  for, 139
optimism, 59
oral communication, for direct patient
  care, 229
organizational capacity
  service innovation project and, 126
organizational readiness phase in integrated service design framework, 152
organizational systems, 260
organizations
  D3.0 driven by, 177
  redesign, 301
  transformation design, 23, 25
Ormandy, Paula, 34
Oslo School of Architecture and
  Design, 313
Ottawa Hospital Research Institute, 69
outcome measures, for operational
  studies, 139
outpatient treatment, 254
Özbekhan, Hasan, 272, 309

P

Palestrant, Daniel, 186
Pangaro, Paul, 93
paper artifacts, 230
paper records, EMRs vs., 209
participant, patient as, 85
participatory design
  dialogue as, 290–296
  methods, 160
  scenarios, 153–155
Pastor, Elizabeth, 22
patiency, 91
patient-centered care model,
  259, 264–266
  goal of, 257
patient-centered healthcare frame, 94
patient-centered medical homes
  (PCMH), 126, 256

patient-centered paradigm, 300
  transition to, 85
patient charts, printed, 222
patient empowerment, 100
patient experience
  in health service, 124–127
patient-focused decision support, 104
patients, 13–14, 40, 317
  as customers, 261
  design goals for health seeker as, 86
  information across services, 163
  information asymmetry for, 127
  as legal designation, 124
  rarity of access, 82
  reframing as agents, 98
  traditional relationship, 89
  value of information, 39
  Western healthcare treatment of, 3
patient scenarios, 32, 86
  ablation procedure, 248–249
  background, 33
  chronic diseases, 208
  health-seeking journey, 5, 85
  health self-service, 124
  peer interaction, 298
  personal health issues, 56
  personal health journey as patient,
    88–89
  supraventricular tachycardia
    (SVT), 168
PatientsLikeMe, 101, 298
Paton, Bec, 281
PDCA (Plan, Do, Check, Act) cycle, 96
PD (Positive Deviance), 204–206
peer interaction, 298
peer-to-peer communications, 220
Pennefather, Peter, 35
Perednia, Douglas, 238
person. See also consumers; patients; users
  shifting focus from product to, 16
personal experiences in healthcare, 19
personal feedback systems, 319
personal health journey, 88–89
personal health, managing as system,
  94–96

solutions
formulation, 203
implementation, 203
speciality medicine
systems view of, 254–257
specialized center, 131
specialty healthcare
residency training for, 192
three horizons in, 310–313
Spohrer, Jim, 142
stakeholders, 12, 271
co-creation, 200–206
in developing design concepts, 157
in dialogic design, 272
engagement methods, 206
influence on organization, 258
map generation, 274
mind map to identify, 315
responsibility for process, 28
standard of care, 66
for clinical professionals or patients vs.
consumers, 139
start-ups, 103
static data, vs. flow, 38
STEEPV (social, technological, economic,
environmental, political, and values)
trend and environmental scan, 310
stories, 77
story narratives, 78
storytelling personas, 78
strange-making, 26
strategic innovation, 220
stress reduction, healthcare environment
and, 137
Structured Dialogic Design (SDD),
272, 292–295
language patterns, 294
subscriber resources, 45
"success to the successful" archetype, 280
supportive design theory on healing
process, 137
supraventricular tachycardia (SVT), 168
sustaining innovations, 186
symptomatic solution, 279
Symptom Triage tool, 71

systemic approach, need for, 18–19
systemic design, 129–130, 283
systemic institutional innovation, 129
systemic risks, 215–217
systemic task design, 223–225
system-level innovation, 275–283
systems
changing behavior, 275–277
designing inside, 267–269
design methods for
innovation, 288–296
dynamics as design
thinking, 277–280
encountering problems, 261–262
problems as, 269–274
reframing methods, 280
systems inquiry theory, 270–271
systems of healthcare, 258–264
systems science, laws of, 262
systems thinking
organization in, 257
rationalizing bias and, 270
systems view of speciality
medicine, 254–257

T

tacit knowing, 157
TAGLab (University of Toronto), 94
task design, systemic, 223–225
task-oriented design approach, 57
Taylor, Robert, 36
team
cognitive aiding of care, 192–193
team-based care practices, 192–193
team system, 306
technical work, 224, 225
technological imperative, 20
technology
impact on healthcare, 8–10
role in health, 100
technology innovation, 10
technology spectrum
for health information, 105
Thackara, John, 276

ACKNOWLEDGMENTS

This book was made possible by the extraordinary community of contributors who supplied ideas, research, case studies, news, perspectives, and feedback in support of the book. Keeping track of everyone was helped by the Designforcare.com online community, whose members numbered 472 at press time.

Special thanks to those who provided case studies, reviews, and contributed high-value work and materials. James Caldwell, designer of visual communications for print and new media, brought the book to life by advising, designing, and rendering the visual content. James had the audacity and skill to create a consistent design language in the book by re-composing the original figures from top designers who provided their materials. I thank the designers who contributed to cases, methods, and concepts, especially Hugh Dubberly, GK VanPatter, Birger Sevaldson, and Liz Sanders.

Innovative physicians and medical experts brought vision and reality to the book. I'm especially grateful to Dr. John Halamka, CIO at Beth Israel Deaconess Medical Center and professor at Harvard Medical School, for his thoughts in the Foreword. Cardiologist Antony Pothoulakis contributed to Elena's medical journey across the book's chapters, and with George Demosthenous, also from uKare, contributed their personal health concept. Special thanks to CICC's Dr. Dante Morra and designer Leslie Beard, now both at Trillium Health Centre, Ontario. Dr. Mike Evans of the Health Design Lab and designer Heather McGaw contributed stories and cases in healthcare innovation. Dr. Sam Basta of Healthcare Innovation by Design has been a supporter from the beginning. Thanks to Dr. Richard Cook and Dr. Chris Nemeth, and to my mentor, Dr. Aleco Christakis.

OCAD University graduate students contributed exemplary work from research and in case contributions. Thanks to Oksana Kachur, Karl Schroeder, Chris Meier, and Jonathan Resnick from our first class of Strategic Foresight and Innovation students; Josina Vink, Martin Ryan, Uma Maharaj, Jessica Mills, Phouphet Sihavong, Jen Chow, and Eric Blais from our second year; and from our third year, George Shewchuck, Michi Komori, Tai Huynh, Jen Recknagel, Jayar Lafontaine, and Ian Moss, as well as other great grad students whose work is in progress. I wish to acknowledge as well the inspiration of many students whose work I could not fit into the final cut.

Several contributors helped significantly at the start of the book project. Special thanks to contributors Min Basadur and Mauro Amoruso. Julie Cabinaw, Becky Reed, Alexandra Carmichael, and Amy Tenderich helped with cases and concepts. Satu Miettinen and Arne van Oosterom from Europe, and Dr. Peter Pennefather and Peter West from Canada, brought great books and papers to my attention.

Toward the end of the project, a great publishing team produced this book and worked impeccably with my writing, research, and revisions. Thanks to JoAnn Simony, my tireless editor; Lou Rosenfeld, my pioneering publisher; and the production staff, Karen Corbett and Danielle Foster.

If I've left someone out that contributed in any way, I'm sorry for the oversight. Please contact me at peter@designforcare.com to contribute to the ongoing publications and posts online.

—Peter Jones, Toronto, March 2013

ABOUT THE AUTHOR

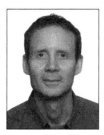 **Peter Jones** is an experienced design research consultant in software and large-scale online information services. He specializes in evidence-based reference services for point of care, clinical education, and clinical practice. In 2001 he founded Redesign, a company specializing in innovation research for knowledge-based services and organizational performance. He leads research into complex social practices and new markets, to help clients design tools and integrated services for all forms of intellectual work. He has designed market-leading information services in healthcare, education, scientific work, and professional practice. He consults with organizations to develop their innovation strategies and service design practices, and publishes his methods and case studies whenever possible.

Peter is an associate professor in the Faculty of Design at OCAD University and teaches in the Strategic Foresight and Innovation graduate program. He is a senior fellow of the Strategic Innovation Lab and coordinates research in dialogic design and scholarly publishing innovation. He publishes research in organizational behavior, strategic innovation, and human information interaction. In 2000 he completed his PhD (Design and Innovation Management) at Cincinnati's Union Institute, and has developed methods and new research from his research on embedded values in innovation processes in large organizations.

Peter also wrote *We Tried to Warn You* (Nimble Books, 2008), a case study in transformative organizational recovery from a systemic market failure leveraging user experience design capacities. His first book, *Team Design: A Practitioner's Guide to Collaborative Innovation*, was revised in 2002, and although showing its age, it remains a valued treatise on classic design facilitation methods.

Peter's articles, posts, and publications are found at designdialogues.com. Peter is also found at: @designforcare and @redesign. Find *Design for Care* online at designforcare.com.